UICC

International Union Against Cancer
Union Internationale Contre le Cancer

Illustrated Tumor Nomenclature

Nomenclature illustrée des Tumeurs

Иллюстрированная номенклатура опухолей

Illustrierte Tumor-Nomenklatur

Nomenclatura ilustrada de los Tumores

Second Revised Edition

Springer-Verlag Berlin Heidelberg New York 1969

The first edition was published with the financial support of the
Calouste Gulbenkian Foundation of Lisbon, Portugal

ISBN-13: 978-3-642-48262-5   e-ISBN-13: 978-3-642-48260-1
DOI: 10.1007/978-3-642-48260-1

Softcover reprint of the hardcover 2nd edition 1969

© by International Union Against Cancer Geneva 1965, and

© by Springer-Verlag, Berlin · Heidelberg 1969.

Library of Congress Catalog Card Number 79—84818

Title No. 1239

2nd Edition: Prepared by

HERWIG HAMPERL, M.D.
Professor of Pathology, Bonn/Rhine, University

LAUREN V. ACKERMAN, M.D.
Professor of Surgical Pathology and Pathology
Washington University School of Medicine, St. Louis, Missouri
Surgical Pathologist-in-Chief to Barnes Hospital
and Associated Hospitals
Consultant to the Armed Forces Institute of Pathology

1st Edition: Prepared by the

Committee on Tumor Nomenclature (Chairman: H. HAMPERL) of the International
Union Against Cancer. On this committee the following served:

Préparée par le Comité pour la Nomenclature des Tumeurs (Président: H. HAMPERL)
de l'Union Internationale Contre le Cancer. Ce comité était composé comme suit:

Подготовлено комитетом по номенклатуре опухолей (председатель: Г.Ф.Гамперль)
Международного Противоракового Союза. Членами комитета были:

Ausgearbeitet vom Komitee für Tumor-Nomenklatur (Vorsitzender: H. HAMPERL)
der Internationalen Union gegen den Krebs. In diesem Komitee haben mitgearbeitet:

Realizada por el Comité para la Nomenclatura de los Tumores (Presidente:
H. HAMPERL) de la Unión Internacional Contra el Cáncer. En este comité han
colaborado:

Prof. Dr. L. V. ACKERMAN
Washington University, Department of Surgical Pathology,
St. Louis, Missouri, USA

Dr. J. CAMPOS
Avenida Alfonso Ugarte 823, Lima, Peru

Dr. J. CLEMMESEN
Cancerregisteret, Strandboulevard 49, Copenhagen, Denmark

Dr. C. DUKES
22 Albermarle Wimbledon, London SW 19, England

Prof. Dr. M. F. GLAZUNOV †, Leningrad, USSR

Prof. Dr. H. HAMPERL
Pathological Institute, Venusberg, Bonn/Rhine, Germany

Prof. Dr. E. KOPPISCH †, Porto Rico, USA

Prof. Dr. CH. OBERLING †, Paris, France

Dr. G. VOGT-HOERNER
Institut Gustave Roussy, Villejuif, Seine, France

Prof. Dr. T. YOSHIDA
Cancer Institute, Nishi-sugamo 2-Chome,
Toshima-ku, Tokyo, Japan

Introduction to the Second Edition

The first edition of this book was the work of the UICC Committee on Tumor Nomenclature. It met with so much interest, that a second edition seemed indicated. To avoid any possible overlap with the program developed by the World Health Organization in the field of histopathological nomenclature of tumors, the UICC decided not to reappoint the Committee whose term of office had expired. The decision to bring out a second edition of the book therefore rested with the publishing house of Springer. The former Chairman of the Committee for Tumor Nomenclature, HERWIG HAMPERL, and one of its members LAUREN ACKERMAN, were asked to prepare the second edition. The editors are grateful to all those who wrote to them; their constructive criticisms have helped them to improve this new edition.

Most of the criticisms were concerned with the quality of some of the illustrations chosen to illustrate the various tumors. This is largely explained by the decision of the original Committee to choose, as far as possible, the figures from among the fascicles of the Tumor-Atlas of the AFIP or from authoritative text-books to illustrate the correct interpretation of a term. On occasion these illustrations were unsatisfactory. In this new edition, the editors decided to abandon this principle and to prepare their own new illustrations to replace unsuitable ones.

As the original preface indicated the purpose of the editors is to illustrate the accepted common neoplasms as they occur in various organs. It is not possible to illustrate rare tumors or debatable tumours for such illustrations are available in more detailed atlases.

It was the aim of the original committee and the present authors to indicate what is believed to be the most acceptable term for a given neoplasm. The other terms commonly used are also indicated. The editors have not invented or recommended any new names. It was the original purpose and continues to be their purpose to make this book on the nomenclature of tumors a book which will unify and clarify the nomenclature of neoplasms as they are used in different countries.

HERWIG HAMPERL   LAUREN V. ACKERMAN

Préface de la Deuxième Edition

La première édition de ce livre, fruit des travaux du Comité de Nomenclature des Tumeurs de l'UICC, a été accueillie avec tant d'intérêt qu'une deuxième édition s'imposait. Afin d'éviter tout empiètement sur le programme de l'Organisation Mondiale de la Santé dans le domaine de la nomenclature histopathologique des tumeurs, l'UICC décida en son temps de ne pas reconduire le mandat du Comité. La décision de publier une deuxième édition était, dès lors, l'affaire exclusive de la maison Springer. Pour la préparation de cette édition, il a été fait appel à MM. Herwig Hamperl et Lauren Ackerman, respectivement Président et Membre de l'ancien Comité de Nomenclature des Tumeurs. Tous deux désirent exprimer ici leur gratitude à ceux qui, par leurs critiques constructives, ont contribué à la préparation de la présente édition améliorée. Parmi les observations formulées, la plupart portaient sur la médiocre qualité de certaines illustrations de tumeurs. Ces imperfections s'expliquent aisément si l'on considère la décision prise par l'ancien Comité de faire un large usage, pour illustrer l'interprétation correcte des termes, des clichés de l'Atlas des Tumeurs de l'AFIP et des autres ouvrages faisant autorité en la matière. Il se trouve que quelques uns de ces clichés n'étaient pas satisfaisants du point de vue technique. Les rédacteurs de la présente édition ont décidé d'abandonner ce principe et d'utiliser leur propre matériel en lieu et place des clichés défectueux. Comme l'indiquait la préface de la première édition, l'objet du présent ouvrage est de définir par voie d'illustrations les néoplasmes couramment reconnus, tels qu'ils apparaissent dans divers organes, à l'exclusion des tumeurs rares ou discutables qui ont leur place toute trouvée dans des atlas plus détaillés.

L'objectif des rédacteurs de la nouvelle édition demeure celui de l'ancien Comité, à savoir proposer pour chaque néoplasme la terminologie la plus adéquate, tout en indiquant également les variantes d'usage courant. Aucune appellation nouvelle n'est créée ou recommandée. Le but des auteurs de ce livre est aujourd'hui comme hier d'encourager l'adoption dans les différents pays d'une nomenclature des néoplasmes claire et uniforme.

Herwig Hamperl   Lauren V. Ackerman

Предисловие ко второму изданию

Первое издание этой книги было результатом деятельности Комитета по номенклатуре опухолей Международного Противоракового Союза. Это издание было встречено с таким большим интересом, что потребовалось второе издание. Чтобы избежать возможного совпадения с программой, разработанной Всемирной Организацией Здравоохранения в области гистопатологической номенклатуры опухолей, Международный Противораковый Союз решил не обиовлать прежнего комитета, срок работы которого истек. Таким образом, решение о выпуске второго издания книги осталось за издательством Шпрингера. Бывшего председателя Комитета по номенклатуре опухолей Гервига Гамперла и одного из членов Комитета Лаурена Аккермана просили взять на себя подготовку второго издания.

Мы благодарны всем кто написали нам и критические замечания которцх помогли улучшить новое издание. Большинство замечаний касалось качества некоторых изображений. Это объясняется решением Комитета отобрать, насколько это возможно, иллюстрации из отдельных выпусков Атласа Опухолей Института Патологии Вооруженных Сил США и авторитетных руководств, чтобы проиллюстрировать правильное толкование терминов. Иногда эти иллюстрации были неудовлетворительными. В новом издании редакторы решили отказаться от этого принципа и дать свои собственные иллюстрации в замень старых недостаточных иллюстраций.

В предисловии к первому изданию указана наша цель — иллюстрировать общепризнанные виды опухолей, встречающихся в разных органах. Мы не имеем возможности иллюстрировать редкие или спорные по своему характеру опухоли, изображения которых можно найти в более подробных атласах.

Целью Комитета и авторов настоящего издания ыло привести наиболее приемлемый термин для обозначения данной опухоли. Приводятся и другие широко применяемые названия. Мы не вводим и не предлагаем каких-либо новых наименований. Первоначальной нашей целью, сохраняющейся и теперь, является создание книги по номенклатуре опухолей, которая будет объединять и вносить ясность в номенклатуру опухолей, применяемую в различных странах.

Гервиг Ф. Гамперль   Лаурен В. Аккерман

Vorwort zur zweiten Auflage

Die 1. Auflage dieses Buches, das Werk des Komitees für Tumor-Nomenklatur der Internationalen Union gegen den Krebs (UICC) wurde mit solchem Interesse aufgenommen, daß eine 2. Auflage angezeigt erschien. Um jede mögliche Überschneidung mit dem von der Weltgesundheitsorganisation entwickelten Programm auf dem Gebiete der histopathologischen Nomenklatur der Tumoren zu vermeiden, beschloß die UICC, ihr Komitee für Tumor-Nomenklatur, dessen Amtszeit zu Ende gegangen war, nicht mehr zu erneuern. Die Entscheidung, eine 2. Auflage des vorliegenden Buches herauszubringen, lag daher beim Verlag Springer. Der Vorsitzende des früheren Komitees für Tumor-Nomenklatur, H. HAMPERL, und eines der Komitee-Mitglieder, L. ACKERMAN, wurden nun vom Verlag aufgefordert, diese 2. Auflage vorzubereiten. Beide Herausgeber sind nunmehr allen denjenigen dankbar, deren konstruktive Kritik dazu verholfen hat, diese Neuauflage zu verbessern.

Die meisten kritischen Bemerkungen betrafen die Qualität einzelner Abbildungen, die ausgewählt worden waren, um die verschiedenen Tumoren darzustellen. Dieser Mangel geht zum größten Teil darauf zurück, daß das ursprüngliche Komitee beschlossen hatte, soweit als irgend möglich, die Illustrationen der Fasciceln des Tumor-Atlas des Armed Forces Institute of Pathology oder von anerkannten Lehrbüchern oder Monographien zu benützen, um eine Tumor-Bezeichnung richtig zu belegen. In der vorliegenden neuen Auflage haben die Herausgeber beschlossen, diesen Grundsatz dort, wo es nötig schien, aufzugeben und dafür ihre eigenen Abbildungen beizubringen.

Wie schon im Vorwort zur 1. Auflage erwähnt wurde, lag dem Buch die Absicht zugrunde, die in den verschiedenen Organen vorkommenden gewöhnlichen Tumortypen durch Bilder zu belegen; nicht jedoch alle, auch die selteneren und in ihrer Deutung noch ungeklärten Tumoren abzubilden — entsprechende Illustrationen wird man in den viel mehr Einzelheiten bringenden Atlanten finden können.

Es war das Bestreben der ursprünglichen Komitee-Mitglieder und der jetzigen Herausgeber, deutlich zu machen, welche Bezeichnung eines gegebenen Tumors sie für die empfehlenswerteste halten; andere gebräuchliche Bezeichnungen sind jedoch ebenfalls immer aufgeführt. Andererseits hat man sich davor gehütet, neue Namen zu erfinden oder zu empfehlen. Die ursprüngliche Absicht bei der Veröffentlichung dieses Buches bleibt auch die der jetzigen Herausgeber, nämlich diese Illustrierte Nomenklatur der Tumoren zu einem Werk zu machen, welches dazu helfen soll, die Benennungen der Tumoren, welche in den verschiedenen Sprachgebieten gebraucht werden, zu verdeutlichen und damit auch einer Einheitlichkeit näherzubringen.

H. HAMPERL   L. V. ACKERMAN

Prefacio a la segunda edición

La primera edición de este libro fué preparada por el Comité que la UICC constituyó para la nomenclatura de los tumores. Fué acogida con un interés tal, que pareció indicado el preparar una segunda edición. La UICC decidió no volver a encargar a dicho Comité, cuyo período de legislación había expirado, con esta tarea, evitando así posibles interferencias con el programa de la Organización Mundial de la Salud en el campo de la nomenclatura histopatológica de los tumores. La casa Springer sigue siendo la editora de la segunda edición. HERWIG HAMPERL, antiguo presidente del Comité para la nomenclatura de tumores, y LAUREN ACKERMAN, uno de sus miembros, se encargaron de preparar la segunda edición. Expresamos nuestro agradecimiento a todos aquéllos que con sus críticas constructivas han contribuído a mejorar esta nueva edición.

La mayor parte de las críticas se han referido a la calidad de ciertas fotografías elegidas para documentar los diversos tumores. Esto se explica suficientemente si se considera que el Comité decidió, en tanto en cuanto fuera posible, elegir las fotografías destinadas a interpretar correctamente un término entre las de los fascículos del Atlas de tumores del AFIP o a partir de libros de texto reconocidos. En ciertos casos la calidad de las fotografías no era totalmente satisfactoria. Los editores de esta nueva edición decidieron abandonar este principio y utilizar su propio material para reemplazar illustraciones insuficientes.

Como indicaba el primer prólogo, nuestro propósito es aportar una documentación iconográfica de los neoplasmas comúnmente aceptados, tal como se presentan en diversos órganos. No nos es posible tratar de los tumores raros o discutidos que se encuentran recopilados en atlas más especializados.

El objetivo del comité que preparó la primera edición y el de los autores de la presente es indicar el término que creemos más aceptable para un determinado neoplasma. También se indican otros términos de uso corriente. No hemos inventado ni recomendado nombres nuevos. El propósito original fué, y continúa siendo, hacer de este libro sobre la nomenclatura de los tumores un libro que unifique y aporte claridad en la nomenclatura de los neoplasmas tal como se usa en los diversos países.

HERWIG HAMPERL   LAUREN V. ACKERMAN

Preface to the First Edition

At the 6th International Cancer Congress held at São Paulo a list of tumors, intended primarily for the purpose of statistical codification, was presented and accepted with slight alterations only. This list had been prepared by the Committee on Tumor Nomenclature and Statistics, of the International Union against Cancer, under the chairmanship of Dr. PERRY. It had also served as a basis for the somewhat simplified code submitted to WHO, which circulated it as document WHO/HS/CANC/24.1. An alphabetical index to the code, mostly based on terms in use in the United States, constitutes part 2 of this document (WHO/HS/CAN/C24.2).

The preparation of a list of descriptive terms which could be used for the coding of tumor statistics was only the first objective of this committee, and it had been intended also that there should have been combined with the statistical code an orderly and scientifically acceptable manual of tumor nomenclature. This second objective, namely an agreed tumor nomenclature, proved difficult to reach in spite of much discussion at special conferences and voluminous correspondence between members of the committee extending over a period of more than four years. Eventually it came to be seen that the main obstacle to agreement arose from an attempt to reach two different objectives at the same time, namely statistical coding and tumor nomenclature. Therefore, at the Cancer Congress held at São Paulo in 1954 it was decided that the committee should be reorganized under the chairmanship of Dr. HAMPERL and that it should in the future direct its activities exclusively to the second goal, namely the histological nomenclature of tumors. It should be pointed out that though the Statistical Code and Manual of Tumor Nomenclature are now each being produced separately there will be no difficulty later in linking them together for reference purposes. In the meantime the new committee has endeavored to produce a simple, generally acceptable tumor nomenclature founded on logical principles of pathology.

A first draft without pictures was published in "ACTA" Vol. XIV No. 3—1958, which is now followed by an illustrated edition. We are greatly indebted to all the authors and publishers for permission to use their illustrations and for providing us with the original prints. Unfortunately it was not possible to obtain the original prints for the figures from the Atlas of Tumor Pathology; we therefore had to use the printed illustrations for reproduction and are grateful to the Armed Forces Institute of Pathology for permission to use them.

The illustrated Tumor Nomenclature, containing as it does many illustrations, could not have been published without help: our thanks go to the Calouste Gulbenkian Foundation of Lisbon for their support which has made this publication possible.

The present unsatisfactory state of affairs with regard to tumor nomenclature is universally recognized. Obviously tumors affecting mankind are basically alike in all parts of the world, yet the names applied to these same tumors differ from country to country. The first task facing the committee therefore was to collect as complete a list as possible of synonymous terms in current use, and then to consider each of these from the point of view of descriptive accuracy and usefulness. Needless to say, they have strenuously resisted any temptation to invent new names and so add to the already existing confusion! Fortunately, for some varieties of tumors only one single histologic designation is now in general use throughout the scientific world; and this is of course the ideal at which to aim. Unfortunately, other varieties of tumors at present have many different histologic designations, so that the same tumor is known by different names in different countries.

XII

When listing tumors which are known by several names the committee has placed first those names which seem to be most logical and most in keeping with general principles and have listed antiquated or objectionable terms last in order. Names which are synonymous are as far as possible grouped together.

There are certain names still applied to tumors which are now in use only in a small and restricted circle. To have included all of them would have added an unnecessary encumbrance to this work. They have therefore been omitted. By the use of a medical dictionary alternative names could easily be discovered.

There are also tumors of which only a few examples may have been described, and the classification and terminology of which has varied from author to author (e.g. Retinal Anlage Tumor or Melanoameloblastoma). Rare tumors of this type have been accepted only if they have already been included in one of the larger text books and wherever possible adequately illustrated. In other words, the committee decided not to rely on the illustrations and descriptions of the original authors but before recognizing claims to the discovery of a new variety of tumor felt compelled to wait until these should have been sifted by the criticism of a second author. This policy will avoid the necessity for frequent revisions of the text.

Terms descriptive of lesions which are not true tumors, such as cysts, granulomas and hyperplasias, have not been accepted for inclusion. Moreover in order to keep this first undertaking within reasonable proportions the so-called premalignant lesions and precancerous changes have also been excluded. For similar reasons most examples of lesions described as "carcinoma in situ" have been omitted. In justification of this it may be pointed out that though some cases of so-called "carcinoma in situ" may eventually prove to be true cancers displacing and replacing normal epithelium, it is also true that the term "carcinoma in situ" may occasionally be used to describe other lesions, the relationship of which to true cancer is not always clearly established. Some of these lesions may even retrogress and disappear. Their inclusion

would be out of place in a manual of tumor nomenclature.

In the choice and selection of acceptable descriptive terms the committee has been guided by the following principles. Designations of tumors should be short and definitive: such names have always been quickly adopted. For this reason simple names have been selected in preference to a long and elaborate terminology, even though this might describe a given tumor more completely.

The fact that so many tumors are linked to the name of the person who first described them is only another expression of a natural wish to find a concise and easily remembered designation. However, in accordance with agreed international conventions it has been decided that all designations based on personal names should be rejected and replaced by appropriate descriptive terms, but, to avoid misunderstanding, the name by which some such tumors have been known in the past is now printed in brackets. In a few instances it proved impossible to replace an eponymous term (e.g. Brenner tumor, Ewing sarcoma) or a term objectionable for other reasons (e.g. hamartoma, chondroma of lung) without inventing a new name.

Obviously, the words carcinoma and sarcoma should be reserved for genuine malignant tumors and adenoma only for benign growths, and as far as possible all mutually contradictory terms such as malignant adenoma should be avoided.

At the present time the functional activity of a tumor, such as its possible endocrine secretion, cannot be determined with certainty from its histologic structure. For this reason designations dependent on the functional relationships of a tumor have been avoided, though histologic differentiations such as mucus production have been taken into account.

Also, there exist well defined tumors whose position is still under discussion, such as malignant nonchromaffin paraganglioma or alveolar soft part sarcoma. The listing of these tumors may be subject to changes in the future.

As we are dealing with a purely histologic classification of a single tumor, terms like "neurofibroma" were included but not "neurofibromatosis", a diagnosis made on the basis of gross or clinical inspection.

Leukemias are included only in so far as they concern lesions of tissues detectable by histologic methods; lesions diagnosed by smears, as in hematology and exfoliative cytology, have not been included.

Terms such as round cell and spindle cell sarcoma have not been included because such diagnoses were thought to be incomplete or of a provisional nature.

Finally, a word of explanation concerning the order adopted. Since every arrangement is bound to be open to some objections it has been the aim of the committee to find the simplest and the least likely to give offence.

Tumors with a histologic structure characteristic of the organ in which they arise are described in sequence, first, tumors of the surface epithelium followed by tumors of glandular organs. As far as possible the order followed has been that of the categories on malignant neoplasms in the International Classification of Diseases (Manual of the International Classification of Diseases, Injuries and Causes of Death, Vol. 1, World Health Organization, Geneva, Switzerland, 1957). The numbers in brackets under the various sites refer to the corresponding three-digit categories for malignant neoplasms in the International Classification. Then follow the tumors derived from melanin-forming tissues, from nerve tissue, from mesenchymal tissues, from the blood and blood-forming organs and finally the teratomas.

The order of tumors in each separate section is so arranged that benign tumors are followed first by tumors of relatively low grade malignancy and then by those of average and high grade malignancy.

At the various conferences of members of the committee it has always proved useful to produce a good illustration which would make definitions and descriptions of a tumor more easily understood. With this experience in mind the committee decided to try to provide representative illustrations which would indicate better than any verbal description what the name is intended to convey, though it was recognized that these illustrations would not represent all the possible variations which might occur in different regions of the tumor. The committee thought that the pictures in the recently published American Atlas of Tumor Pathology would be especially suitable for illustrations as well as certain others from authoritative text books published in other countries.

Thus, the illustrated Tumor Nomenclature in question is calculated to give representative illustrations of the most frequent tumors where an agreement between the different language groups is already in existence. As the text is printed in English, French, Russian, German, Spanish and Latin the illustrated Tumor Nomenclature should be able to further this mutual understanding: a pathologist may easily find how a given tumor is designated in other languages. The illustrated Tumor Nomenclature will also help the pathologist in isolated areas of the globe, as more than 90% of the tumors he sees will be listed and illustrated in it. This illustrated Tumor Nomenclature will therefore not infringe on the work of the reference centers set up by the World Health Organization. It is hoped that the World Health Organization reference centers will contribute to a better understanding of the remaining debatable tumors which have been purposely omitted from the listing in the illustrated tumor nomenclature.

The names given to the different tumors listed represent the opinion of the committee as a group. They are therefore at times a compromise between the opinions of different members of the committee and should be viewed with this in mind. The discussion of the proper names and the selection of the best illustrations has occupied the deliberations of the committee for almost a decade.

In spite of this, the members of the Committee on Tumor Nomenclature recognize that their production is far from complete and that it is certainly not in its final form, but they regard it simply as "the end of the beginning" and as a preliminary draft which they venture to think may serve as a basis for fruitful discussions.

Préface de la Première Edition

Au 6ᵉ Congrès International du Cancer à São Paulo, une liste de tumeurs, destinée primitivement à servir de code pour les usages de statistique, a été présentée et acceptée avec seulement de légères modifications. Cette liste avait été préparée par le Comité de Nomenclature et de statistique de l'Union Internationale contre le Cancer, comité qui était alors présidé par le Docteur PERRY. Cette liste a servi comme base pour le code un peu simplifié soumis à l'Organisation Mondiale de la Santé, qui l'a diffusé comme document WHO/HS/Cancer/24.1. Un index alphabétique du code, basé principalement sur les termes utilisés aux Etats-Unis, constitue la deuxième partie de ce document (WHO/HS/Cancer/24.2).

La préparation d'une liste de termes descriptifs pouvant servir à la codification statistique des tumeurs n'avait été que le but initial de ce comité; l'idée était de compléter ce répertoire à l'usage des statisticiens par une nomenclature des tumeurs, satisfaisante du point de vue logique et scientifique. Ce second objectif, c'est-à-dire l'établissement d'une nomenclature des tumeurs universellement acceptable s'est révélé difficile à realiser, malgré bien des discussions au cours d'une série de réunions spécialement organisées et malgré une volumineuse correspondance échangée entre les membres du comité, s'étendant sur une période de plus de quatre ans. Il fut finalement reconnu, que l'accord avait été impossible à réaliser parce que deux objectifs différents étaient visés à la fois: une codification à l'usage de la statistique et une nomenclature des tumeurs acceptable par les pathologistes. Pour cette raison, il a été décidé au Congrès du Cancer tenu à São Paulo en 1954 que le comité devait être réorganisé sous la présidence du Docteur HAMPERL et qu'il devait, à l'avenir, orienter son activité exclusivement vers le deuxième but, c'est-à-dire vers la nomenclature histologique des tumeurs. Or, quoique le Code Statistique et la Nomenclature des Tumeurs soient, à l'heure actuelle, préparés séparément,

il n'y aura pas de difficultés, pensons-nous, à les réunir ultérieurement. Ceci nous tenons expressément à le souligner. En attendant, le nouveau comité s'est efforcé d'établir une nomenclature simple, adaptée à l'usage général et basée sur des principes logiques de la pathologie.

Un premier projet sans illustrations avait été publié dans ACTA Vol. XIV—N° 3—1958, auquel fait suite cette nomenclature histologique illustrée.

Nous adressons nos remerciements à la Fondation GULBENKIAN qui nous accorda son aide financière pour l'impression de cette monographie.

Nous voudrions ensuite remercier tous les auteurs et éditeurs qui nous ont permis d'utiliser leurs documents et ont mis gracieusement à notre disposition leurs photographies originales. Malheureusement il ne nous a pas été possible de disposer des originaux de l'Atlas of Tumor Pathology dont les illustrations imprimées ont dû nous servir de modèles pour les reproductions.

Tout le monde reconnaît que l'état actuel de la nomenclature des tumeurs n'est pas satisfaisant. Les tumeurs affectant l'humanité sont manifestement semblables dans leur essence; pourtant les noms des mêmes tumeurs diffèrent de pays à pays. Le premier devoir du comité était donc de réunir une liste, aussi complète que possible, de termes synonymes d'usage courant, de les évaluer ensuite quant à leur exactitude descriptive et à leur utilité. Bien entendu le comité s'est biengardé de forger de nouveaux noms et d'ajouter ainsi à la confusion déjà existante.

Heureusement, il y a quelques tumeurs pour lesquelles une seule appellation histologique est utilisée dans le monde scientifique et c'est là, naturellement, l'idéal vers lequel il faut tendre. Les autres, malheureusement, sont désignées par des termes très divers et souvent la même tumeur est connue sous des noms différents dans les pays différents.

Certains termes, proposés à un moment donné mais dont l'utilisation est restée limitée à un cercle plus ou moins restreint ont été éliminés. Leur inclusion aurait encombré la nomenclature inutilement. A l'aide d'un dictionnaire médical, il sera toujours facile de retrouver tous ces noms.

Pour classer les termes s'appliquant à une seule et même tumeur, le comité a toujours placé au premier rang le nom qui lui paraissait le plus logique et le plus conforme aux principes généraux de la nomenclature. Les noms démodés ou discutables ont été rejetés en fin de liste. Les termes synonymes ont été autant que possible groupés ensemble.

Il existe aussi des tumeurs dont on n'a décrit que peu de cas et dont la classification et la terminologie ont varié suivant les auteurs (par exemple: Retinal Anlage Tumor ou mélano-améloblastome). Les rares tumeurs de ce genre n'ont été acceptées que si elles étaient déjà mentionnées dans un des grands traités, autant que possible avec une illustration adéquate. En d'autres mots, le comité a décidé de ne pas reconnaître comme définitivement acquises les descriptions et illustrations originales de variétés tumorales nouvelles, mais d'attendre qu'une certaine décantation se fasse afin d'éviter de trop fréquentes révisions du texte.

Les lésions qui ne sont pas de vraies tumeurs comme les kystes, granulomes et hyperplasies, n'ont pas été prises en considération. En outre, pour tenir ce premier essai dans des limites raisonnables, les lésions dites prémalignes ou précancéreuses ont été, elles aussi, exclues. Pour des raisons similaires, la plupart des lésions décrites comme «épithélioma in situ» ont été éliminées. En effet, si certains cas d'«épithélioma in situ» peuvent se révéler ultérieurement comme de vrais cancers déplaçant et remplaçant l'épithélium normal, d'autres auxquels le même terme est appliqué, répondent à des lésions dont la relation avec un vrai cancer n'est pas établie avec certitude. Certaines de ces lésions peuvent même régresser et disparaître. Leur inclusion dans une nomenclature de tumeurs ne serait donc pas justifiée.

Quelques principes, qui ont guidé le comité dans le choix et la sélection des termes descriptifs, méritent encore d'être brièvement signalés. La dénomination d'une tumeur doit être courte et caractéristique; les noms répondant à ces désiderata ont toujours été rapidement adoptés. Pour cette raison des noms simples ont été sélectionnés de préférence à une terminologie compliquée, même si celle-ci donnait une définition plus parfaite de la tumeur.

Le fait que tant de tumeurs sont désignées d'après le nom de la personne qui les a décrites pour la première fois n'est qu'une autre expression du désir naturel de trouver une appellation concise et facile à retenir. Cependant, en accord avec les conventions internationales, il a été décidé de rejeter les noms propres et de les remplacer par des termes descriptifs appropriés. Pour éviter des malentendus, le nom sous lequel de telles tumeurs ont été connues dans le passé a été indiqué entre parenthèses. En quelques rares occasions il a été impossible de remplacer des termes éponymes (par exemple: tumeur de Brenner, sarcome d'Ewing) ou des termes qui pour d'autres raisons sont discutables (par exemple: hamartome, chondrome du poumon). Naturellement, les noms d'épithélioma et de sarcome doivent être réservés aux tumeurs malignes véritables, le terme d'adénome aux tumeurs bénignes et, dans la mesure du possible, des termes contradictoires comme «adénome malin» devraient être évités.

Actuellement, l'activité fonctionnelle d'une tumeur, comme par exemple sa sécrétion endocrine éventuelle, ne peut pas être déduite de sa structure histologique. Pour cette raison, les appellations impliquant une signification fonctionelle ont été évitées autant que possible, alors que des différenciations histologiques, comme la muciparité, qui ont été prises en considération.

Il existe des tumeurs bien définies dont la position est encore discutée comme le paragangliome malin non chromaffine ou le sarcome alvéolaire des parties molles. La terminologie de ces tumeurs peut encore changer dans l'avenir.

Etant donné qu'il s'agit d'une classification purement histologique d'entités tumorales, des termes comme «neurofibrome» ont été inclus, alors que celui de «neurofibromatose», basé sur des notions macroscopique et clinique, a été éliminé.

Les leucémies sont incluses seulement dans la mesure où elles créent des lésions tissulaires décelables par des méthodes histologiques; des lésions pour le diagnostic desquelles il faut recourir à des frottis, comme en hématologie ou en cytologie exfoliative, ont été écartées.

Les termes comme «sarcome à cellules rondes» ou «fusiformes» n'ont pas été inclus parce que de tels diagnostics ont été considérés comme incomplets ou de nature provisoire.

Un mot, enfin, pour expliquer l'ordre adopté. Etant donné qu'aucun classement n'est à l'abri des critiques, le comité a toujours adopté celui qui lui paraissait le plus simple et le moins apte à susciter des objections.

Les néoplasmes ayant une structure histologique caractéristique du tissu dans lequel ils se développent sont énumérés successivement, d'abord les tumeurs provenant des épithéliums de surface, ensuite celles des organes glandulaires. Autant que possible l'ordre suivi a été celui du chapitre relatif aux tumeurs malignes dans la Classification Internationale des Maladies (Manuel de la C assification Statistique Internationale des Maladies, Traumatismes et Causes de Décès, Vol. 1, Organisation Mondiale de la Santé, Genève, Suisse, 1957). Les numéros entre parenthèses qui suivent l'indication des divers sièges se rapportent aux rubriques correspondantes à trois chiffres utilisés pour les tumeurs malignes dans la Classification International. La suite est réservée aux tumeurs dérivées des tissus mélanogènes, nerveux, mésenchymateux, du sang, des organes hémopoïétiques et enfin aux tératomes.

La succession de l'énumeration des tumeurs dans chaque section est telle que les tumeurs bénignes sont suivies par les tumeurs à degrés de malignité croissante.

L'utilité d'une bonne illustration s'est affirmée à toutes les réunions du comité, chaque fois qu'il s'est agi notamment d'obtenir la définition précise et concise d'une tumeur. Fort de cette expérience, le comité a décidé de fournir des figures représentatives, caractéristiques pour le type histologique des tumeurs destinées à être incluses ultérieurement dans la Nomenclature Histologique, figures qui indiqueront mieux que n'importe quelle description verbale ce que le terme proposé a l'intention de représenter. Bien entendu, ces figures ne sauraient intégralement illustrer toutes les variations possibles qui peuvent exister dans les différentes régions de la même tumeur.

Le comité a pensé que les figures de l'American Atlas of Tumor Pathology publié récemment seraient particulièrement appropriées pour de telles illustrations, de même que certaines autres provenant de traités connus, publiés dans d'autres pays.

Cette nomenclature illustrée des tumeurs a pour but de définir les aspects histologiques caractéristiques des tumeurs les plus fréquemment observées et pour lesquelles a été établie une concordance entre les différents groupes linguistiques. Le texte, rédigé en plusieurs langues (Anglais — Français — Russe — Allemand — Espagnol et Latin) favorisera une compréhension réciproque. Un pathologiste pourra aisément, pour une tumeur déterminée, trouver le nom correspondant dans les autres langues. Cette nomenclature illustrée pourra également être utile aux multiples pathologistes isolés dans les diverses parties du globe puisque plus de 90 % des tumeurs pour lesquelles il est appelé à établir le diagnostic y sont énumérées et illustrées.

Cette brochure ne fait en aucune manière double emploi avec les «Centres de Références» institués par l'Organisation Mondiale de la Santé, qui, nous l'espérons, contribueront toujours à faciliter la classification de certaines tumeurs encore controversées qui ne figurent pas, pour cette raison, dans cette nomenclature.

Les termes choisis pour les différentes tumeurs l'avis reflètent de l'ensemble du comité de nomenclature. Ils résultent donc d'un compromis entre les différents membres du comité ce qui ne doit pas être oublié lorsque l'on porte un jugement sur cette nomenclature. Le choix de meilleurs termes et celui d'illustrations plus représentatives fut l'objet pendant près d'une décennie des réunions du comité et malgré celà, ses membres reconnaissent le caractère incomplet et provisoire de leur travail.

Les membres de la Commission pour la Nomenclature des tumeurs reconnaissent que ce premier travail est loin d'être parfait et ils n'ont nullement la prétention d'avoir fait une œuvre définitive. Pour eux c'est la «fin d'un début» et en tout cas un résultat préliminaire. Ils pensent néanmoins que cette nomenclature pourra servir de base à des discussions fructueuses, et c'est dans cet esprit qu'ils la soumettent à leurs collègues.

Предисловие к первому изданию

Уже на УI конгрессе по раку в Сан-Пауло был предложен и принят с незначительными изменениями перечень опухолей, имевший целью в первую очередь удовлетворить потребности их кодификации. Этот перечень был подготовлен комитетом по номенклатуре и статистике опухолей под председательством д-ра Перри (США), созданным Международным Союзом против рака. В дальнейшем, на основе этого перечня, был выработан несколько упрощенный код, переданный Всемирной Организации Здравоохранения (ВОЗ), которая ввела его в обращение как документ ВОЗ/ХС/Рак/24.1: алфавит к этому коду, построенный преимущественно на терминах, применяемых в США, составляет вторую часть этого документа (ВОЗ/ХС/Рак/24.2).

Составление перечня описательных терминов для статистической кодификации было лишь первой целью Комитета. С самого начала существовало намерение одновременно со статистическим кодом создать номенклатуру опухолей, логически выдержанную и приемлемую с научной точки зрения. Достичь этой второй цели оказалось однако трудной задачей, как выяснилось из многочисленных дискуссий и объемистой корреспонденции между членами Комитета за больше чем 4-х летний период его деятельности. Следует учесть, наконец, что главное препятствие для достижения единогласия состояло в стремлении в одно и то же время достичь двух целей — создания статистического кода и логически выдержанной номенклатуры опухолей. Поэтому на Международном Конгрессе в Сан-Пауло было решено реорганизовать Комитет, возложив председательство в нем на проф. Г. Гамперля; целью работы комитета в будущем было выполнение второй задачи, а именно, создание гистологической номенклатуры опухолей. Таким образом, хотя в настоящее время статистический код и гистологическая номенклатура опухолей будут разрабатываться и опубликовываться отдельно, все же — это следует подчеркнуть, не существует трудностей их объединения для нужд практики. Обновленный Комитет стремился выработать номенклатуру, которая, будучи построенной на

логических основах общей патологии, могла бы повсюду найти применение.

Первый набросок, без иллюстраций, был опубликован в АКТА том ХІУ, № 3, 1958; сейчас представляется иллюстрированная номенклатура опухолей. Мы благодарим фонд Гульбенкиана за предоставление средств для издания этой монографии. Кроме того мы приносим благодарность всем авторам и издательствам за разрешение использовать их иллюстрации и предоставление оригиналов для репродуцирования. К сожалению не было возможности получить оригиналы иллюстраций из Атласа патологии опухолей; поэтому мы должны были воспользоваться самими иллюстрациями для изготовления репродукций. Современное положение с общей номенклатурой опухолей признано повсюду совершенно неудовлетворительным, и все же нет сомнений в том, что опухоли человека повсюду одинаковы и только называются в различных странах по-разному. Поэтому первой задачей Комитета было составить по возможности полный перечень применяемых в настоящее время синонимов, проверив в дальнейшем все ли эти термины действительно точно характеризуют определенную опухоль и пользуются применением. Само собой понятно, что Комитет энергично отверг попытку ввести новые термины, что могло бы внести еще больше путаницы в существующее положение. [Если в прилагаемом перечне все же встречаются названия, которые непривычны или совсем новы для немцев (и для русских), то причиной этого является перевод (транскрипция) терминов, употребляемых в английской и французской литературе. Однако, почти везде, рядом с термином, переведенным с иностранного, указан применяемый в немецком (и русском) языке, как напр. «светлоклеточный рак почки» и «гипернефроидный рак почки» — Примечание издателя].

К счастью, для многих родов опухолей во всем научном мире применяется единственный гистологический термин, что, так сказать, является идеалом, к которому нужно стремиться. К несчастью, для других родов опухолей в различных странах употребляются самые разнообразные термины, или на одном и том же языке имеется несколько терминов для одной и той же опухоли.

Из разных для одной и той же опухоли терминов Комитет ставил на первое место тот, который ему казался самым логичным и отвечающим общим предпосылкам; устаревшие и не безупречные термины приведены на последнем месте. Синонимы сколько возможно были объединены.

Существуют термины, которые применяются для известных опухолей в небольшом кругу патологов. Приводить их все было бы бесполезной перегрузкой. Поэтому такие термины совсем не упомянуты; для каждого названия, которого можно избежать, всегда можно найти общеупотребительный термин в медицинском словаре.

Существуют однако опухоли, которые описаны в единичных экземплярах, классификация и номенклатура которых меняется от автора к автору, как напр. «опухоль из зачатка ретины» или «мелано-амелобластома». Такого рода редкие опухоли включены в список только тогда, когда они по меньшей мере подтверждены и по возможности воспроизведены в крупных руководствах. Иными словами: Комитет решил не основываться на иллюстрациях и терминах оригинальных работ; он считал себя обязанным обождать впредь до признания нового рода опухоли другим критичным исследователем. Такой путь представлялся наилучшим, чтобы избежать необходимости чересчур часто исправлять номенклатуру опухолей.

Не включены в список кроме того названия не истинных опухолей, включая все т. н. псевдоопухоли, как-то: кисты, грануломы и гиперплязии в общепринятом смысле этих терминов. Не упомянуты также т. н. предраковые изменения во избежание чрезмерного разбухания списка опухолей. Из тех же соображений в нем отсутствуют изменения, именуемые обычно «раком на месте», поскольку в таких случаях дело идет или об истинном раке, сместившем нормальный эпителий и занявшем его место, т. е. об особой форме роста рака, которая может быть охарактеризована иначе; или это процесс особого рода, существующий сам по себе, или могущий подвергнуться обратному развитию или, наконец, перейти в истинный рак; в последнем случае можно говорить самое большее о предраке, который в данной номенклатуре не учитывается.

При выборе и оценке названий Комитет придерживался следующего принципа: установлено, что для того, чтобы термин вошел в обиход, он должен быть кратким и впечатляющим. Такому термину всегда отдавалось предпочтение по сравнению с более длинным и сложным, даже если последний характеризовал опухоль полнее и лучше.

Тот факт, что многие опухоли называются именем описавшего их, выражает стремление пользоваться более кратким и впечатляющим термином. В соответствии с международной договоренностью, в данной номенклатуре названия опухолей по фамилии автора заменялись наиболее подходящими другими. Чтобы избежать недоразумений одновременно с последним приводится в кавычках фамилия описавшего. В некоторых случаях найти такой заменяющий термин оказалось невозможным, как, например, для «опухоли Бреннера» или «саркомы Юинга», или таких, вошедших по другим мотивам терминов, как, например, «гамартома» или «хондрома» легкого.

Названия «карцинома» и «саркома» применялись только для действительно злокачественных опухолей, «аденома» же — только для доброкачественных. Внутренние противоречивые термины, как например, »злокачественная аденома«, очевидно исключены.

В настоящее время гистология не всегда в состоянии предсказать функцию опухоли на основании микроскопической картины. Поэтому избегались все названия, включавшие в себе функциональную характеристику опухоли. Гистологически же констатируемые формы функционирования, как напр. слизеобразование, должны быть отражены в термине.

Существуют также характерные по своему микроскопическому строению опухоли, тканевая природа которых пока что остается спорной — например нехромаффинная параганглиома (альвеолярная саркома) мягких тканей. Включение ее в определенную рубрику данной номенклатуры очевидно может претерпеть изменения в будущем.

Так как в основу данной номенклатуры положен гистологический критерий, то в ней напр. применено название «нейрофиброма», а не «нейрофиброматоз»: последний диагноз может быть поставлен только на основании макроскопических или клинических данных.

Лейкэмии учитываются постольку, поскольку они сопровождаются изменениями тканей, уловимыми гистологическими методами; изменения, диагносцируемые с помощью мазков или цитодиагностически, не учитываются.

Названия вроде «круглоклеточные» или «веретеноклеточные саркомы» отвергнуты, так как подобные диагнозы следует считать предварительными или неполноценными.

Наконец, несколько слов о построении перечня опухолей. Любой из них имеет свои недостатки: целью Комиссии было найти наиболее простое и наименее дискутабельное решение задачи.

Опухоли, имеющие гистологическое строение, характерное для исходного органа, расположены так, что сначала перечисляются опухоли эпителиев, покрывающих поверхности, затем опухоли отдельных железыстых органов. Расположение злокачественных опухолей соответствует насколько возможно тому, как это сделано в соответствующем разделе Международной классификации болезней (Руководство по международной классификации болезней, повреждений и причин смерти, т. I, ВОЗ, Женева, 1957). Цифра в скобках под названием различных органов относится к соответствующей категории этой международной классификации. Дальше следуют опухоли из тканей, образующих меланин, затем нервной системы, мезенхимных тканей, крови и кроветворных органов, наконец тератомы.

В каждом разделе опухоли распределены так, что сначала стоят доброкачественные, затем умеренной степени злокачественности и наконец более злокачественные.

На различных совещаниях Комиссии постоянно отмечалась большая польза ссылок на хорошие иллюстрации, что облегчало бы определение и описание опухоли. Основываясь на этом опыте, Комиссия решила сопроводить каждый термин ссылкой на иллюстрацию, опубликованную в руководствах и пособиях. Такие иллюстрации говорят больше, чем слова о содержании того или другого названия опухоли. Следует однако признать, что вряд ли представится возможность показать таким образом все варианты той или другой опухоли.

Комитет был того мнения, что для этих целей помимо иллюстраций из известных руководств и учебников, особенно подходящим был бы американский атлас патологии опухолей.

Таким образом настоящая иллюстрированная номенклатура опухолей ставит себе целью дать демонстративные иллюстрации наиболее частых опухолей, по поводу которых уже достигнуто согласие между представителями различных языковых групп. Так как текст подан на английском, французском, русском, немецком, испанском и латинском языках, то данная иллюстрированная номенклатура опухолей должна способствовать взаимопониманию: патологу будет легко найти как именуется данная опухоль на других языках. Иллюстрированная номенклатура опухолей будет полезна также патологам отдаленных местностей, поскольку в ней приведены и изображены больше чем 90% опухолей, с которыми приходится встречаться в жизни.

Иллюстрированная номенклатура опухолей ни в какой мере не предназначена затруднить деятельность референц-центров, которые будут создаваться Всемирной Организацией Здравоохранения. Следует надеяться, что эти центры могут достичь лучшего понимания тех спорных опухолей, которые намеренно не внесены в иллюстрированную номенклатуру опухолей.

Названия, приведенные для различных опухолей, отражают мнения всех членов комитета по номенклатуре опухолей. Однако, иногда они являлись результатом компромисса между разными членами комитета, что следует учесть при критическом рассмотрении представляемой номенклатуры. Дискуссия по поводу наилучших и наиболее подходящих терминов и отбор наиболее показательных иллюстраций занял у членов комитета по номенклатуре опухолей почти декаду времени. Несмотря на это они хорошо сознают, что их работу нельзя считать законченной и, тем более, вылившейся в окончательную форму. Они смотрят на нее как на конец начала, как на набросок, который, они надеются, послужит основой для дальнейших плодотворных дискуссий.

Vorwort zur ersten Auflage

Schon auf dem VI. Internationalen Krebs-Kongreß in São Paulo wurde eine Liste der Tumoren vorgelegt und mit geringen Abänderungen angenommen, die in erster Linie für Zwecke einer statistischen Kodifizierung der Tumoren bestimmt war. Diese Liste war vorbereitet worden durch das von der Internationalen Union gegen den Krebs eingesetzte Komitee für Tumor-Nomenklatur und Statistik unter dem Vorsitz von Dr. I. PERRY (USA). In der Folgezeit wurde ein auf Grund dieser Liste ausgearbeiteter, etwas vereinfachter Code der Weltgesundheits-Organisation übergeben, die ihn als Dokument WHO/HS/CAN/24.1 in Umlauf brachte; ein alphabetischer Index zu diesem Code, der sich hauptsächlich auf die in den Vereinigten Staaten gebräuchlichen Termini stützt, bildet den zweiten Teil dieses Dokumentes (WHO/HS/CAN/24.2).

Die Aufstellung einer Liste von beschreibenden Termini für die statistische Kodifizierung stellte aber nur das erste Ziel des Komitees dar. War es doch von Anfang an die Absicht gewesen, zugleich mit dem statistischen Code eine logisch geordnete und wissenschaftlich annehmbare Tumor-Nomenklatur zu schaffen. Dieses zweite Ziel zu erreichen, erwies sich jedoch als schwierig, wie sich bei vielen Diskussionen und in einer umfangreichen Korrespondenz zwischen den Mitgliedern des Komitees im Laufe von mehr als 4 Jahren herausstellte. Schließlich mußte man einsehen, daß das Haupthindernis für eine Übereinstimmung daher kam, daß man gleichzeitig zwei Ziele erreichen wollte, nämlich einen statistischen Code und eine logische Tumor-Nomenklatur. Deshalb wurde auch auf dem Internationalen Krebs-Kongreß in São Paulo beschlossen, das Komitee unter dem Vorsitz von Dr. H. HAMPERL zu reorganisieren: Es sollte in Zukunft seine Tätigkeit ausschließlich dem zweiten Ziel widmen, nämlich der Ausarbeitung einer histologischen Nomenklatur der Tumoren. Obwohl also jetzt der statistische Code und die histologische Tumor-Nomenklatur getrennt bearbeitet und herausgegeben

werden, besteht doch — wie ausdrücklich betont werden soll — keine Schwierigkeit, sie später einmal auch für den praktischen Gebrauch zu verbinden. Inzwischen hat das erneuerte Komitee getrachtet, eine einfache, überall anwendbare Tumor-Nomenklatur aufzustellen, die auf den logischen Grundsätzen der allgemeinen Pathologie beruht.

Ein erster Entwurf ohne Bilder wurde in den ACTA Band XIV No. 3 1958 veröffentlicht, welchem nun die illustrierte Tumor-Nomenklatur folgt. Wir danken allen den verschiedenen Verfassern und Verlagen dafür, daß sie uns die Verwendung ihrer Abbildungen erlaubten und uns ihre Originalaufnahmen zur Reproduktion zur Verfügung stellten. Leider war es nicht möglich, die Originale der Abbildungen aus dem Atlas für Tumorpathologie zu erhalten; wir mußten daher die Abbildungen selbst als Vorlagen für die Reproduktionen verwenden und danken dem Armed Forces Institute of Pathology für die Erlaubnis, sie zu benützen.

Diese illustrierte Tumor-Nomenklatur hätte ohne eine Unterstützung nicht gedruckt werden können. Wir danken der Calouste Gulbenkian-Foundation in Lissabon für die Hilfe, die erst die Veröffentlichung ermöglichte.

Die gegenwärtige, ganz unbefriedigende Lage hinsichtlich einer allgemeinen Tumor-Nomenklatur ist allgemein bekannt, und doch kann kein Zweifel darüber bestehen, daß die beim Menschen vorkommenden Tumoren letzten Endes überall dieselben sind — sie werden bloß in den verschiedenen Ländern und Sprachgruppen verschieden benannt. Die erste Aufgabe, der sich das Komitee gegenübersah, bestand darin, eine möglichst vollständige Liste der derzeit gebräuchlichsten synonymen Bezeichnungen aufzustellen und dann die einzelnen Bezeichnungen daraufhin zu prüfen, ob sie wirklich einen bestimmten Tumor genau umschreiben und brauchbar sind. Selbstverständlich hat das Komitee energisch der Versuchung widerstanden, neue Namen zu erfinden und auf diese Weise die bereits bestehende Verwirrung noch zu vermehren. (Wenn trotzdem in der folgenden Liste Bezeichnungen erscheinen, die im deutschen Sprachgebiet ungewohnt oder gar neu sind, so geht das darauf zurück, daß es sich dabei um die Übersetzung eines in englischer oder französischer Sprache gebräuchlichen Terminus handelt. Fast überall ist aber neben der aus der Fremdsprache übersetzten Bezeichnung noch die entsprechende im deutschen Sprachgebiet übliche angegeben, wie z. B. „Klarzell-Carcinom der Niere" und „Hypernephrom". — Anmerkung der Herausgeber.)

Glücklicherweise wird für manche Tumorarten in der ganzen wissenschaftlichen Welt eine einzige histologische Bezeichnung gebraucht — das ist sozusagen der Idealzustand, dem wir zustreben sollten. Leider sind aber für andere Tumorarten in den verschiedenen Ländern ganz verschiedene, manchmal auch mehrere Bezeichnungen in ein und demselben Sprachgebiet üblich.

Bei der Anführung von Bezeichnungen für Tumoren, die unter verschiedenen Namen bekannt sind, hat das Komitee diejenige Bezeichnung an die erste Stelle gesetzt, welche ihm als die logischste und die am meisten den allgemeinen Grundsätzen entsprechende erschien, und hat die veralteten und nicht einwandfreien Bezeichnungen zuletzt angeführt. Synonyme Bezeichnungen wurden, soweit als möglich, zusammengefaßt.

Es gibt gewisse Bezeichnungen, die bloß in einem kleinen Kreis von Pathologen und in sehr beschränktem Umfang immer noch für gewisse Tumoren angewendet werden. Sie alle anzuführen, hätte die auszuarbeitende Zusammenstellung nur unnütz belastet. Sie wurden deshalb ganz weggelassen, weil man sicher für jede Bezeichnung, die man eventuell vermissen könnte, durch Benützung eines medizinischen Lexikons leicht den allgemein gebräuchlichen Namen finden kann, der in der Liste auch aufgeführt ist.

Nun gibt es aber Tumoren, die erst in wenigen Exemplaren beschrieben wurden und deren Einordnung und Benennung daher von Verfasser zu Verfasser schwankt, wie z. B. der „Retinalanlage-Tumor" bzw. „Melano-Amelo-

blastom". Derartige seltene Tumoren wurden nur dann aufgenommen, wenn sie zumindest in einem der größeren Sammelwerke bestätigt und womöglich einwandfrei abgebildet wurden. Mit anderen Worten: Das Komitee war entschlossen, sich nicht auf die Bilder und Benennungen der originalen Beschreibung zu verlassen, sondern fühlte sich verpflichtet, auf die Anerkennung einer neuen Tumorart durch einen kritischen, zweiten Verfasser zu warten. Es glaubte dadurch am besten der Notwendigkeit zu entgehen, die Liste der Tumoren allzuoft korrigieren zu müssen.

Nicht aufgenommen sind ferner Bezeichnungen, die keine echten Tumoren betreffen, darunter alle sog. Pseudo-Tumoren, wie Cysten, Granulome und Hyperplasien im üblichen Sinne. Auch die prämalignen bzw. sog. präcancerösen Veränderungen wurden nicht erwähnt, um diesen ersten Versuch einer Nomenklatur nicht allzusehr anschwellen zu lassen. Aus ähnlichen Gründen konnten die meisten der als „Carcinoma in situ" bezeichneten Veränderungen keinen Platz finden: Entweder handelt es sich um einen echten Krebs, der normales Epithel verdrängt hat, in dem er sich an seine Stelle setzt — dann läge bloß eine besondere Wuchsform eines auch anderweitig zu charakterisierenden Krebses vor; oder es handelt sich um eine Veränderung, die als solche bestehen bleibt, ja sich vielleicht sogar zurückbilden kann oder aber in echten Krebs übergeht — im letzteren Falle läge also höchstens eine Präcancerose vor, die ja nicht zu berücksichtigen war.

Bei der Auswahl und Beurteilung der Bezeichnungen hat sich das Komitee von folgenden Grundsätzen leiten lassen: Immer wieder hat es sich gezeigt, daß Bezeichnungen, um sich einzubürgern, kurz und prägnant sein müssen. Deshalb wurde stets ein einfacher Name vorgezogen vor zusammengesetzten, langen Benennungen, und zwar auch dann, wenn diese einen Tumor besser und vollständiger charakterisierten.

Die Tatsache, daß viele Tumoren mit dem Namen eines Beschreibers verbunden werden, drückt auch nur den Zug zu einer kurzen, einprägsamen Benennung aus. Entsprechend dem internationalen Übereinkommen wurden aber alle auf Personennamen beruhenden Bezeichnungen vermieden und gegebenenfalls durch andere treffende Bezeichnungen ersetzt. Um Mißverständnisse zu vermeiden, ist vielfach der Eigenname, unter dem ein solcher Tumor bis jetzt bekannt ist, doch noch in Klammern beigefügt. In einigen wenigen Fällen erschien es unmöglich, die eponyme Bezeichnung, wie z. B. „Brenner-Tumor" oder „Ewing-Sarkom", oder eine aus anderen Gründen nicht einwandfreie Bezeichnung, wie z. B. Hamartom oder Chondrom der Lunge, zu ersetzen, ohne einen neuen Namen zu erfinden, was ja vermieden werden sollte.

Die Bezeichnungen Carcinom und Sarkom sind den wirklich bösartigen Tumoren vorbehalten, Adenom nur den gutartigen. Sich selbst widersprechende Bezeichnungen, z. B. malignes Adenom, verbieten sich daher von selbst.

Zur Zeit ist der Histologe nicht immer imstande, mit Sicherheit vom morphologischen Bild auf die Funktion eines Tumors bzw. seine endokrine Tätigkeit zu schließen. Deshalb wurden alle Bezeichnungen vermieden, in denen solche funktionellen Bestimmungen enthalten waren; histologisch erkennbare Differenzierungen, wie z. B. Schleimproduktion, konnten jedoch berücksichtigt werden.

Es gibt auch wohlgekennzeichnete Tumoren, deren Einordnung noch umstritten ist, wie z. B. der Tumor, der als malignes, nicht chromaffines Paragangliom oder als alveoläres Weichteilsarkom bezeichnet wird. Die Einordnung solcher Tumoren in die vorliegende Liste mag deshalb in der Zukunft Änderungen unterworfen sein.

Da wir es mit einer rein histologischen Einteilung einzelner Tumoren zu tun haben, wurden Bezeichnungen wie „Neurofibrom" aufgenommen, nicht aber „Neurofibromatose", eine Diagnose, die erst auf Grund einer makroskopischen oder klinischen Untersuchung gestellt werden kann.

Leukämien sind nur insoweit berücksichtigt, als sie Gewebsveränderungen setzen, die mit histologischen Methoden zu erfassen sind; Veränderungen, die aus Abstrichen diagnostiziert werden, wie z. B. in der Hämatologie und Cytologie, wurden nicht aufgenommen.

Bezeichnungen wie Rundzellsarkom und Spindelzellsarkom wurden nicht aufgenommen, da derartige Diagnosen als unvollständig oder vorläufig anzusehen sind.

Schließlich noch ein Wort zur Anordnung unserer Liste. Da jede Anordnung angreifbar ist, handelte es sich darum, eine möglichst wenig anstoßende und einfache zu finden.

Tumoren mit einer histologischen Struktur, die kennzeichnend für das Ausgangsorgan ist, wurden so angeordnet, daß zuerst die Tumoren der Oberflächenepithelien aufgezählt werden, dann die Tumoren der einzelnen drüsigen Organe. Soweit als möglich entspricht die Anordnung der der malignen Neoplasmen in der internationalen Klassifikation der Krankheiten (Manual of the International Classification of Diseases, Injuries and Causes of Death, Vol. 1, World Health Organization, Geneva, Switzerland, 1957). Die Zahl in Klammern bei den verschiedenen Organen bezieht sich auf die entsprechenden Kategorien dieser internationalen Klassifikation. Dann folgen die Tumoren, die von den melaninbildenden Geweben abstammen, weiter die des Nervengewebes, der mesenchymalen Gewebe, des Blutes und der blutbildenden Gewebe sowie schließlich die Teratome.

Die Tumoren sind in jedem einzelnen Abschnitt so angeführt, daß die gutartigen Tumoren zuerst stehen, dann folgen die Tumoren von verhältnismäßig geringer Bösartigkeit und schließlich diejenigen größerer Bösartigkeit.

Bei den verschiedenen Beratungen der Kommission hat es sich immer als sehr nützlich erwiesen, wenn man auf eine gute Abbildung verweisen konnte, welche Definition und Beschreibung eines Tumors leichter verständlich machte. Im Hinblick auf diese Erfahrung beschloß das Komitee zu versuchen, auf repräsentative Illustrationen von Tumoren hinzuweisen, die dann besser als viele Worte sagen, was eine Bezeichnung bedeuten solle, wobei freilich zuzugeben ist, daß solche Abbildungen kaum je alle möglichen Abwandlungen eines Tumors aufzeigen können, die einem schon das einfachste histologische Präparat vermitteln kann.

Das Komitee war der Ansicht, daß neben Bildern aus anerkannten Lehrbüchern die Bilder in dem eben erscheinenden amerikanischen

Atlas der Tumorpathologie für eine solche Bebilderung besonders geeignet wären.

So beabsichtigt also die vorliegende illustrierte Tumor-Nomenklatur, repräsentative Abbildungen der häufigsten Tumoren zu geben, hinsichtlich derer bereits eine Übereinstimmung zwischen den verschiedenen Sprachgruppen besteht. Da der Text in Englisch, Französisch, Russisch, Deutsch, Spanisch und in lateinischer Sprache wiedergegeben ist, sollte diese illustrierte Tumor-Nomenklatur fähig sein, diese gegenseitige Verständigung weiter zu fördern: Ein Pathologe dürfte leicht imstande sein, herauszufinden, wie ein gegebener Tumor in anderen Sprachen bezeichnet wird. Die illu-

strierte Tumor-Nomenklatur will aber auch dem Pathologen in den vielen abgeschiedenen Teilen der Welt nützlich sein, da ja wohl mehr als 90% der Tumoren, mit denen er es zu tun hat, hier angeführt und abgebildet sind.

Die illustrierte Tumor-Nomenklatur beabsichtigt dementsprechend, in keiner Weise die Tätigkeit der Referenzzentren zu beeinträchtigen, die von der Weltgesundheits-Organisation eingerichtet werden. Es ist vielmehr zu hoffen, daß diese Zentren zu einem besseren Verständnis derjenigen strittigen Tumoren beitragen werden, die mit Absicht in der illustrierten Tumor-Nomenklatur nicht berücksichtigt wurden.

Prefacio de la primera edición

En el 6° Congreso de Cancerología en São Paulo fué presentada una lista de tumores, destinada en primer lugar a la codificación estadística. Esta lista, aceptada con pequeñas modificaciones, fue preparada por un Comité para la Nomenclatura de Tumores, bajo la presidencia del Dr. I. Perry (E.E.U.U.), designado por la Unión Internacional Contra el Cáncer. Sobre la base de esta lista fue presentado un código algo simplificado a la Organización Mundial de la Salud, la cual lo puso en circulación como documento WHO/HS/CANC/24.1. Un índice alfabético basado en la terminología habitual en los Estados Unidos constituye la segunda parte de dicho documento (WHO/HS/CANC/24.2).

La elaboración de una lista de términos descriptivos que pudiera ser usada con el código de estadística de tumores constituyó la primera meta del Comité, pero desde el principio se tuvo la intención de crear, aparte del código científico, una nomenclatura tumoral lógicamente ordenada y científicamente aceptable. Esta segunda meta presentó un sin número de dificultades pese a las numerosas discusiones en conferencias especiales y a la correspondencia mantenida durante 4 años entre los miembros del Comité. Por fin tuvo que reconocerse que la principal dificultad residía en la intención de alcanzar simultáneamente las dos metas: un código estadístico y la nomenclatura tumoral. Por esta razón en el mencionado Congreso de Cancerología reunido en São Paulo en 1954, se resolvió que el Comité debería reorganizarse bajo la dirección del Dr. H. Hamperl y que en el futuro sería solamente perseguida una meta, es decir la nomenclatura tumoral histológica. A pesar de que esta nomenclatura y el código estadístico son elaborados y publicados en forma separada, no existen dificultades, como se ha manifestado expresamente, en coordinarlos ulteriormente para su uso práctico. Este Comité ha tratado mientras tanto de crear una nomenclatura tumoral, basada en los principios lógicos de la patología general.

Una primera versión sin figuras fue publicada en "ACTA" Vol. XIV, N° 3—1958, la cual es ahora seguida por una edición ilustrada. Agradecemos a la Fundación Gulbenkian por proveer fondos para la impresión de esta monografía. Estamos muy agradecidos a todos los autores y casas editoras por su autorización para usar sus ilustraciones y habernos proporcionado sus originales. Desgraciadamente no fue posible obtener los moldes originales de las figuras del Atlas de Patología Tumoral; por lo tanto tuvimos que reproducir las ilustraciones impresas.

Es bien conocida la actual situación insatisfactoria, en lo que a la nomenclatura tumoral se refiere. A pesar de que no existen dudas de que los tumores humanos son básicamente semejantes en todas partes del mundo, los nombres aplicados a los mismos tumores difieren en los distintos países e idiomas. Por esto, la primera tarea enfrentada por el Comité fue reunir en la forma más completa posible, las denominaciones sinónimas actualmente en uso y considerar luego su utilidad y exactitud descriptiva. Desde luego, el Comité ha evitado crear nuevos nombres y aumentar de esta manera la confusión ya reinante. (Si a pesar de todo aparecen nombres nuevos, no usuales en el idioma español, se debe a que fueron traducidos del inglés o francés, idiomas en los cuales son de uso común. Casi siempre se ha publicado, aparte de esta denominación traducida, el término habitual en el idioma español.)

Afortunadamente existen tumores en los cuales se usa una sola denominación en todo el mundo científico; estos son casos ideales a los cuales deberíamos tender. Desgraciadamente también tenemos tumores con distintas denominaciones, aún para un mismo idioma, por lo que un mismo tumor es conocido con diferentes nombres en diferentes países.

Cuando se hizo la relación de tumores conocidos con varios nombres, el Comité colocó primero los nombres que parecen ser más lógicos y de acuerdo con los principios básicos generales. Los términos considerados anticuados o no del todo correctos son mencionados al final; los sinónimos, en lo posible, son presentados en forma conjunta.

Existen nombres de tumores que son usados por un grupo pequeño de patólogos. Estas denominaciones no fueron mencionadas en la presente lista, ya que ello hubiera significado un recargo de trabajo. Por otro lado, estos términos pueden ser identificados fácilmente por medio de un diccionario médico.

Existen tumores que son descritos excepcionalmente y cuya clasificación varía de un autor a otro. Tal ocurre por ejemplo con el "Retinalanlage-Tumor" o con el "Melanoameloblastoma". Tumores raros de este tipo fueron incorporados en la presente lista solamente si fueron publicados en alguno de los principales libros de texto, especialmente si fueron adecuadamente ilustrados. En otras palabras, el Comité decidió no basarse en las figuras y descripciones de las publicaciones originales, sino en el trabajo ulterior de un autor crítico. De esta manera se ha esperado evitar la necesidad de corregir repetidas veces la lista de tumores.

Términos descriptivos de lesiones que no son tumores verdaderos, tales como quistes, granulomas e hiperplasias no fueron considerados. Tampoco son mencionados las alteraciones premalignas o precancerosas con el fin de evitar un recargo en el presente trabajo. Por semejantes razones fueron omitidas las alteraciones conocidas como "carcinoma in situ"; en justificación de esta política puede señalarse que, aunque algunos casos del así llamado "carcinoma in situ" pueden eventualmente probar ser cánceres verdaderos, desplazando y reemplazando al epitelio normal, es también cierto que el término "carcinoma in situ" puede ocasionalmente ser usado para describir otras lesiones cuya relación con el cáncer verdadero no siempre está claramente establecida; algunas de estas lesiones pueden retroceder y desaparecer por lo que su inclusión en un manual de nomenclatura de tumores estaría fuera de lugar.

En la elección de las distintas denominaciones, el Comité se ha basado en lo siguiente: un término debe ser corto y definidor para encontrar aceptación general. Por esta razón se han preferido los nombres sencillos a los nombres largos y compuestos, aún cuando estos pueden describir mejor y en forma más completa un tumor.

El hecho de que numerosos tumores lleven un nombre propio –el del autor que los describió– confirma la tendencia natural de usar denominaciones breves. Sin embargo, como consecuencia de un acuerdo internacional, se ha decidido rechazar todas las designaciones basadas en nombres propios y reemplazarlas por términos descriptivos apropiados; pero para evitar errores de interpretación se ha agregado entre paréntesis el nombre propio, que era usado en el pasado. En raras ocasiones no se ha podido reemplazar los nombres propios (por ejemplo, para el sarcoma de Ewing, el tumor de Brenner) o términos objetables por otras consideraciones como por ejemplo el hamartoma del pulmón, que no podrían reemplazarse sin introducir un nuevo nombre.

Obviamente, las denominaciones carcinoma y sarcoma son usadas solamente para tumores realmente malignos y la de adenoma para los benignos. Términos contradictorios, como por ejemplo adenoma maligno, han sido evitados. En el momento presente, la actividad funcional de un tumor, por ejemplo la actividad endocrina, no puede ser siempre determinada por su cuadro histológico. Por esta razón se han evitado las denominaciones que se refieren a la actividad de una neoplasia, aunque se han conservado los términos que expresan una diferenciación histológica, por ejemplo tumor muco-productor.

Existen tumores bien conocidos cuya clasificación es todavía discutida, tal es el caso del paraganglioma cromafín maligno, o del sarcoma alveolar de partes blandas. La clasificación de estos tumores está sujeta a modificaciones futuras.

Como estamos tratando con una clasificación puramente histológica se han incorporado denominaciones como neurofibroma; en cambio términos deducidos del examen macroscópico o clínico, como "neurofibromatosis", no lo han sido. Las leucemias fueron incluidas solamente en relación a las lesiones de las tejidos, reconocibles por medios histológicos; en cambio no son mencionadas las alteraciones que son diagnosticadas solamente por frotis (hematología o citología exfoliativa).

Los términos sarcoma de células redondas o fusocelulares, no han sido incluídos por representar diagnósticos incompletos o provisionales.

Finalmente, debemos decir unas palabras en relación con el orden que ha sido adoptado. Como toda clasificación está abierta a la crítica, se ha tratado de crear una lista sencilla y adaptable, con posibilidades mínimas de provocar resentimientos.

Los tumores que por su arquitectura histológica permiten reconocer su origen son mencionados en el siguiente orden: en primer lugar los tumores originados en las superficies epiteliales, en segundo lugar los tumores de órganos glandulares; luego siguen los tejidos formadores de melanina, los tumores de sistema nervioso, los del mesenquima, de la sangre y órganos hematopoyéticos y finalmente los teratomas. En lo posible se ha seguido el orden de las categorías de neoplasias malignas de la Clasificación Internacional de Enfermedades, Injurias y Causas de Muerte (Vol. I. Organización Mundial de la Salud. Ginebra, Suiza, 1957). Los números entre paréntesis corresponden a los números que señalan la categoría de las neoplasias malignas de la Clasificación Internacional.

Los tumores han sido ordenados de tal manera, que en cada sección aparecen en primer lugar las neoplasias benignas, luego las de malignidad relativamente baja y luego las neoformaciones altamente malignas.

Durante las discusiones del Comité se ha observado que una buena ilustración ha sido la forma más sencilla de definir y describir un tumor. En consecuencia, el Comité resolvió proporcionar ilustraciones representativas, que mejor que cualquier descripción verbal defina un tumor dado, aunque se reconoció que estas ilustraciones no podrían representar todas las variaciones posibles de un tumor, como lo demuestra mejor la lámina histológica más sencilla.

El Comité pensó que las fotografías del Atlas de Patología Tumoral, publicado por el Instituto de Patología de las Fuerzas Armadas de los Estados Unidos, serían especialmente convenientes para ilustrar esta clasificación, así como otras de autorizados libros de textos de otros países.

Así, la Nomenclatura Ilustrada de Tumores ha sido proyectada con el propósito de mostrar figuras representativas de los tumores más frecuentes, sobre los que ya existe acuerdo entre los diferentes grupos idiomáticos. Como el texto está impreso en inglés, francés, ruso, alemán y latín, la Nomenclatura Ilustrada de Tumores debe ampliar este entendimiento mutuo: un patólogo puede encontrar fácilmente como un tumor determinado es designado en otros idiomas. La Nomenclatura Ilustrada de Tumores también ayudará al patólogo que trabaja en áreas aisladas del globo, dado que más del 90 por ciento de tumores, con los cuales ha de tratar, estan en la lista y serán ilustrados. Por lo tanto la Nomenclatura Ilustrada de Tumores no interfiere con el trabajo de los Centros de Referencia establecidos por la Organización Mundial de la Salud. Se espera que estos Centros de Referencia contribuirán al mejor conocimiento de los tumores todavía en litigio que deliberadamente han sido omitidos en la presente Nomenclatura.

Los nombres que se han dado a los diferentes tumores en este nomenclatura, representan la opinión del Comité, en su conjunto. Por lo tanto hay casos que constituyen una avenencia o compromiso entre los diferentes miembros del Comité y deben ser considerados con este criterio. La discusión de los nombres más apropiados y la selección de las mejores ilustraciones ha sido motivo de deliberaciones entre los miembros del Comité durante casi una década.

Pese a lo expuesto, los miembros del Comité para la Nomenclatura de Tumores, reconocen que el producto de su trabajo dista de ser completo y que ciertamente no constituye la forma definitiva; ellos lo consideran simplemente como el "fin del comienzo" y como un proyecto preliminar, que se atreven a esperar puede servir como base para discusiones fructíferas.

Contents

Table des matières

Содержание

Inhalt

Indice

Index

Source of Illustrations

The illustrations quoted in the text are referred to by letters indicating the author (e.g. M = Masson) and by two numbers, one denoting the page and the other the illustration.

e.g. F 14 33–24 means:

Fascicle 14 of the Atlas of Tumor Pathology, page 33, Figure 24.

Origine des figures

Les figures citées dans le texte sont marquées par des lettres indiquant l'auteur (par exemple M = Masson) et par des chiffres représentant les pages et des numéros les figures.

Par exemple: F 14 33–24 veut dire:

Fascicule 14 de l'Atlas of Tumor Pathology, page 33, figure 24.

Источники иллюстраций

Указанные в тексте рисунки отмечаются буквой для автора (напр. М=Массон) и двумя цифрами, из которых первая относится к странице источника, а вторая — к номеру рисунка: напр. В 14, 33–24 означает — Выпуск 14 Атласа патологии опухолей, стр. 33, рисунок 24.

Quellenangabe der Abbildungen

Die im Text angegebenen Abbildungen wurden mit Buchstaben für den Autor (z. B. M = MASSON) und zwei Zahlen für Seite und Abbildung bezeichnet; so bedeutet z. B. F 14 33–24: Faszikel 14 des Atlas of Tumor Pathology, Seite 33, Abbildung 24.

Procedencia de las figuras

La procedencia de las figuras citadas en el texto fue expresada por medio de letras para el autor (M = MASSON) y dos cifras para la página y la figura; por ejemplo: F 14 33–24 significa: Fascículo 14 del "Atlas of Tumor Pathology", página 33, figura 24.

A   = Ackerman, L. V. Surgical Pathology (C. V. Mosby Company St. Louis, 1959).

A-R = Ackerman, L. V., and del Regato, J. A. Cancer-Diagnosis Treatment and Prognosis (C. V. Mosby Company, St. Louis, 1962).

v. A. = v. Albertini, A. Histologische Geschwulstdiagnostik (Georg Thieme Verlag Stuttgart, 1955).

F   = Fascicle of the Atlas of Tumor Pathology — and number of it (Armed Forces Institute of Pathology, Washington, D.C.).

Glaz = Glazounoff, M. F. Tumors of the Ovary (Medgis Leningrad, 1961).

H   = Hamperl, H. Lehrbuch der allgemeinen Pathologie und pathologischen Anatomie, 24. und 25. Auflage (Springer Verlag, Berlin, Göttingen, Heidelberg, 1960).

K   = Kraus F. T. Gynecologic Pathology (C. V. Mosby Company St. Louis 1967).

M   = Masson, P. Tumeurs Humaines (2e édit. Librairie Maloine, Paris, 1956).

Z   = Zülch, K. J. Biologie und Pathologie der Hirngeschwülste; in: Handbuch der Neurochirurgie, 3. Bd. (Springer Verlag, Berlin, Göttingen, Heidelberg, 1956).

A   = Аккерман, Л. В. Хирургическая патология (Мосби, Сан Луи, 1959).

A-R = Аккерман, Л. В. и дель Регато, Ю. А.: Рак-: Диагнозиз и прогнозиз (Мосби, Сан Луи, 1962).

v. A. = Ф. Альбертини, А. Гистологическая диагностика опухолей (Тиме, Штутгарт, 1955).

F   = Выпуск Атласа патологии опухолей (Ин-т патологии вооруженных сил, Вашингтон, США).

Glaz = Глазунов, М. Ф. Опухоли яичников (Медгиз, Ленинград, 1961).

H   = Гамперль, Г. Учебник общей патологии и патологической анатомии 24 и 25 изд. (Шпрингер: Берлин, Гёттинген, Гейдельберг, 1960).

K   = Краус Ф. Т. Гинекологическая Патология (Мосби, Сан Луи, 1967)

M   = Массон, П. Опухоли человека (2 изд., Малуан, Париж, 1956).

Z   = Цюльх, К. Ю. Биология и патология опухолей мозга. В: Руководство по неврохирургии, т. 3 (Шпрингер: Берлин, Гёттинген, Гейдельберг, 1956).

I.

Epithelial tumors of general distribution

Tumeurs épithéliales en général

Эпителиальные опухоли без специфической локализации

Epitheliale Tumoren ohne spezifische Lokalisation

Tumores epiteliales en general

Tumores epitheliales sine locatione specifica

Adenoma — *a benign tumor derived from glandular epithelium, which may be further classified into:*

Adénome — *tumeur bénigne, dérivée d'un épithélium glandulaire, que l'on peut subdiviser en:*

Аденома — *доброкачественная опухоль, исходящая из железистого эпителия; подразделяется на:*

Adenom — *ein gutartiger, vom drüsenbildenden Epithel ausgehender Tumor, der weiter unterteilt werden kann in:*

Adenoma — *tumor benigno derivado de epitelio glandular, que se puede subdividir como sigue:*

1	Trabecular adenoma Solid adenoma	Adénome trabéculaire	Трабекулярная Аденома Солидная Аденома
	Trabeculäres Adenom Solides Adenom	Adenoma trabecular Adenoma sólido	Adenoma trabeculare Adenoma solidum
2	Tubular adenoma	Adénome tubuleux	Тубулярная Аденома
	Tubuläres Adenom	Adenoma tubular	Adenoma tubulare
3	Acinar adenoma Alveolar adenoma Follicular adenoma	Adénome acineux Adénome alvéolaire Adénome folliculaire	Ацинозная Аденома Альвеолярная Аденома Фолликулярная Аденома
	Acinöses Adenom Alveoläres Adenom Follikuläres Adenom	Adenoma acinoso Adenoma alveolar Adenoma folicular	Adenoma acinosum Adenoma alveolare Adenoma folliculare

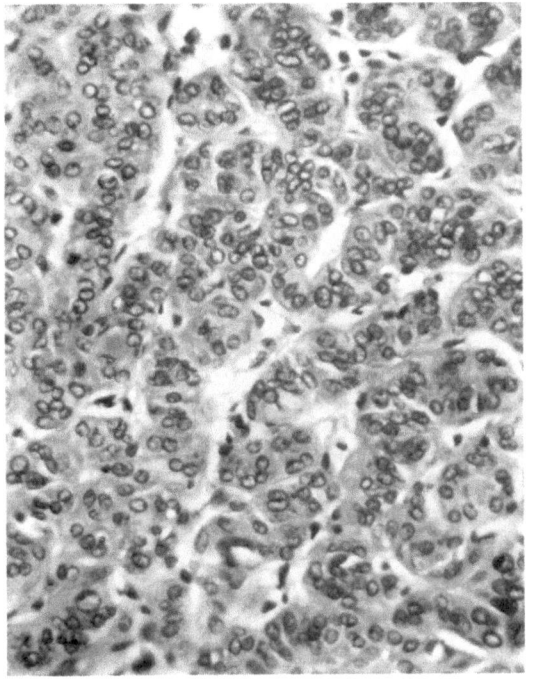 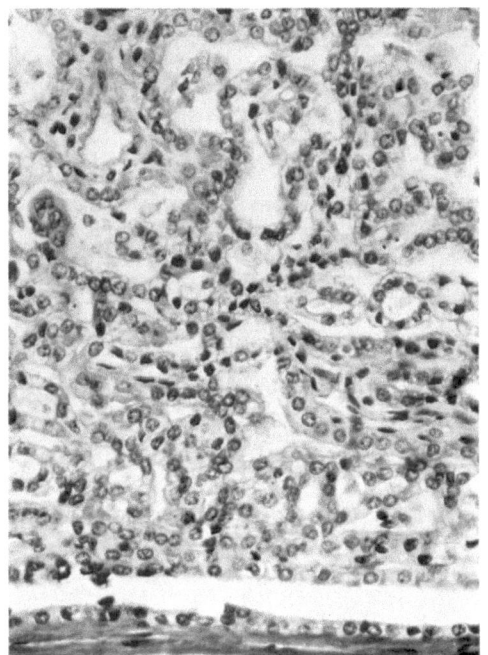

Fig. 1. × 275.   F 14 33—24   Fig. 2. × 300.

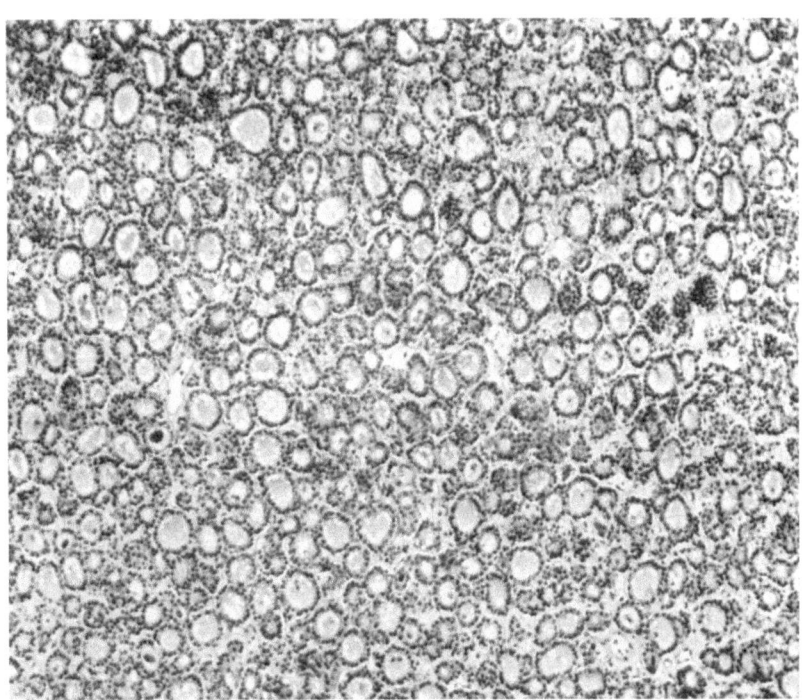

Fig. 3. × 90.   F 15 43—27

1*

4 Cystic adenoma	Adénome kystique	Кистозная Аденома
Cystadenoma	Cystadénome	Кистаденома
Glandular cystoma		Гляндулярная кистома
Cystisches Adenom	Adenoma quístico	Adenoma cysticum
Cystadenom	Cistoadenoma	Cystadenoma
Glanduläres Cystom	Cistoma glandular	Cystoma glandulare

5 Papillary adenoma	Adénome papillaire	Папиллярная Аденома
Papilläres Adenom	Adenoma papilífero	Adenoma papilliferum

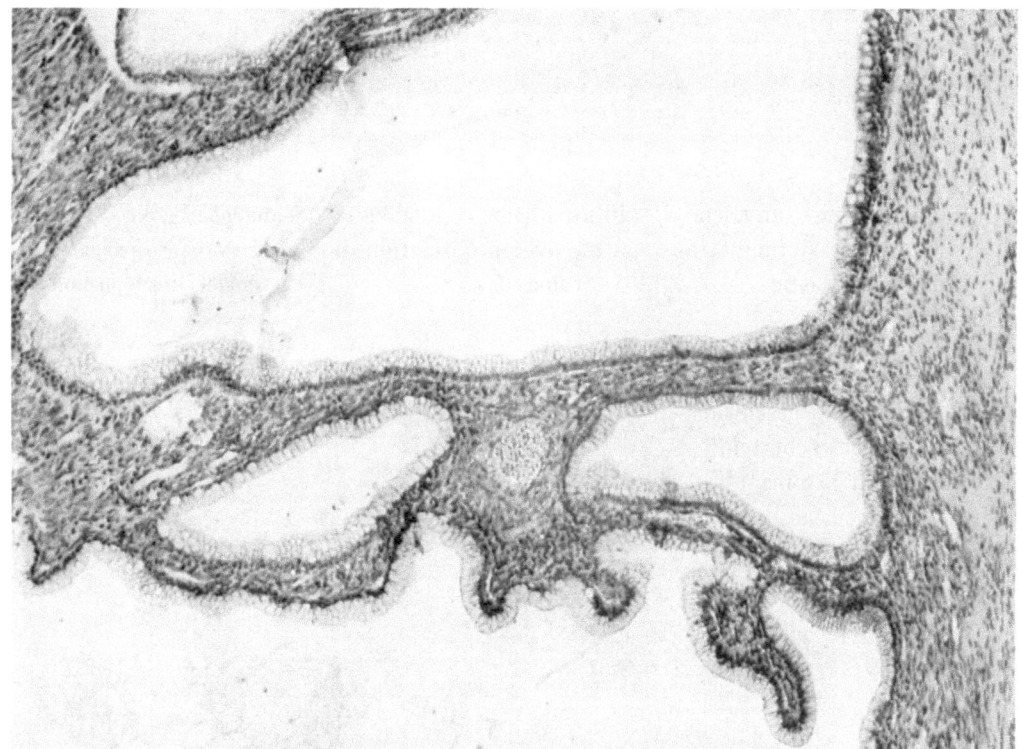

Fig. 4. × 50.   F 33/3 97—87

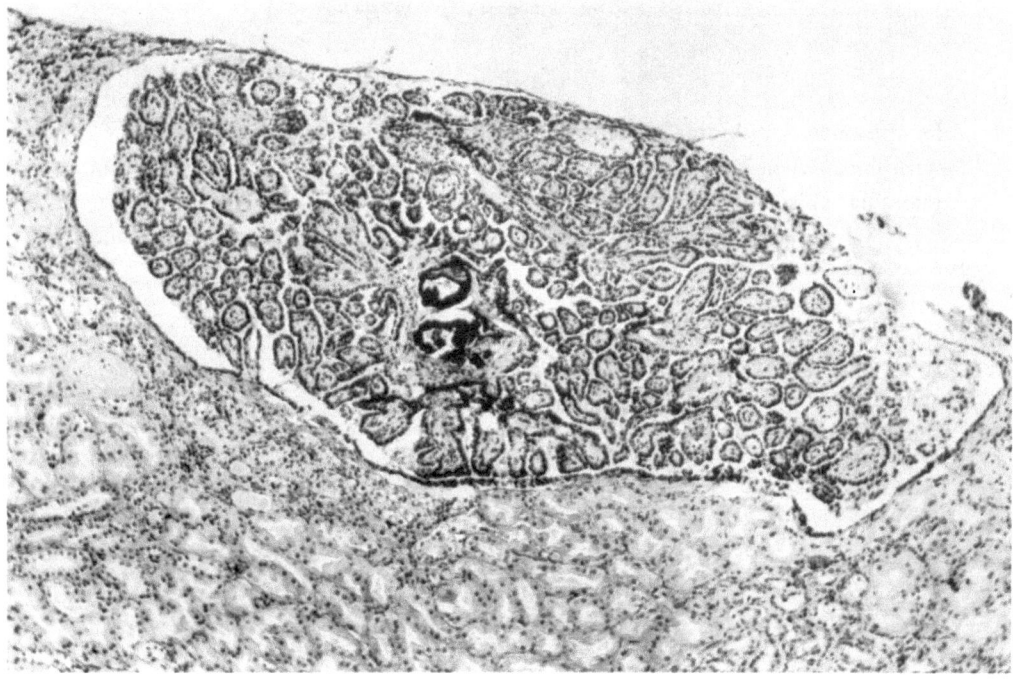

Fig. 5. × 90.   F 30 31—6

6 Fibroadenoma—an adeno-
ma, whose fibrous stro-
ma is neoplastic

Fibro-adénome — adéno-
me avec prolifération du
stroma

Фиброаденома — аденомас
опухолево разраста-
ющейся фиброзной стро-
мой

Fibroadenom — ein Ade-
nom mit geschwulst-
mäßig gewuchertem
fibrösem Stroma

Fibroadenoma — un ade-
noma cuyo estroma fi-
broso es neoplásico

Fibroadenoma

7 Adenofibroma — a fibroma
with enclosed neoplastic
glandular epithelium

Adéno-fibrome — fibrome
contenant des structures
glandulaires qui font
partie de la tumeur

Аденофиброма — фиброма
с включенными в нее
опухолево разрастающи-
мися железистыми
трубками

Adenofibrom — ein Fibrom
mit eingeschlossenen ge-
schwulstmäßig neugebil-
deten Drüsenschläuchen

Adenofibroma — un fibro-
ma que alberga prolife-
ración glandular neo-
plásica

Adenofibroma

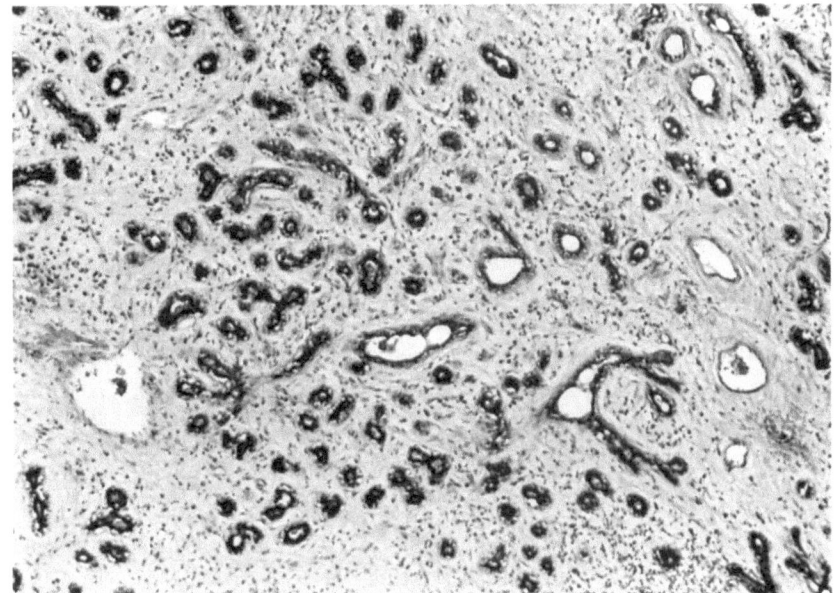

Fig. 6. × 60.

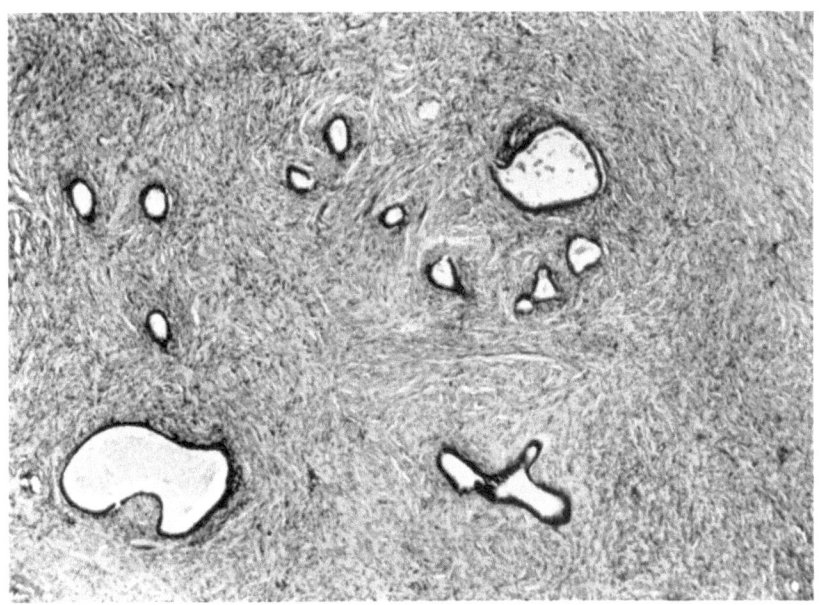

Fig. 7. × 38.

Polyp — *gross descriptive term for an outgrowth of a mucosal surface (not of skin) to be specified histologically e.g.:*

Polype — *terme macroscopique pour désigner une masse exubérante siégeant à la surface d'une muqueuse (non de la peau) devant être spécifiée histologiquement, par exemple:*

Полип — *описательный термин для обозначения экзофитных разрестаний слизистой оболочки (не кожи), которые гистологически могут быть ближе охарактеризованы как:*

Polyp — *makroskopische Bezeichnung für eine Wucherung einer Schleimhautoberfläche, die histologisch näher bestimmt werden kann, z. B.:*

Pólipo — *término macroscópico, descriptivo, para tumores exofíticos de superficies mucosas (no de la piel) que será especificado histológicamente, como sigue:*

8	Adenomatous polyp	Polype adénomateux	Аденоматозный Полип
	Glandular polyp	Polype glandulaire	Железистый Полип
	Adenomatöser Polyp	Pólipo adenomatoso	Polypus adenomatosus
	Glandulärer Polyp	Pólipo glandular	Polypus glandularis

9	Papillary polyp	Polype papillaire	Папиллярный Полип
	Papilloma	Papillome	Папиллома
	Papillärer Polyp	Pólipo papilífero	Polypus papillaris
	Papillom	Papiloma	Papilloma

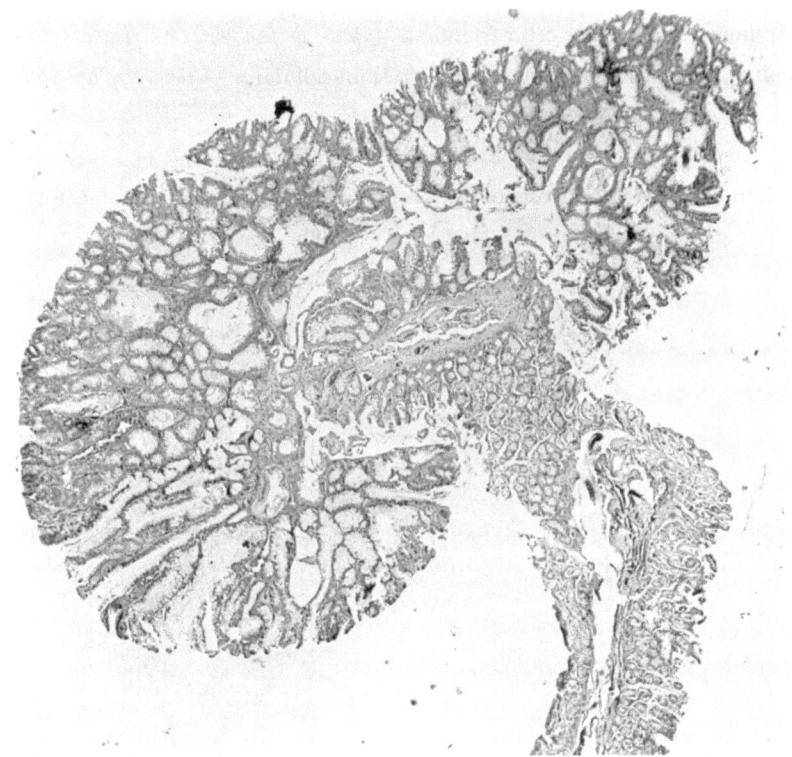

Fig. 8. × 15.

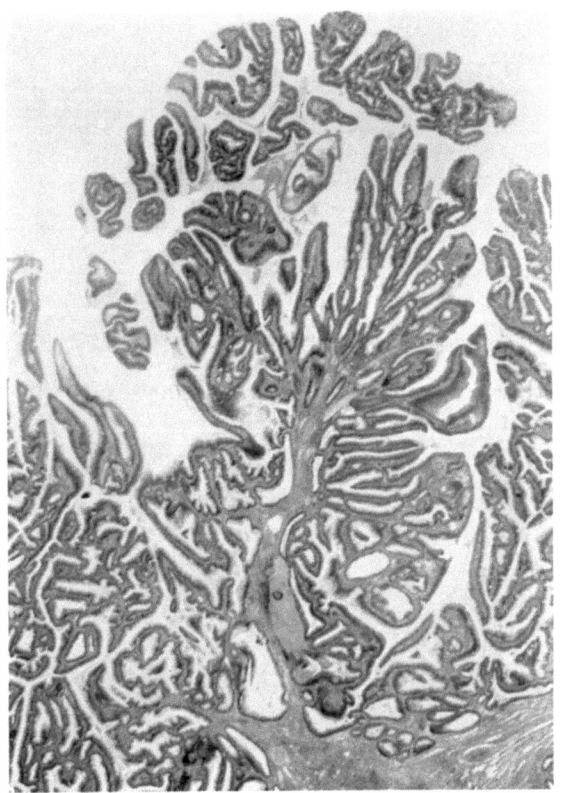

Fig. 9. × 13.   v. A. 121--90

Epidermoid carcinoma, Squamous cell carcinoma — *may be further classified into:*

Epithélioma épidermoïde, Epithélioma malpighien spinocellulaire — *peut être subdivisé en:*

Эпидермальный рак, Плоскоклеточный рак, — *подрдазеляется на:*

Epidermoidcarcinom, Plattenepithelcarcinom — *zu unterteilen in:*

Carcinoma epidermoide, Carcinoma escamoso, Carcinoma malpighiano o espinocelular — *que puede ser subdividido como sigue:*

10	Keratinizing type	Type kératinisant	Ороговевающий
	Malignant acanthoma	Acanthome malin	Злокачественная акантома
	Cancroid	Cancroide	Канкроид
	Verhornendes Platten-epithelcarcinom	Tipo queratinizante	Typus cornescens
	Malignes Acanthom	Acantoma maligno	Acanthoma malignum
	Cancroid	Cancroide	Tumor cancroides

11	Non-keratinizing type	Type non kératinisant	Неороговевающий
	Nichtverhornendes Platten-epithelcarcinom	Tipo no queratinizante	Typus non-cornescens

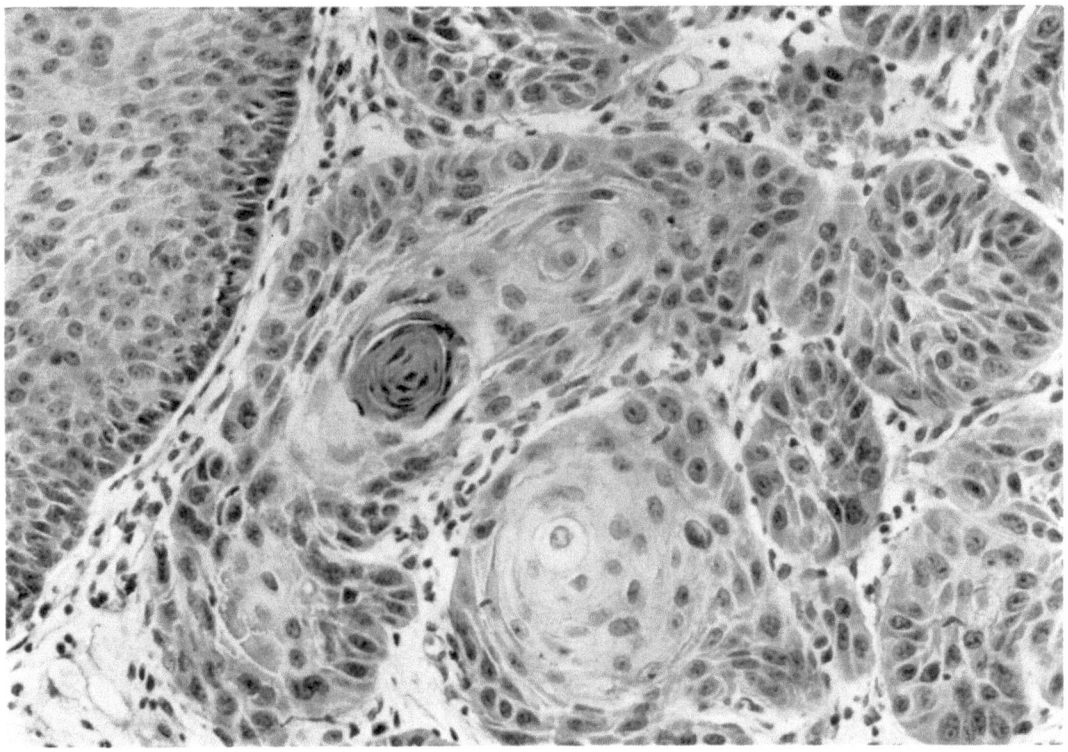

Fig. 10. × 154.

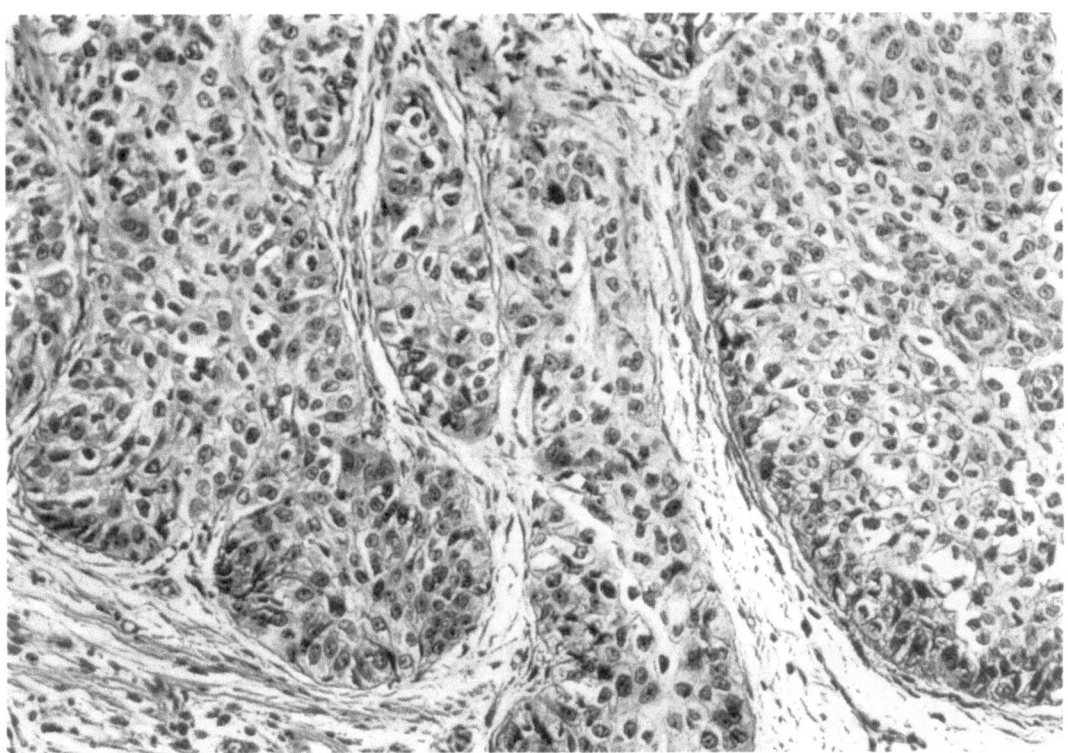

Fig. 11. × 186.

12

Adenocarcinoma — *carcinoma of glandular structure which may be further classified on the basis of predominant histological pattern in the following terms or combinations of these:*

Epithélioma glandulaire (adénocarcinome) — *épithélioma de structure glandulaire qui, suivant le type histologique prédominant, peut présenter les formes ou combinaisons de formes suivantes:*

Аденокарцинома (железистый рак) — *рак железистого строения, который на основании преобладающей гистологической структуры или комбинации их, подразделяется на:*

Adenocarcinom („Drüsenkrebs") — *Carcinom des drüsenbildenden Gewebes, das auf Grund des im histologischen Schnitt vorherrschenden Gewebsanteils oder Kombination von solchen weiter eingeteilt werden kann in:*

Adenocarcinoma — *carcinoma de estructura glandular que puede clasificarse, según el cuadro histológico predominante, con los siguientes términos o con una combinación de ellos:*

12	Tubular adenocarcinoma	Epithélioma glandulaire tubuleux	Тубулярная аденокарцинома
	Tubuläres Adenocarcinom	Adenocarcinoma tubular	Adenocarcinoma tubulare

13	Alveolar adenocarcinoma Acinous adenocarcinoma	Epithélioma alvéolaire Epithélioma acineux	Альвеолярная аденокарцинома Ацинозная аденокарцинома
	Alveoläres Adenocarcinom Acinöses Adenocarcinom	Adenocarcinoma alveolar Adenocarcinoma acinoso	Adenocarcinoma alveolare Adenocarcinoma acinosum

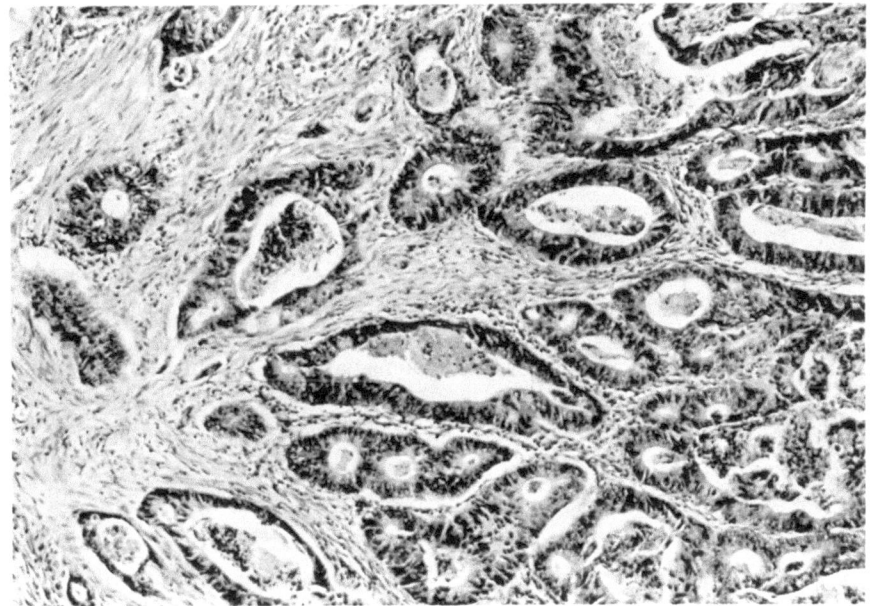

Fig. 12. × 75.

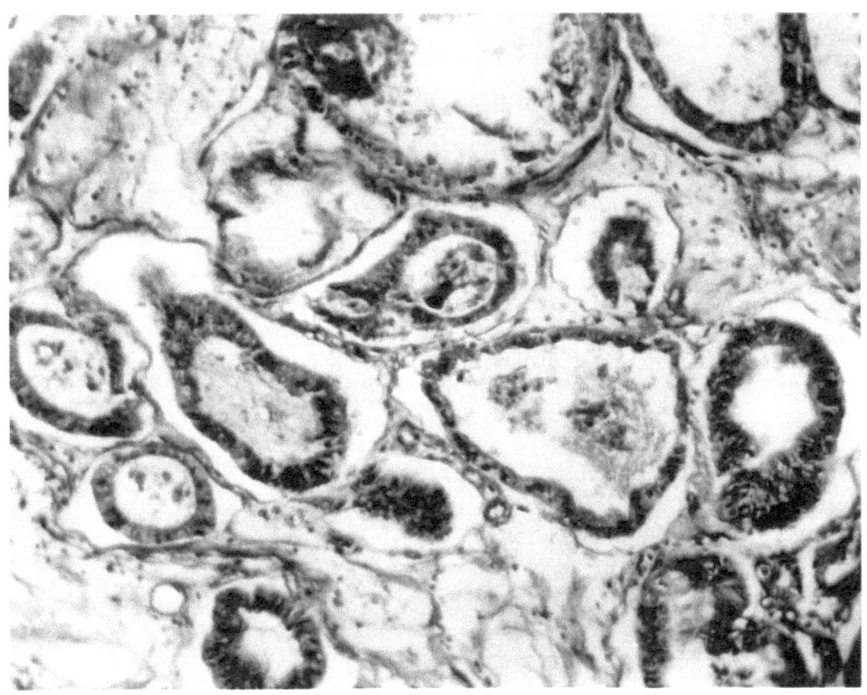

Fig. 13. × 165.

F 32 153—114

14 Papillary adenocarcinoma Epithélioma glandulaire Папиллярная
          papillaire   аденокарцинома

  Papilläres Adenocarcinom Adenocarcinoma papilífero Adenocarcinoma papilli-
                    ferum

15 Mucus producing adeno- Epithélioma glandulaire Слизеобразующая
  carcinoma   sécrétant   аденокарцинома

  Schleimbildendes Adeno- Adenocarcinoma muco Adenocarcinoma mucoides
  carcinom   productor

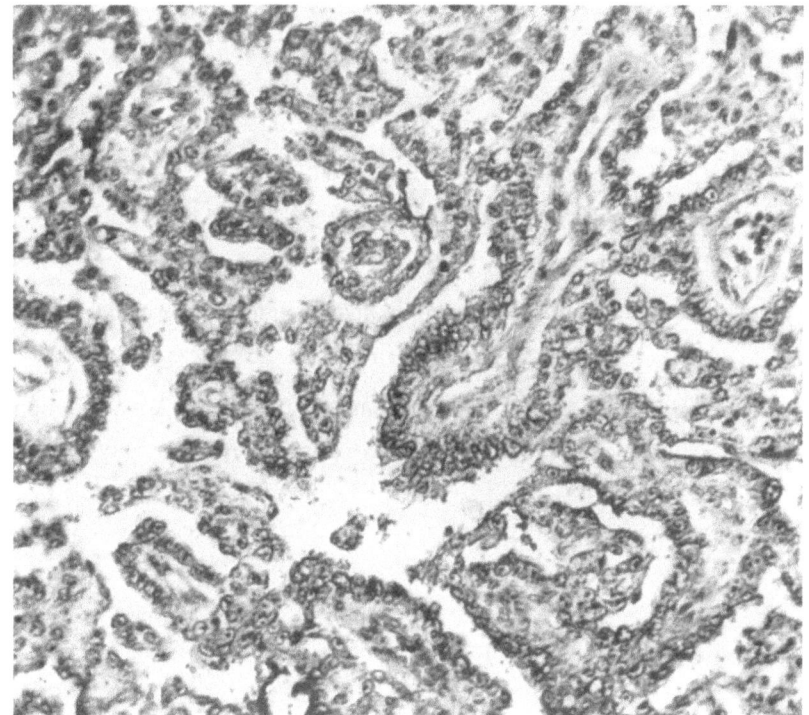

Fig. 14.   × 240.   F 24 123—89

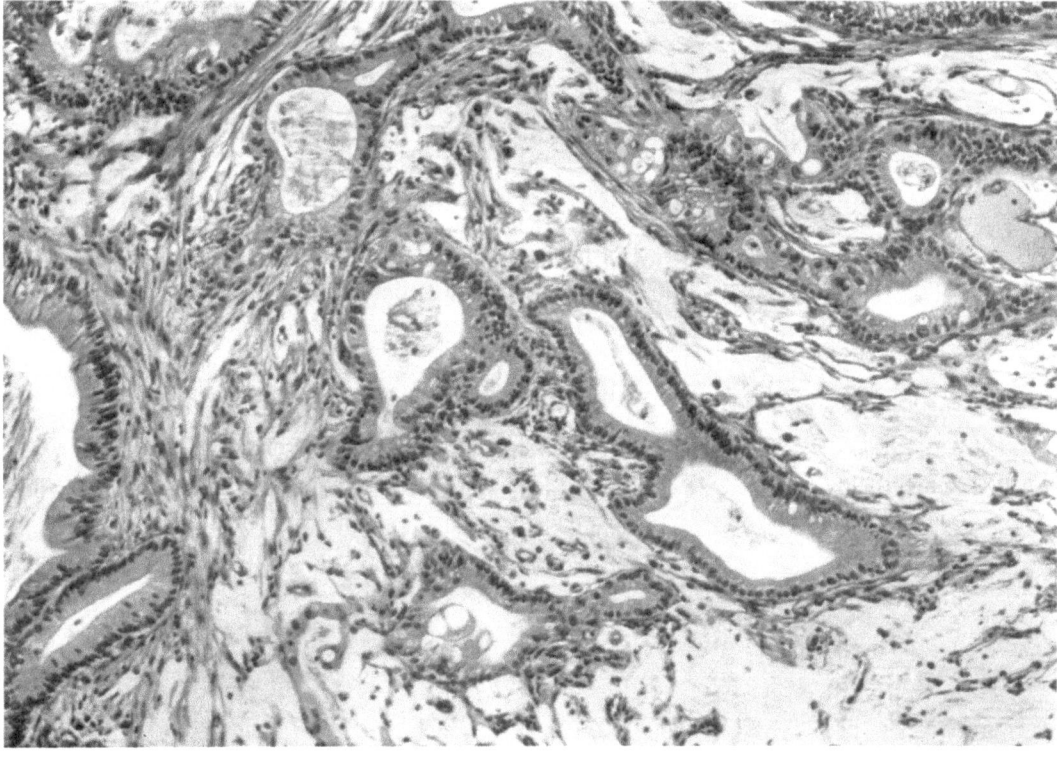

Fig. 15.   × 110.   F 33/2 153—126

16   Anaplastic adenocarcinoma   Epithélioma anaplasique   Анапластическая
                                                                             аденокарцинома

      Anaplastisches Adeno-   Adenocarcinoma anaplá-   Adenocarcinoma anaplasti-
        carcinom   sico   cum

17   Adenocarcinoma with   Epithélioma glandulaire   Аденокарцинома с
        squamous metaplasia   avec métaplasie   плоскоклеточной
      Adenoacanthoma   malpighienne   метаплязией
      Adenocancroid   Adénoacanthome   Аденоакантома
                                    Adénocancroïde   Аденоканкроид

      Adenocarcinom mit Plat-   Adenocarcinoma con meta-   Adenocarcinoma cum
        tenepithelmetaplasie   plasia escamosa   metaplasia epidermoide
      Adenoakanthom   Adenoacantoma   Adenoacanthoma
      Adenocancroid   Adenocancroide   Tumor adenocancroides

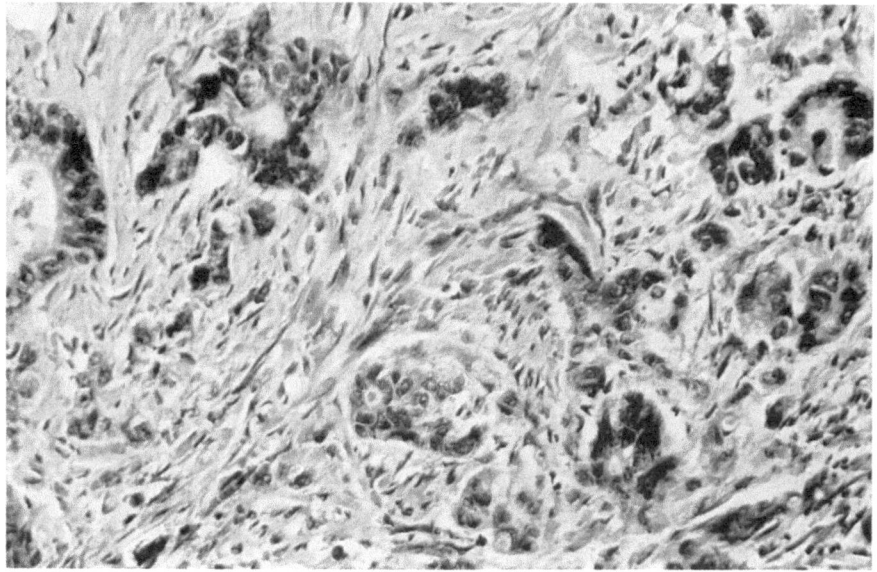

Fig. 16. × 350.

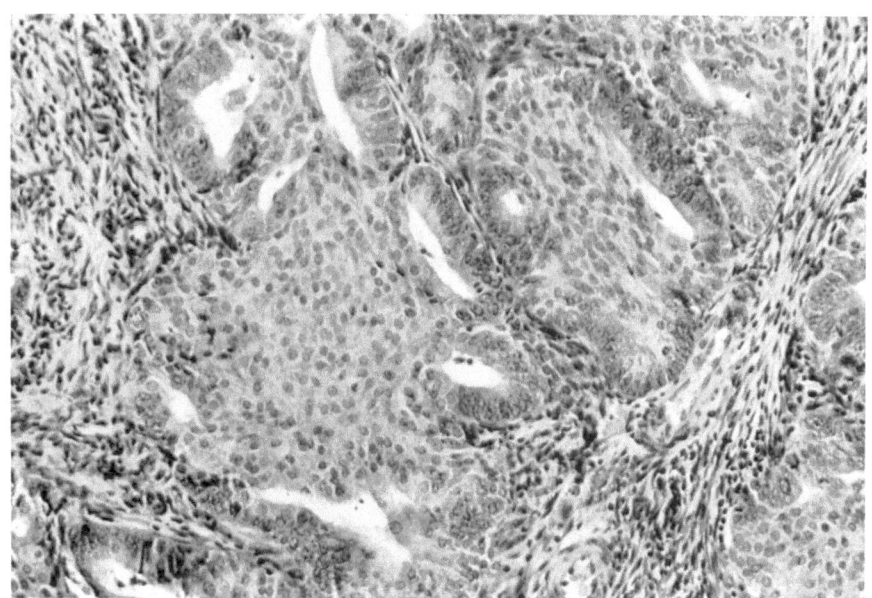

Fig. 17. × 50.

18

18 Mucinous carcinoma — a carcinoma with excessive production of mucin
Mucoid carcinoma
Gelatinous carcinoma
Colloid carcinoma

Muköses Carcinom („Schleimkrebs") — ein Carcinom mit überreichlicher Schleimbildung
Mucoidcarcinom
Gallertcarcinom

Epithélioma muqueux — épithélioma avec production excessive de mucus
Epithélioma colloïde

Carcinoma mucinoso — carcinoma con producción excesiva de mucina
Carcinoma mucoide
Carcinoma gelatinoso
Carcinoma coloide

Слизистая карцинома (слизистый рак) — рак с избыточным слизеобразованием
Мукоидная карцинома
Коллоидный рак

Carcinoma mucoides
Carcinoma gelatinosum
Carcinoma colloides

19 Signet ring cell carcinoma — a particular anaplastic type of mucinous carcinoma characterized by accumulation of intracellular and extracellular mucus

Siegelringzellen-Carcinom ein besonderer Typ eines Schleimkrebses, charakterisiert durch intra- und extracelluläre Anhäufung von Schleim

Epithélioma sigillocellulaire (à cellules en bague à châton) type anaplasique particulier de l'épithélioma muqueux, caractérisé par l'accumulation intra- et extracellulaire de mucus

Carcinoma de células en anillo de sello — este es un tipo especial, anaplásico, de carcinoma mucinoso caracterizado por acúmulos de mucina intra- y extracelular

Перстневидноклеточный рак — особая форма слизистого рака, характеризующаяся внутри и внеклеточным скоплением слизи

Carcinoma sigillocellulare

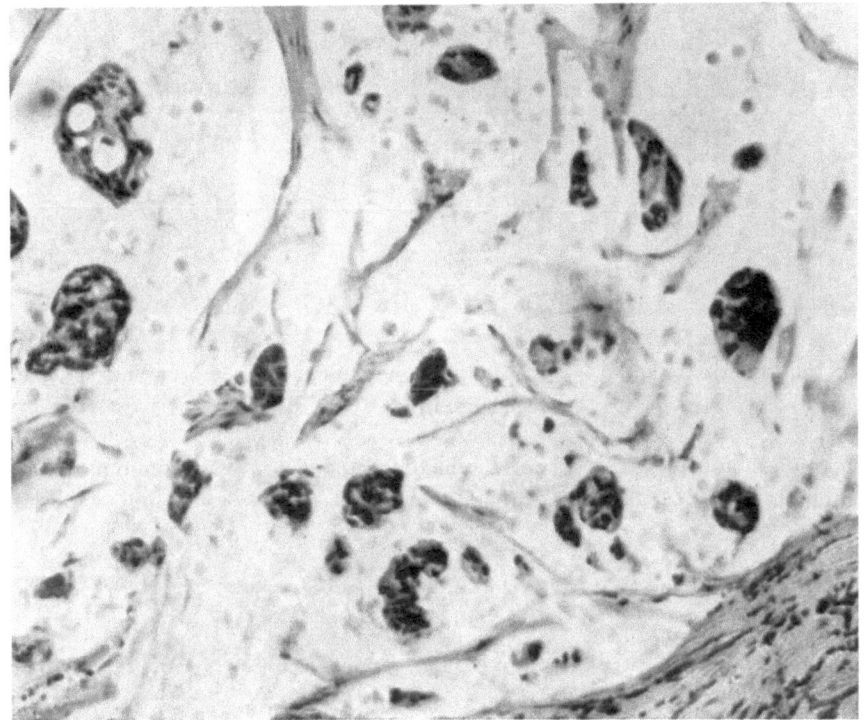

Fig. 18.

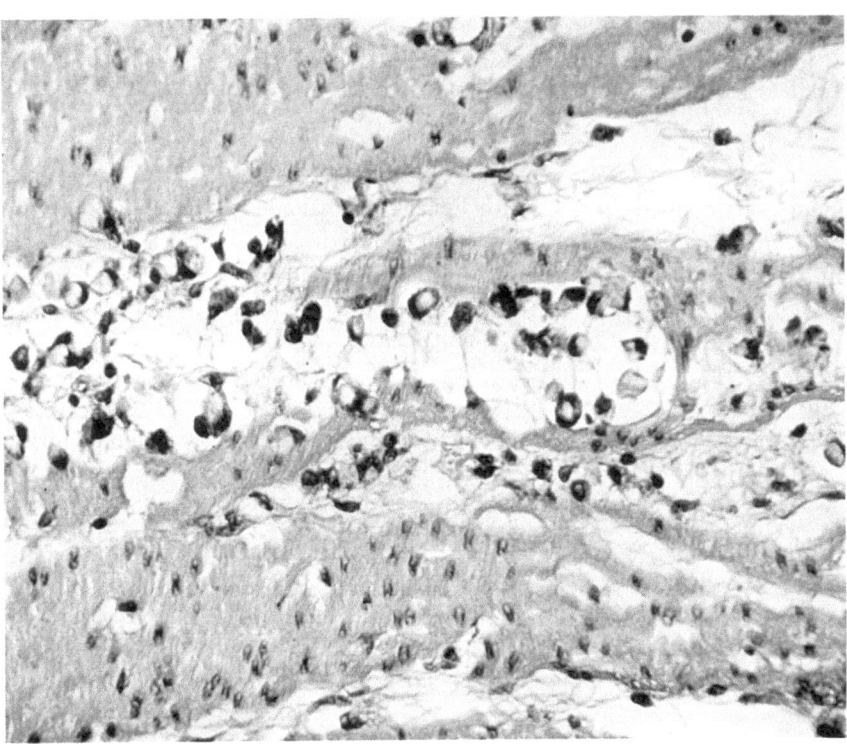

Fig. 19. × 350.

20 Mucoepidermoid carcinoma

Epithélioma «muco-épi-
dermoïde»

Мукоэпидермоидный рак

Mukoepidermoides
Carcinom

Carcinoma mucoepider-
moide

Carcinoma mucoepider-
moides

21 Medullary carcinoma —
term for carcinomas of
soft consistency due to
scarcity of stroma

Epithélioma encéphaloïde
— terme pour désigner
un épithélioma de con-
sistance molle due au
faible développement du
stroma

Медуллярный рак —
название для рака
особенно мягкой
консистенции, бедного
стромой

Medulläres Carcinom—Be-
zeichnung für Carcinome
von besonders weicher
Konsistenz infolge des
geringen Stromaanteils

Carcinoma medular — tér-
mino para carcinomas de
consistencia blanda por
lo escaso de su estroma

Carcinoma medullare

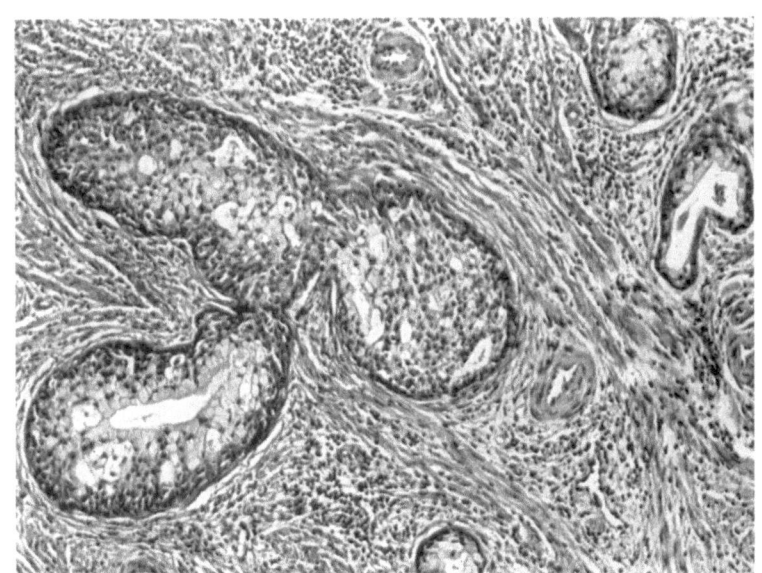

Fig. 20. × 90.   F 33/2 149—119

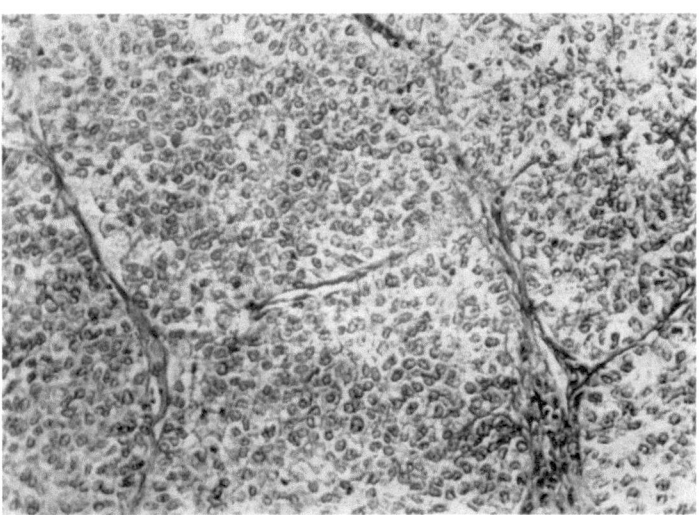

Fig. 21.   F 11 117—154

22 Scirrhus — term for carci-
    nomas of hard consisten-
    cy due to excessive col-
    lagenous (fibrous)
    stroma

    Scirrhus — Bezeichnung
    für Carcinome von be-
    sonders harter Konsi-
    stenz infolge überwiegen-
    den bindegewebigen
    (fibrösen) Stromas

Squirrhe — désigne des épithéliomas de consistance
ferme due à la produc-
tion excessive d'un stro-
ma collagène (fibreux)

Escirro — término para
carcinomas de consisten-
cia firme por su excesivo
estroma colágeno
(fibroso)

Скирр — рак особенно
плотной консистенции
вследствие богатства
соединительнотканной
(фиброзной) стромой

Scirrhus

23 Trabecular carcinoma
    Solid carcinoma

    Trabeculäres Carcinom
    Solides Carcinom

Epithélioma trabéculaire

Carcinoma trabecular
Carcinoma sólido

Трабекулярный рак
Солидный рак

Carcinoma trabeculare
Carcinoma solidum

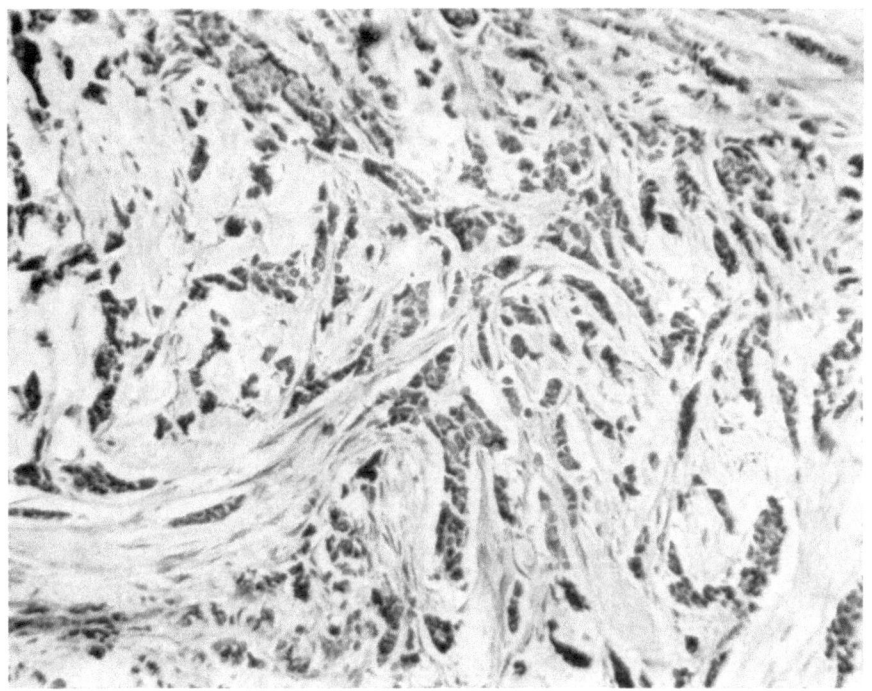

Fig. 22.   F 34 37—18

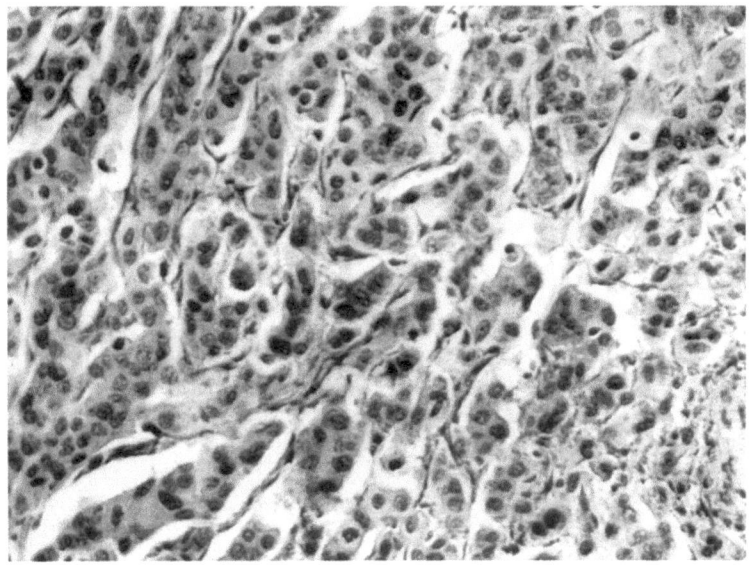

Fig. 23.   F 11 117—156

II.

Tumors of exo- and endocrine glands and epithelial surfaces*

Tumeurs des glandes exo- et endocrines et des surfaces épithéliales*

Опухоли экзо- и эндокринных желез, а также эпителиальных поверхностей *

Tumoren der exo- und endokrinen Drüsen
sowie der epithelialen Oberflächen*

Tumores de glándulas exo- y endócrinas y de superficies epiteliales*

Tumores glandularum exo- et endocrinium et tunicarum mucosarum

---

* In chapter 2, tumors of exo- and endocrine glands and epithelial surfaces are subdivided according to their anatomical sites viz. (1) salivary glands, (2) oral cavity, etc. For economy of description the anatomical site is assumed and not repeated, unless the histological structure of a tumor is exclusive to a particular organ, as for instance in "scirrhous carcinoma of stomach".

* Dans le chapitre 2, les tumeurs des glandes exo- et endocrines et des épithéliums de surface sont subdivisées selon leur siège anatomique, c'est-à-dire (1) glandes salivaires, (2) cavité buccale, etc. Pour abréger la description, le site anatomique n'est pas répété, sauf si la structure histologique de la tumeur est exclusive à un organe particulier, comme par exemple dans le case de «l'épithélioma squir-rheux de l'estomac» (linite plastique).

* В этом отделе опухоли подразделены соответственно их анатомическому положению, напр. (1) слюнных желез, (2) ротовой полости и т. д. Анатомическое положение повторяется только для таких опухолей, которые характерны для определенного органа.

* In diesem Abschnitt sind die Tumoren der exo- und endokrinen Drüsen und der epithelialen Ober-flächen unterteilt entsprechend ihrem anatomischen Sitz, z. B. (1) Mundspeicheldrüsen, (2) Mundhöhle usw. Der Kürze wegen wird jeweils bei einem Tumor der anatomische Sitz vorausgesetzt und nicht wiederholt, außer wenn die histologische Struktur eines Tumors ausschließlich für ein ganz bestimmtes Organ zutrifft, wie z. B. beim „scirrhösen Magencarcinom".

* En el capítulo 2, se subdividen estos tumores de acuerdo con su situación anatómica, por ej.: (1) glándulas salivares, (2) cavidad oral, etc. Para abreviar la descripción, no se repite la situación anatómica a menos que la estructura histológica de un tumor sea exclusiva para un órgano en particular, como sucede con el "carcinoma escirro del estómago".

1. Salivary glands   Glandes salivaires   Слюнные железы

Mundspeicheldrüsen   Glándulas salivares   Glandulae salivales   (142)

24 Adenolymphoma
    Papillary cystadenoma
      lymphomatosum
    Lymphomatous adenoma
    Warthin's tumor

    Adenolymphom
    Papilläres lymphomatöses
      Cystadenom
    Lymphomatöses Adenom
    Warthin's Tumor

    Adénolymphome
    Cystadéno-lymphome
      papillaire
    Adénome lymphomateux
    Tumeur de Warthin

    Adenolinfoma
    Cistoadenoma linfomatoso
      papilífero
    Adenoma linfomatoso
    Tumor de Warthin

    Аденолимфома
    Папиллярная лимфо-
      матозная цистаденома
    Лимфоматозная аденома
    Опухоль Варсина

    Adenolymphoma
    Cystadenoma papilliferum
      lymphomatosum
    Adenoma lymphomatosum
    Tumor Warthin

25 Tubular Adenoma
    Tubuläres Adenom

    Adénome tubuleux
    Adenoma tubular

    Тубулярная аденома
    Adenoma tubulare

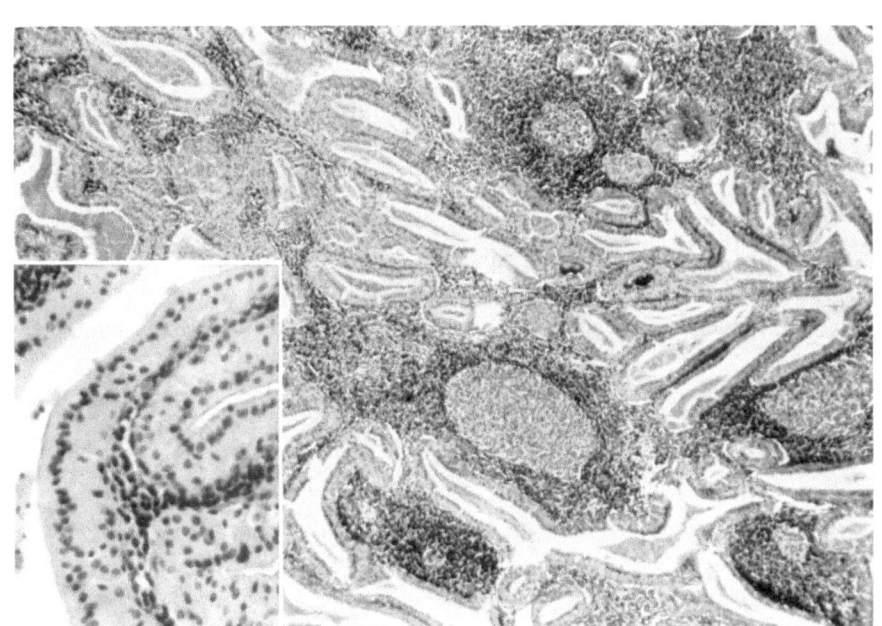

Fig. 24. × 38.   F 11 135—174

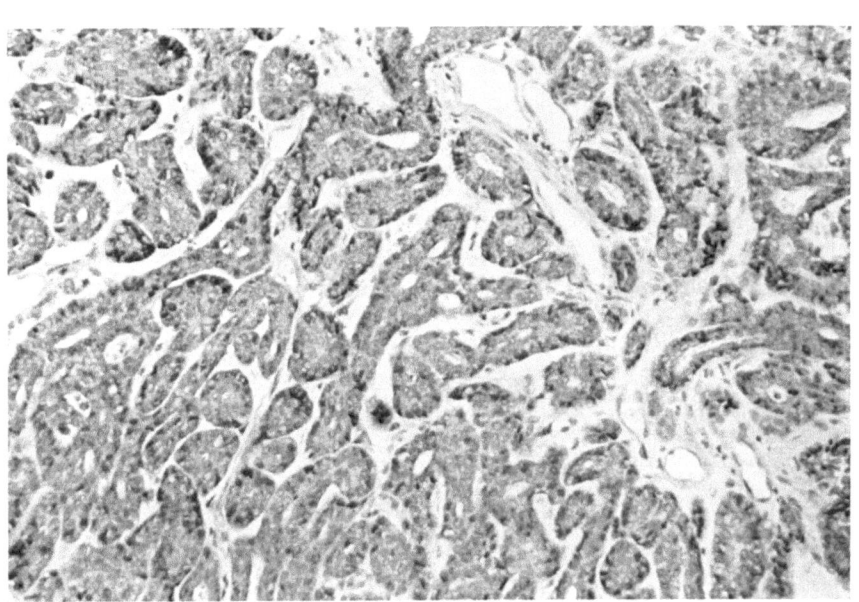

Fig. 25. × 150.

26 Acinic Cell Adenoma Adénome a cellules acineuses Ацинозная альвеолярная аденома

Azinuszell Adenom Adenoma acinocelular Adenoma acinocellulare

27 Trabecular adenoma Adénome trabéculaire Трабекулярная Аденома

Trabeculäres Adenom Adenoma trabecular Adenoma trabeculare

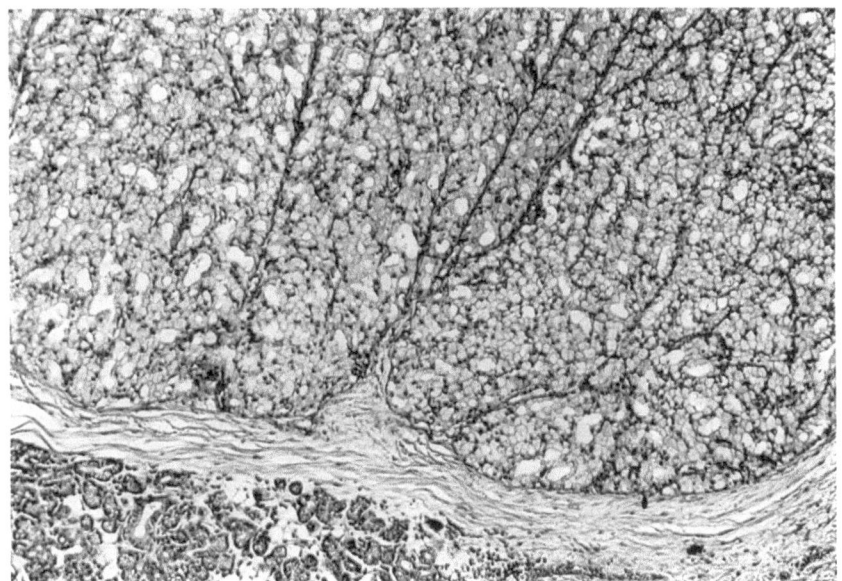

Fig. 26. × 60.

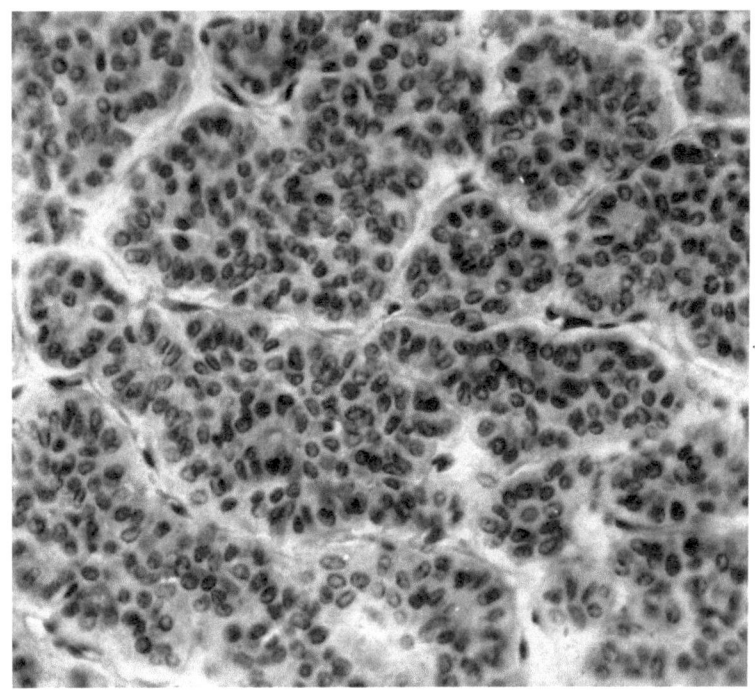

Fig. 27. × 86.

v. A. 160—143

28 Onkocytoma
Onkocytic adenoma
Oxyphil cell adenoma

Oncocytome
Adénome oncocytaire
Adénome à cellules acido-
philes

Онкоцитома
Онкоцитарная аденома
Оксифильноклеточная
аденома

Onkocytom
Onkocytisches Adenom
Acidophiles Adenom

Oncocitoma
Adenoma oncocítico
Adenoma de células oxífilas

Onkocytoma
Adenoma onkocyticum
Adenoma acidophile

29 Sebaceous gland-like
adenoma

Adénome de type sébacé

Аденома типа сальной
железы

Talgdrüsenähnliches
Adenom

Adenoma de tipo glándulas
sebáceas

Adenoma sebaceocellulare

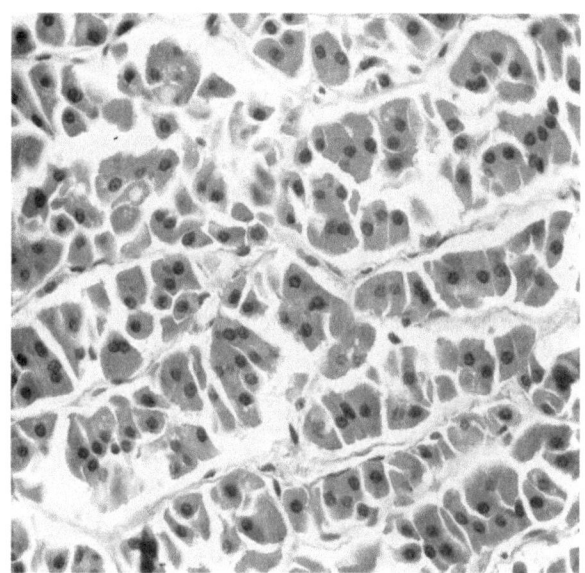

Fig. 28. ×263.   v. A. 161—146

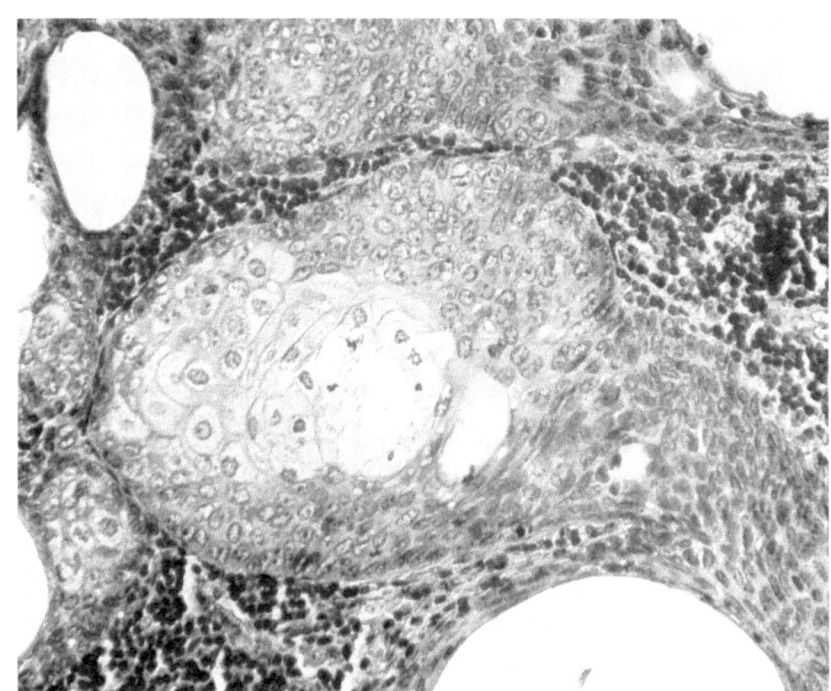

Fig. 29. × 300.

30 Papillary cystadenoma	Cystadénome papillaire	Папиллярная цистаденома
Papilläres Cystadenom	Cistoadenoma papilífero	Cystadenoma papilliferum

31 Mixed tumor	Tumeur mixte	Смешанная опухоль
Mischtumor	Tumor mixto	Tumor mixtus

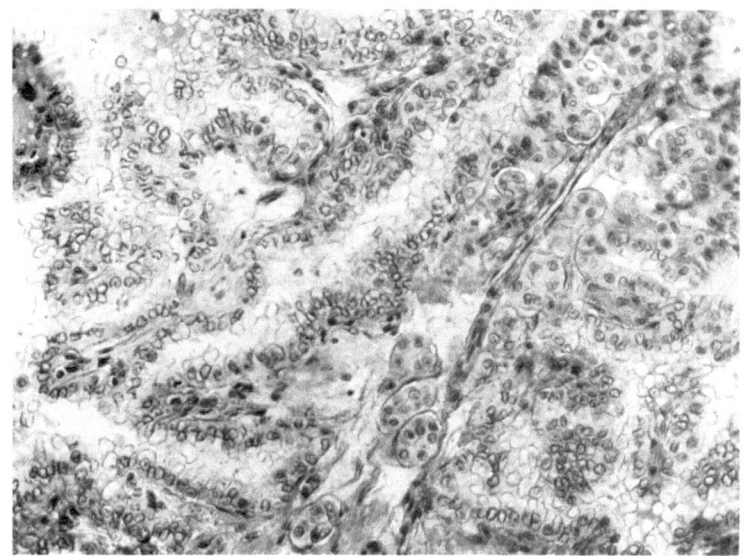

Fig. 30.　× 140.　　　　　　　　　　v. A. 163—151

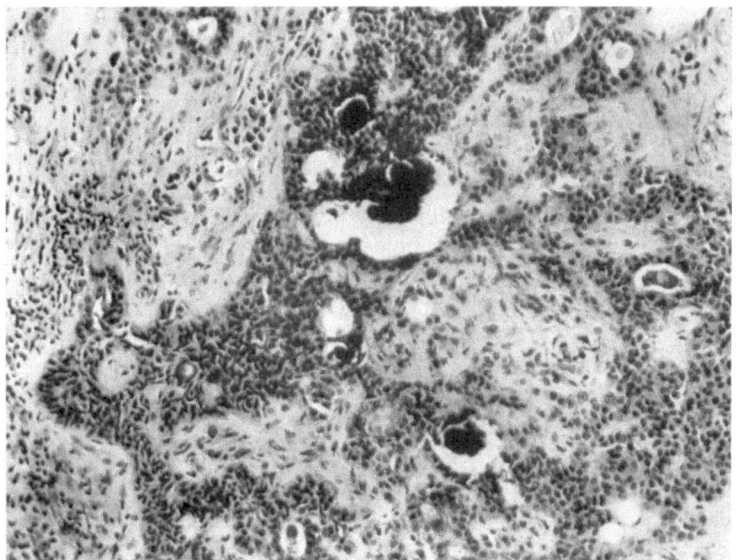

Fig. 31.　　　　　　　　　　　　F 11 21—9

32 Adenoid cystic carcinoma Adenocarcinoma of cylin- dromatous type Cylindroma	Epithélioma glandulaire cylindromateux Cylindrome	Аденоидно-кистозная карцинома Цилиндроматозная аденокарцинома Цилиндрома
Cylindromatöses Adeno- carcinom Cylindrom	Carcinoma adenoide quístico Adenocarcinoma de tipo cilindromatoso Cilindroma	Adenocarcinoma cylindro- matosum Cylindroma

33 Mucoepidermoid carcinoma	Epithélioma muco-épi- dermoïde	Мукоэпидермоидная карцинома
Mucoepidermoides Carci- nom	Carcinoma mucoepider- moide	Carcinoma mucoepider- moides

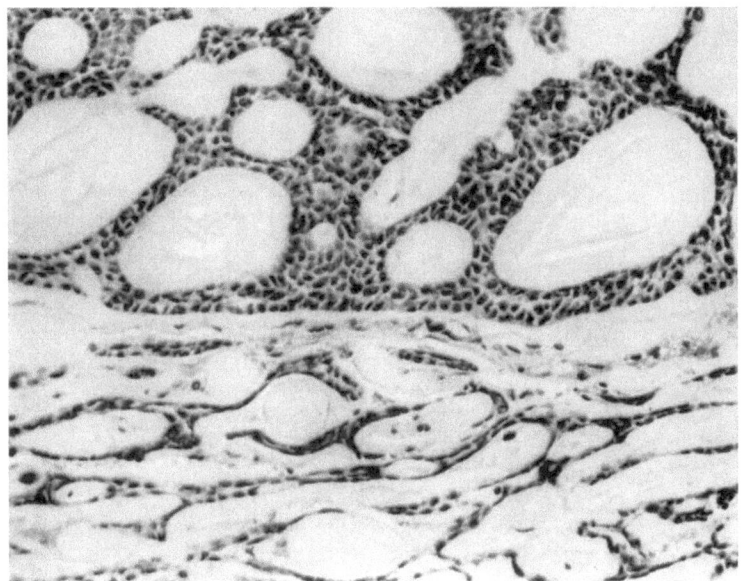

Fig. 32. F 11 111—147

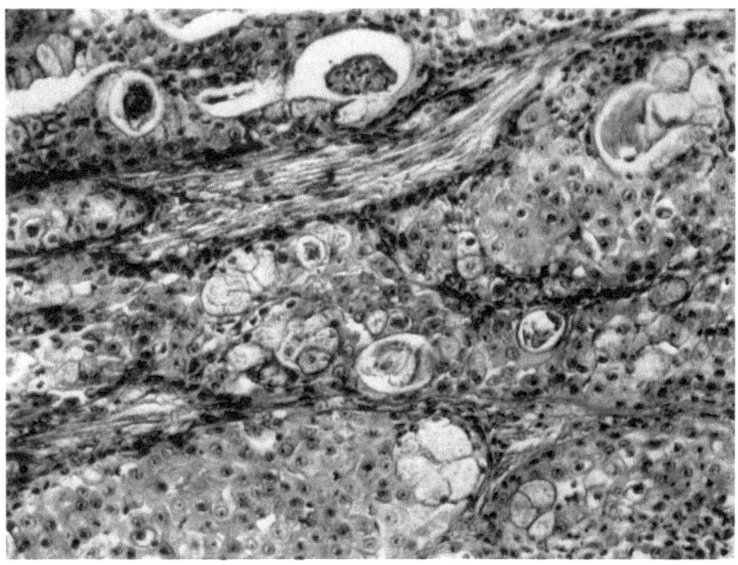

Fig. 33. F 11 89—123

34 Trabecular carcinoma   Epithélioma trabéculaire   Трабекулярная карцинома

    Trabeculäres Carcinom   Carcinoma trabecular   Carcinoma trabeculare

35 Acinic cell adenocarcinoma   Epithélioma acineux   Ациноцеллюлярная
                                                                 аденокарцинома

    Acinocelluläres Adeno-   Adenocarcinoma de   Adenocarcinoma acino-
        carcinom   células acinosas   cellulare

Carcinomas of common types (see I) arising in mixed tumors should be called according to their type.

Les épithéliomas de type commun (voir I), se développant dans les tumeurs mixtes, doivent être désignés selon leur type.

Раки обычных типов (см. I), происходящие из смешанных опухолей, называются соответственно их строению.

Carcinome gewöhnlicher Typen (s. I), wie sie auch in Mischtumoren entstehen, sollten jeweils nach ihrem Typ benannt werden.

Los carcinomas de tipo común (ver I) que se desarrollan en tumores mixtos, deberán clasificarse según su tipo.

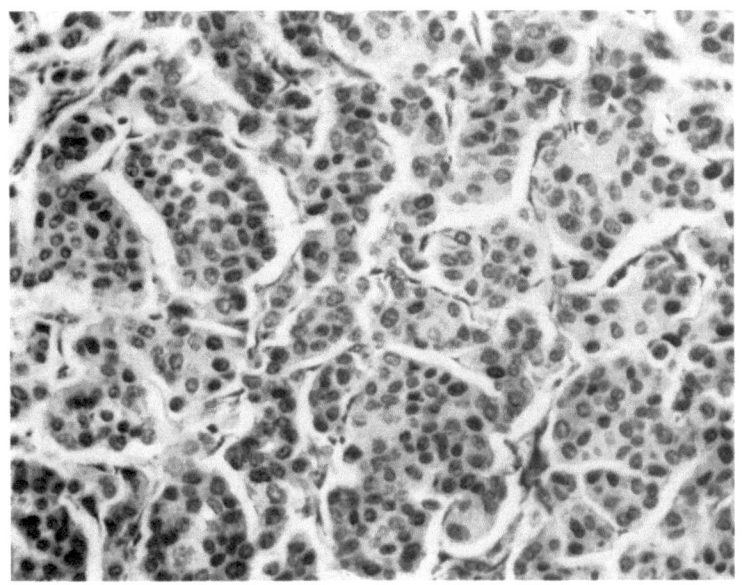

Fig. 34.   F 11 117—155

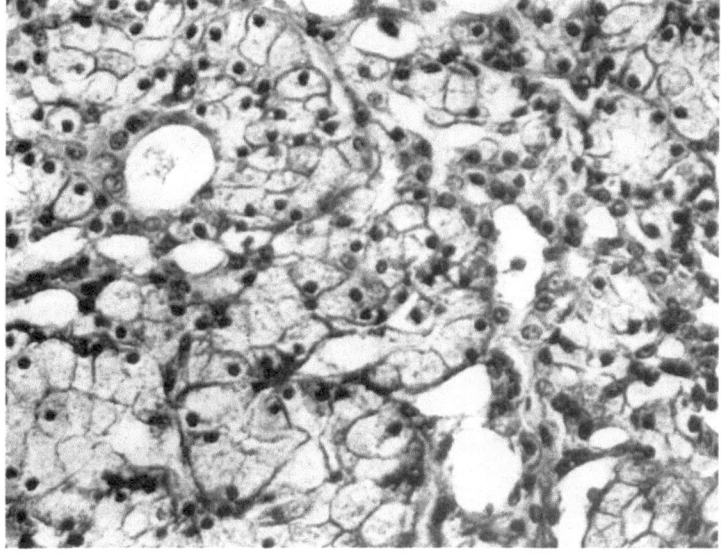

Fig. 35.   F 11 127—170

2. **Oral cavity** Cavité buccale **Ротовая полость** (143—145)

   Mundhöhle   Cavidad oral   Cavum oris

---

36 Ameloblastoma   Améloblastome   Амелобластома
  Adamantinoma   ·Adamantinome   Адамантинома

  Ameloblastom   Ameloblastoma   Ameloblastoma
  Adamantinom   Adamantinoma   Adamantinoma

37 Adeno-Ameloblastoma Adéno-Améloblastome Аденоамелобластома
  Ameloblastic adenomatoid Tumeur améloblastique Амелобластическая
   tumor   adénomateuse   аденоматоидная
                опухоль

  Adenoameloblastom Adeno-Ameloblastoma Adeno-ameloblastoma
         Tumor ameloblástico
         adenomatoso

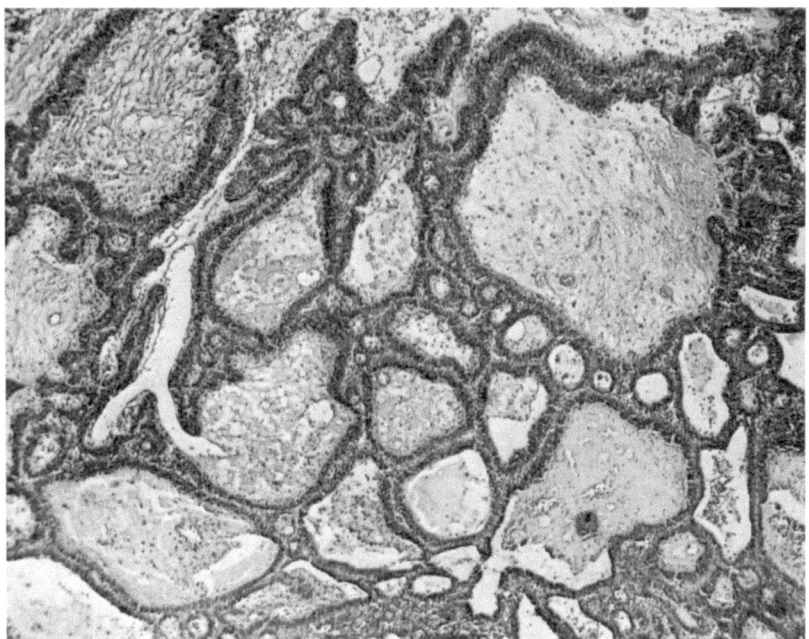

Fig. 36. ×48.   F 10a 37—30

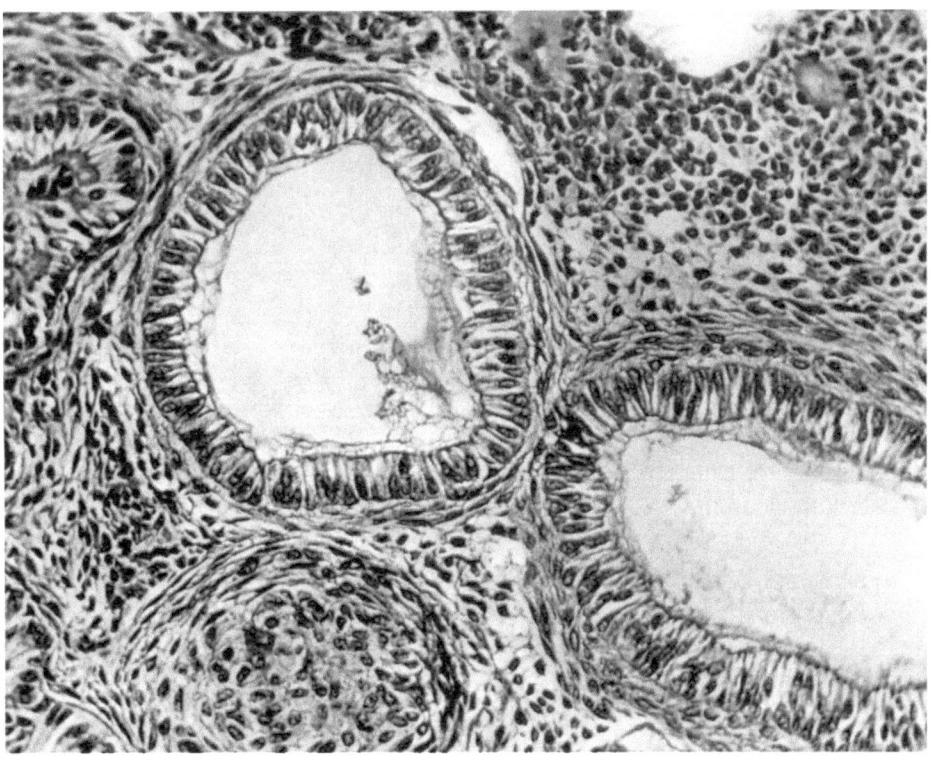

Fig. 37. ×150.   F 10a 41—36

38 Ameloblastic fibroma   Fibrome améloblastique   Амелобластическая
                                                             фиброма

Ameloblastisches Fibrom   Fibroma ameloblástico   Fibroma ameloblasticum

39 Ameloblastic odontoma   Odontome améloblastique   Амелобластическая
   "Soft odontoma"   «Odontome mou»   одонтома
                                                             «Мягкая одонтома»

Ameloblastisches Odontom   Odontoma ameloblástico   Odontoma ameloblasticum
   ,,weiches Odontom"   "odontoma blando"   ,,Odontoma molle"

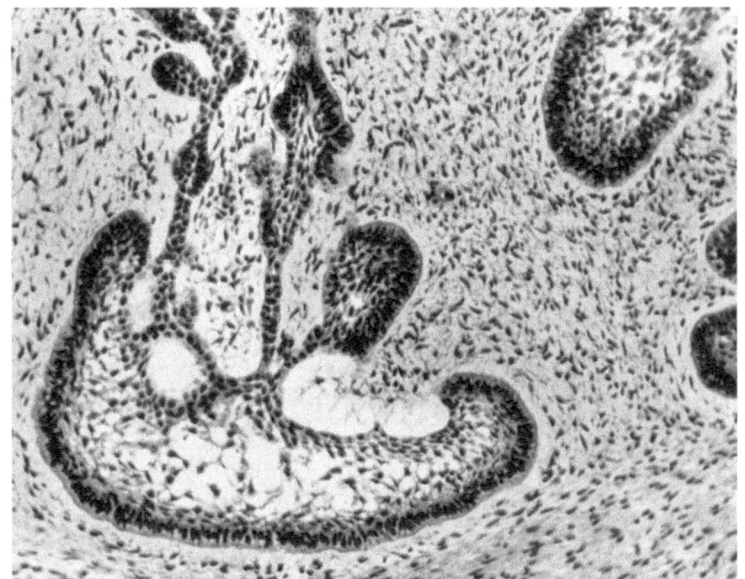

Fig. 38. × 165.   F 10a 55—58

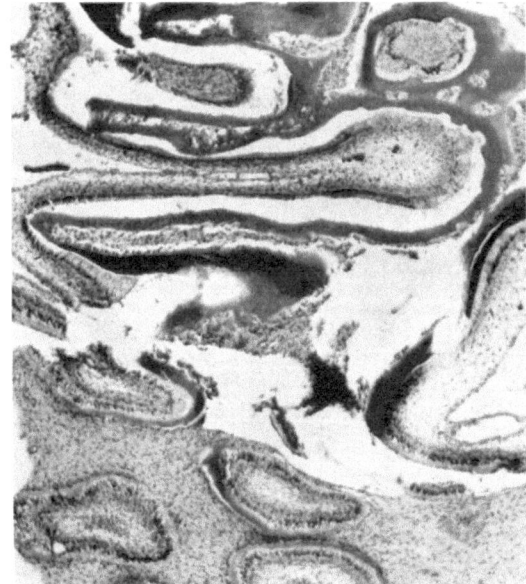

Fig. 39a. × 50.   F 10a 57—60   Fig. 39b. × 165.   F 10a 57—61

40 Melanotic Neurectodermal Tumor	Tumeur melanique neuro-ectodermique	Меланотическая нейроэкто-дермальная опухоль
Melanotischer neurectomaler Tumor	Tumor melanotico neuro-ectodermico	Tumor melanoticus neuroectodermalis

41 Dentinoma	Dentinome	Дентинома
Dentinom	Dentinoma	Dentinoma

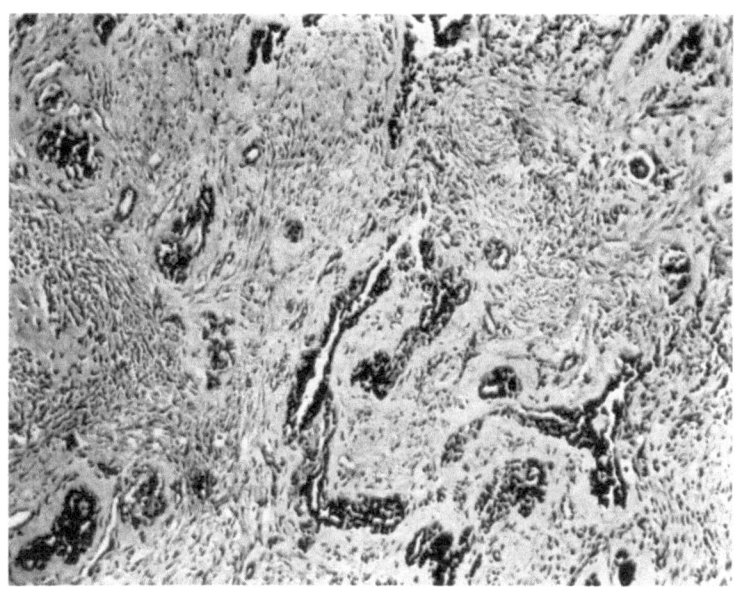

Fig. 40. × 75.   F 10a 43—40

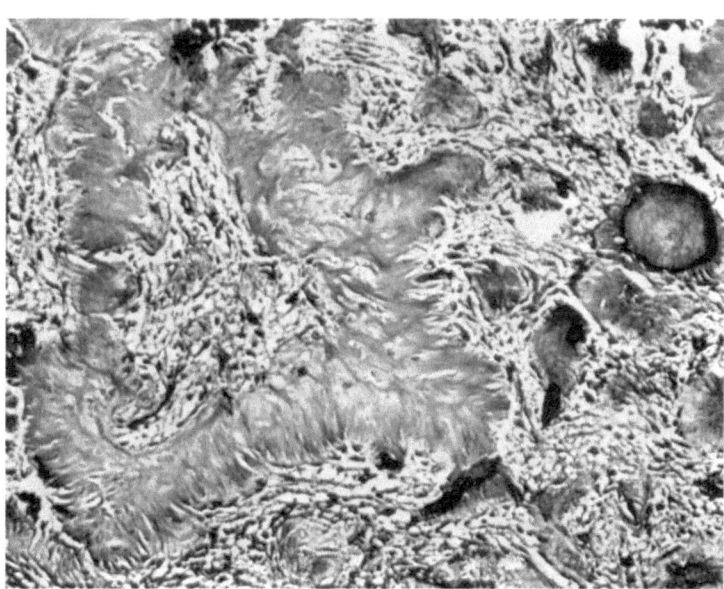

Fig. 41. × 250.   F 10a 49—46

44

42 Calcifying odontoma   Odontome calcifié   Объизвествлевающаяся
    Complex odontoma   Odontome complexe   одонтома
    "Hard odontoma"   «Odontome dur»   Сложная одонтома
                                                            «Твердая одонтома»

    Verkalkendes Odontom   Odontoma calcificante   Odontoma calcificans
                                 Odontoma complejo
                                 (odontoma duro)

43 Cementoma   Cémentome   Цементома

    Zementom   Cementoma   Cementoma

44 Cementifying fibroma   Fibrome avec élaboration   Цементирующаяся
                                    de cément   фиброма

    Fibrom mit Zementbildung   Fibroma cementificante   Fibroma cementificans

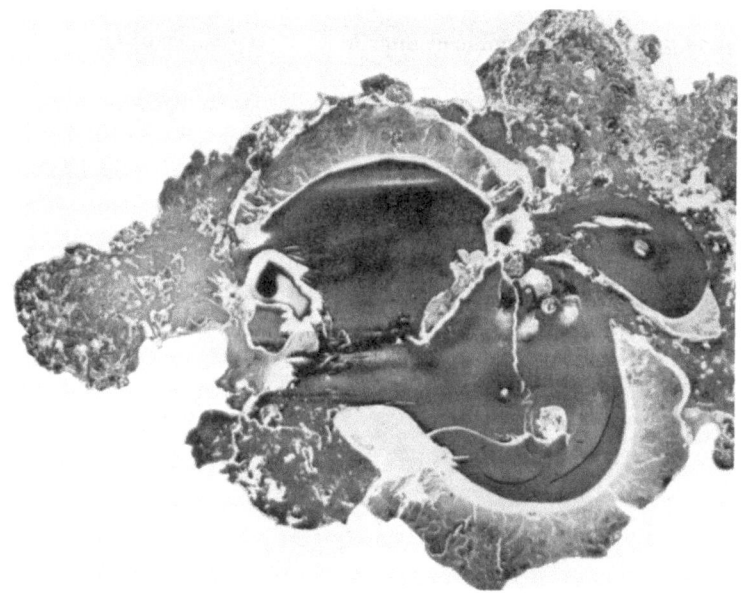

Fig 42. ×8.   F 10a 57—62

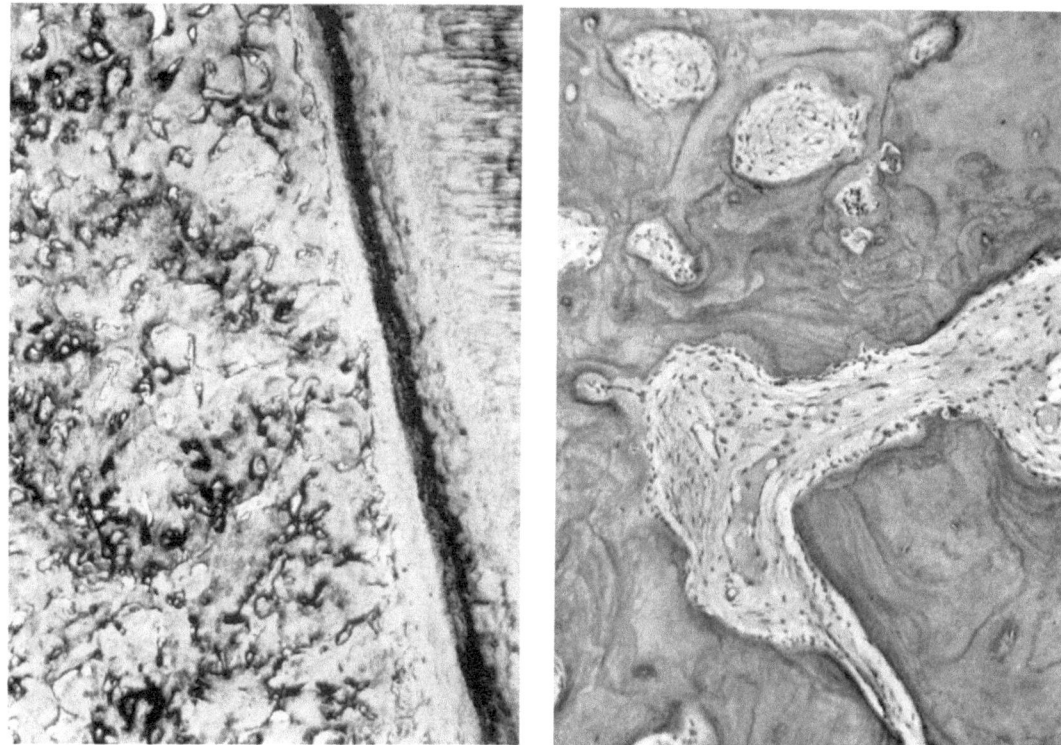

Fig. 43. ×275.   F 10a 53—52   Fig. 44. ×125.   F 10a 53—53

3. Stomach and intestine Estomac et intestin Желудочно-кишечный тракт

Magen-Darmtrakt Estómago e intestinos Tractus gastrointestinalis (151—154)

45 Adenomatous polyp of
stomach

Adenomatöser Polyp des
Magens

Polype adénomateux de
l'estomac

Pólipo adenomatoso del
estómago

Аденоматозный полип
желудка

Polypus adenomatosus
ventriculi

46 Adenomatous polyp of
intestine

Adenomatöser Polyp des
Dünndarms

Polype adénomateux de
l'intestin

Pólipo adenomatoso del
intestino

Аденоматозный полип
тонкой кишки

Polypus adenomatosus
intestini

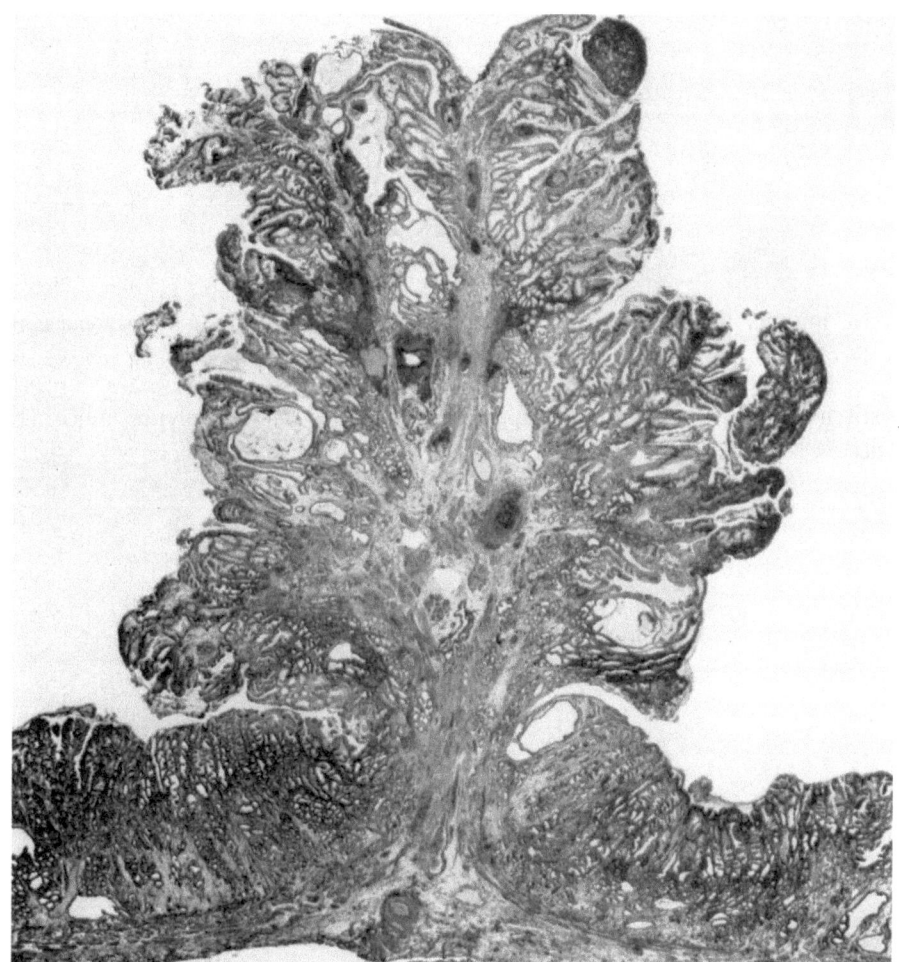

Fig. 45.   F 21 25—8

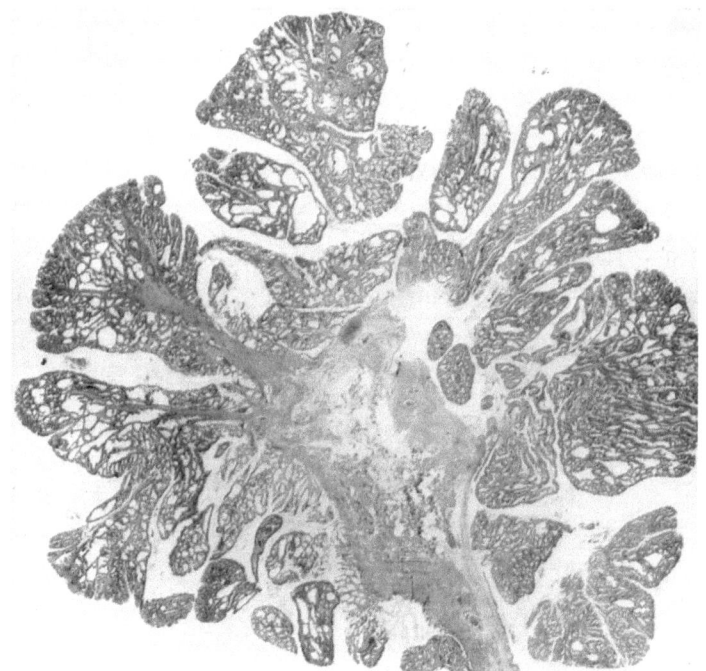

Fig. 46.   A 394—405

47 Cystic mucous polyp
    of colon

    Cystisch-muköser Polyp
    des Dickdarms

Polype muqueux du colon

Pólipo mucoso quístico del
colon

Кистозный слизистый
    полип толстой кишки

Polypus mucosus cysticus
coli

48 Papillary polyp
    Villous tumor

    Papillärer Polyp
    Zottentumor
    Papillom

Polype papillaire
Tumeur villeuse

Pólipo papilífero
Pólipo velloso

Папиллярный полип
Ворсинчатая опухоль

Polypus papillaris
Tumor villosus

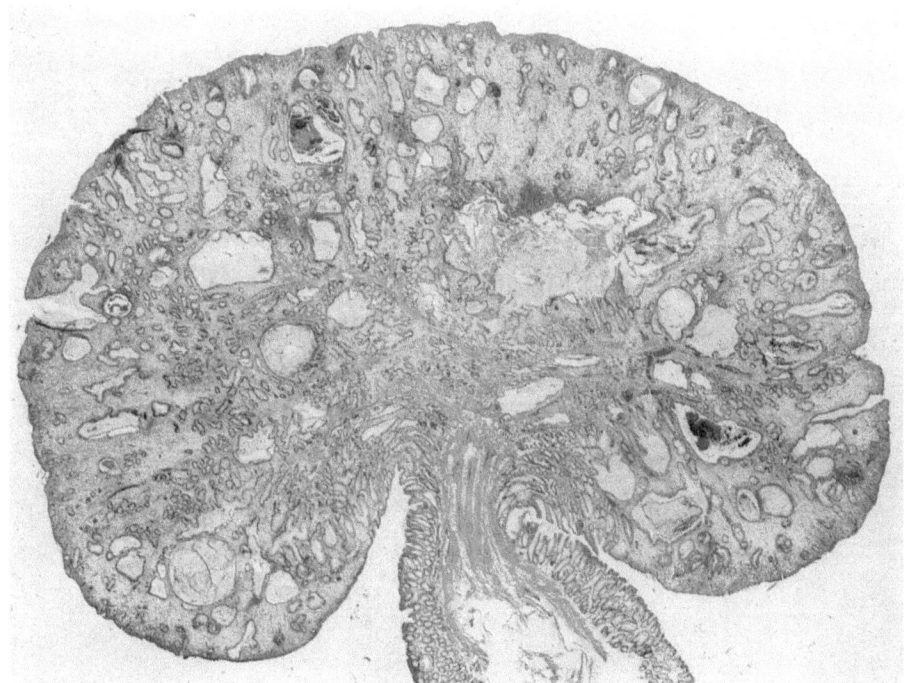

Fig. 47.   A 395—408

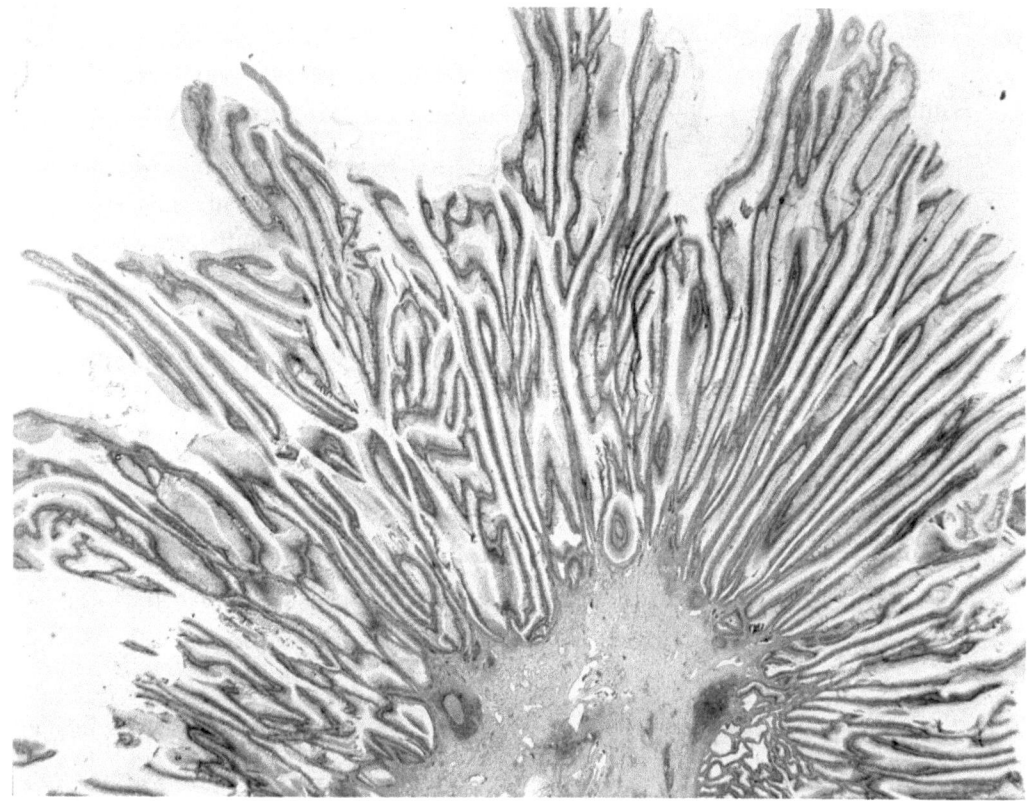

Fig. 48. × 10.

49 Carcinoid tumor	Carcinoïde	Карциноид
Argentaffinoma	Argentaffinome	Аргентаффинома
Carcinoid	Carcinoide	Tumor carcinoides
Argentaffinom	Argentafinoma	Argentaffinoma

50 Scirrhous carcinoma of stomach	Epithélioma squirrheux de l'estomac	Скиррозный рак желудка Пластический линит
Linitis plastica	Linite plastique	
Scirrhöses Carcinom des Magens	Carcinoma escirro del estómago	Carcinoma scirrhosum ventriculi
Linitis plastica	Linitis plástica	Linitis plastica

For other very frequent types of tumor see I: "Adenocarcinoma" with all subgroups.

Pour d'autres types très fréquents de tumeurs voir I «Epithélioma glandulaire» avec les sous-groupes.

Другие очень частые типы опухоли см. I: «Аденокарцинома» со всеми ее подгруппами

Andere sehr häufige Tumoren s. unter I, z. B. ,,Adenocarcinom" mit allen Untergruppen.

Para otros tipos de tumores muy frecuentes ver I: "Adenocarcinoma", con sus distintos subgrupos.

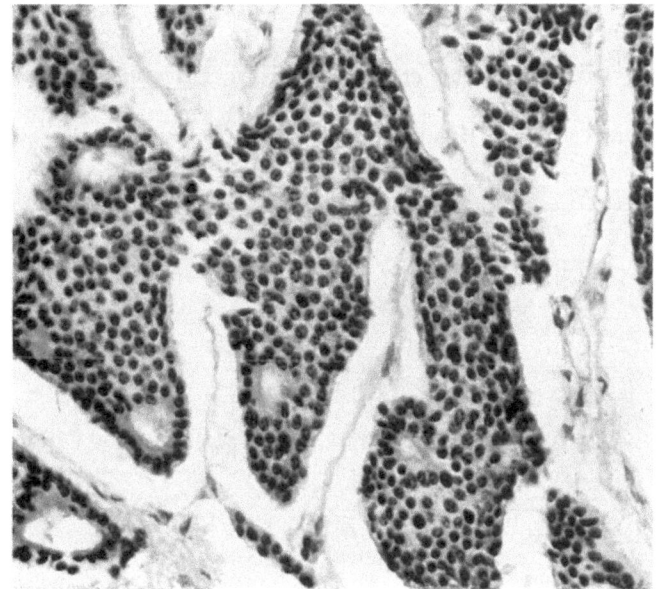

Fig. 49. × 263.   v. A. 129—98 a

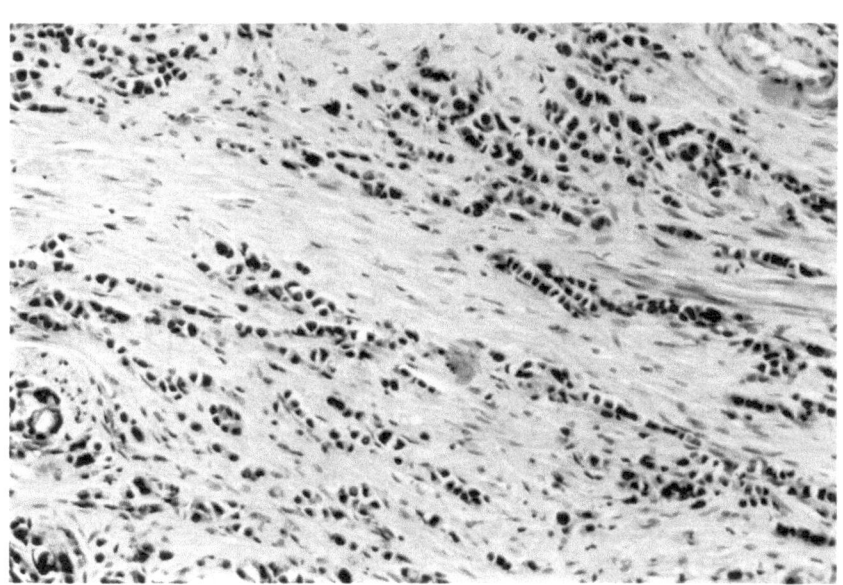

Fig. 50. × 150.

4*

4. Liver and biliary passages   Foie et voies biliaires   Печень и желчные пути

  Leber und Gallenwege   Hígado y vías biliares   Hepar et viae biliares   (155/156)

51 Liver cell adenoma   Adénome à cellules   Гепатоцеллюлярная
  Benign hepatoma   hépatiques   аденома
          Hépatome bénin   Доброкачественная
                гепатома

  Leberzelladenom   Adenoma de células hepáti-   Adenoma hepatocellulare
  Gutartiges Hepatom   cas (hepatocelular)   Hepatoma benignum
          Hepatoma benigno

52 Bile duct adenoma   Adénome biliaire   Аденома из желчных
  Benign cholangioma   Cholangiome bénin   протоков
                Доброкачественная
                холангиома

  Gallengangsadenom   Adenoma de vías biliares   Adenoma biliare
  Gutartiges Cholangiom   Colangioma benigno   Cholangioma benignum

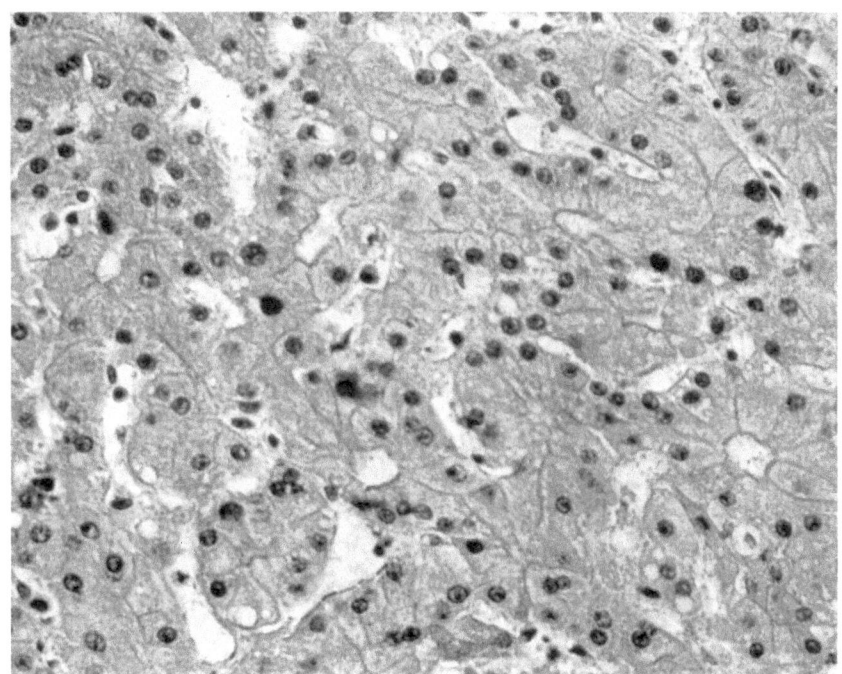

Fig 51. ×625.   F 25 23—9

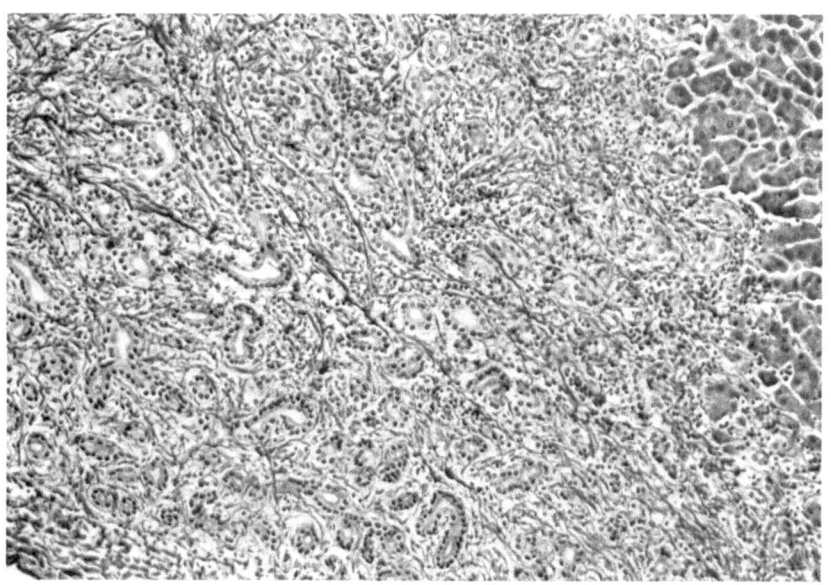

Fig. 52. × 120.

53   Liver cell carcinoma   Epithélioma à cellules   Гепатоцеллюлярный рак
       Malignant hepatoma   hépatiques   Злокачественная гепатома
                                 Hépatome malin

       Leberzellcarcinom   Carcinoma de células hepá-   Carcinoma hepatocellulare
       Bösartiges Hepatom   ticas (hepatocelular)   Hepatoma malignum
                                 Hepatoma maligno

54   Bile duct carcinoma   Epithélioma biliaire   Рак из желчных протоков
       Malignant cholangioma   Cholangiome malin   Злокачественная
                                               холангиома

       Gallengangscarcinom   Carcinoma de vías biliares   Carcinoma biliare
       Bösartiges Cholangiom   Colangioma maligno   Cholangioma malignum

55   Embryonal carcinoma of   Epithélioma embryonnaire   Эмбриональный рак печени
         liver   du foie   Эмбриональная гепатома
       Embryonal hepatoma   Hépatome embryonnaire   Гепатобластома
       Hepatoblastoma   Hépatoblastome   Смешанная опухоль печени
       Mixed tumor of liver   Tumeur mixte du foie

       Embryonales Carcinom der   Carcinoma embrionario de   Carcinoma embryonale
         Leber   hígado   Hepatoma embryonale
       Embryonales Hepatom   Hepatoma embrionario   Hepatoblastoma
       Hepatoblastom   Hepatoblastoma   Tumor mixtus
       Mischtumor der Leber   Tumor mixto de hígado

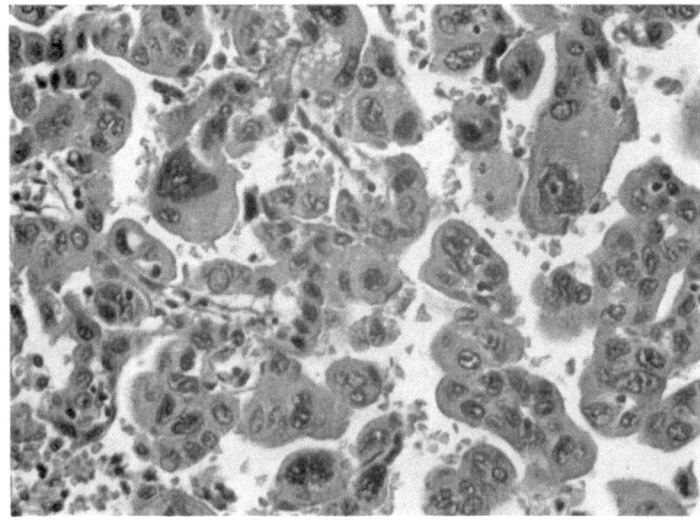

Fig. 53. × 320.   F 25 69—50

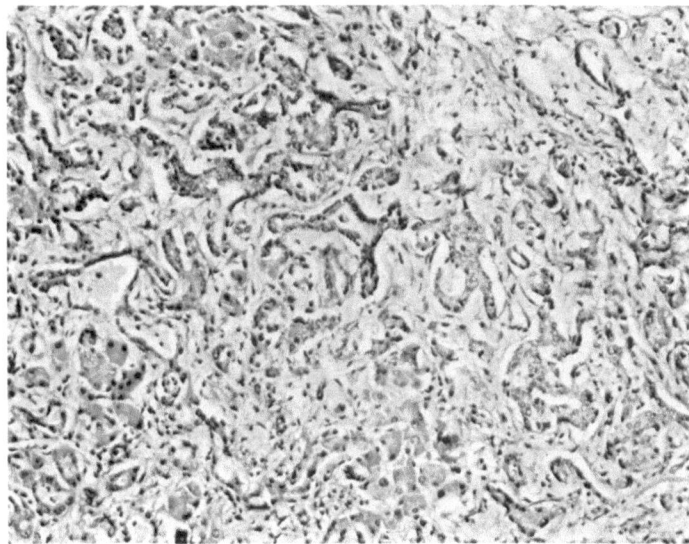

Fig. 54. × 120.

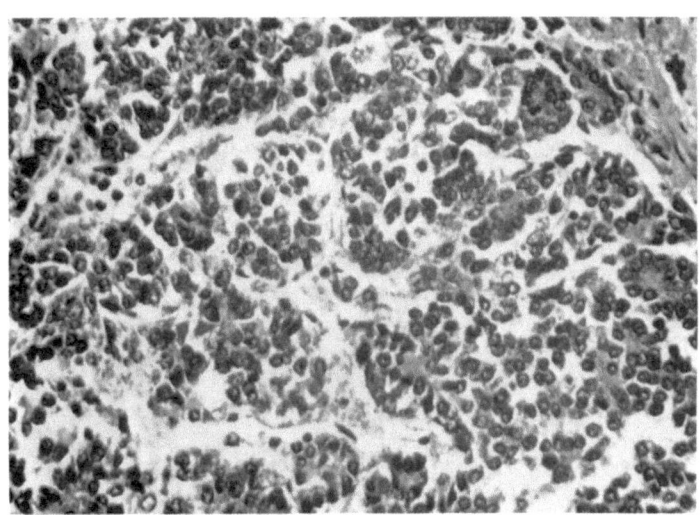

Fig. 55. × 250.   F 25 101—90

5.	**Pancreas**	**Pancréas**	**Поджелудочная железа**
	Bauchspeicheldrüse	**Páncreas**	**Pancreas**	(157)

56	Cystadenoma	Cystadénome	Кистаденома
	Cystadenom	Cistoadenoma	Cystadenoma

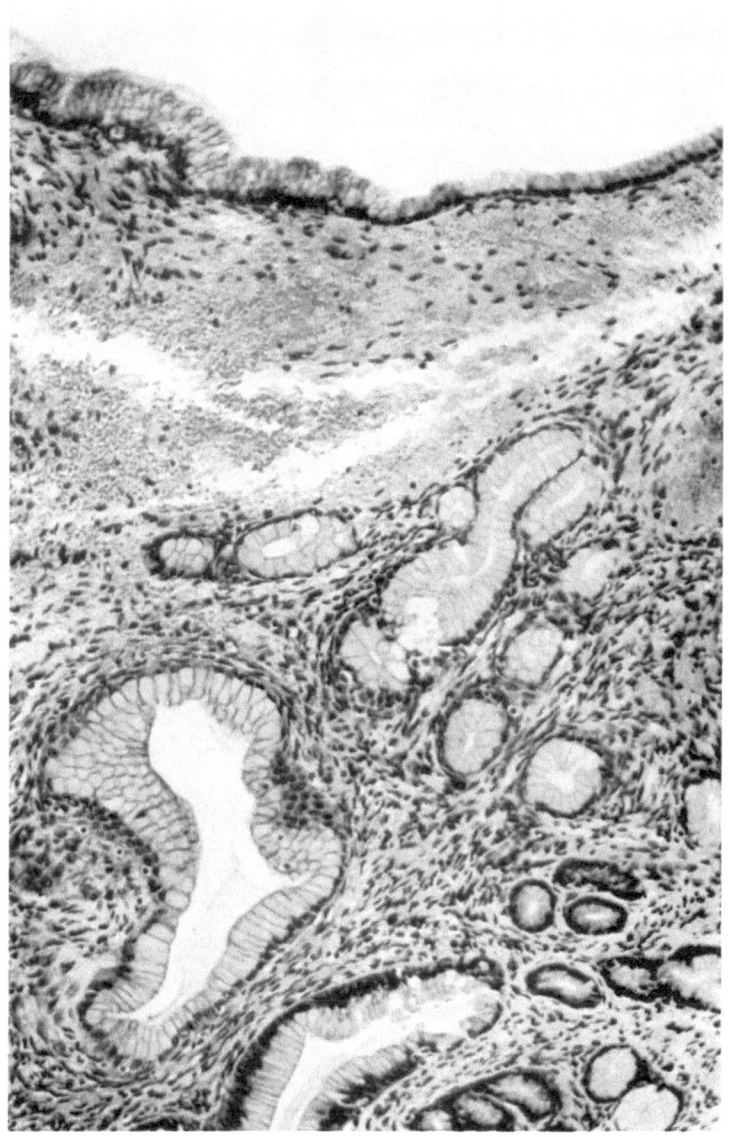

Fig. 56.   F 27/28 31—10

57 Islet cell adenoma
    Benign insuloma

    Inselzelladenom
    Gutartiges Insulom

Adénome insulaire
Nésidioblastome bénin

Adenoma de células de los
    islotes
Insuloma benigno

Островковая аденома
Доброкачественная
    инсулома

Adenoma insulocellulare
Insuloma benignum

58 Islet cell carcinoma
    Malignant insuloma

    Inselzellcarcinom
    Bösartiges Insulom

Epithélioma insulaire
Nésidioblastome malin

Carcinoma de células de los
    islotes
Insuloma maligno

Рак из островковых клеток
Злокачественная инсулома

Carcinoma insulocellulare
Insuloma malignum

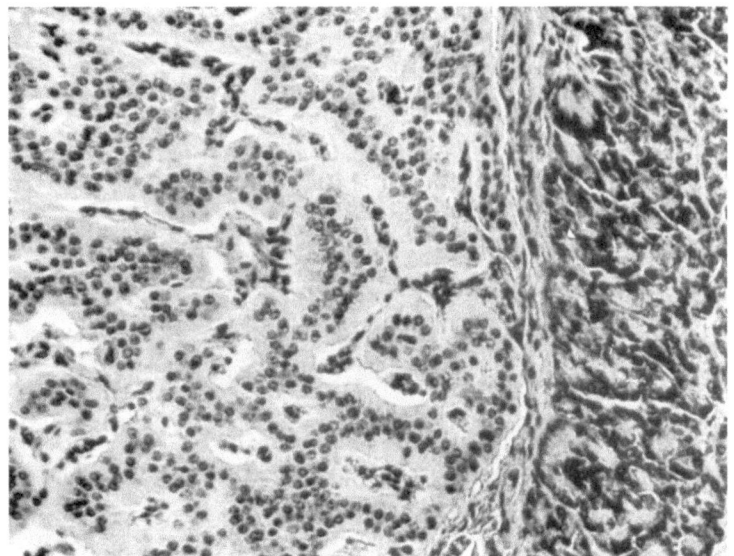

Fig. 57.   F 27/28 109—58

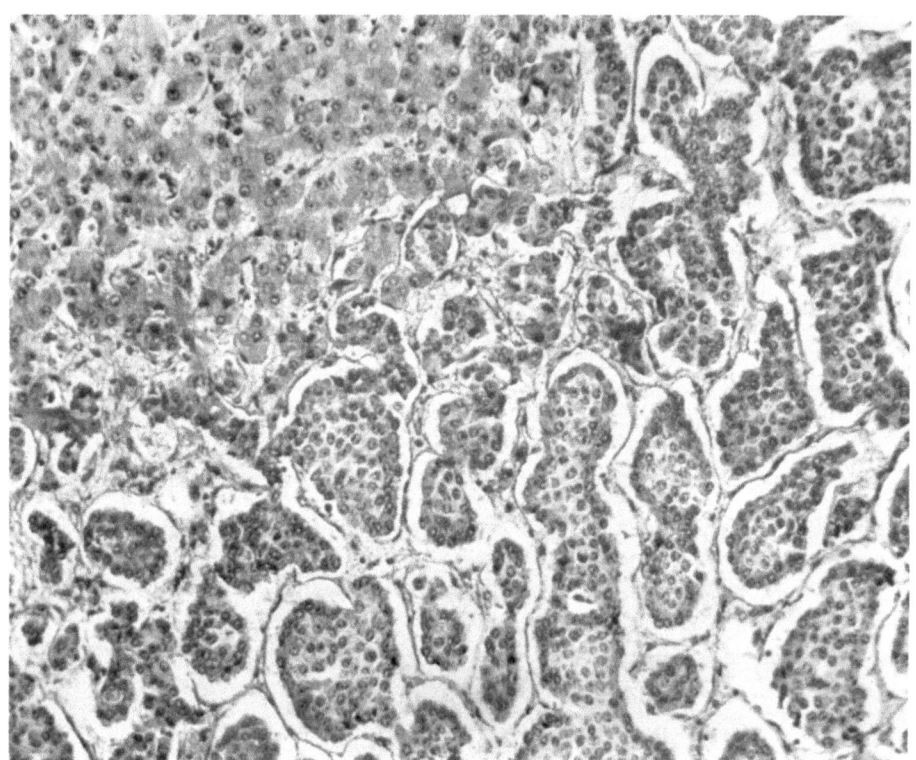

Fig. 58.   F 26/27 133—87

6.   **Respiratory tract**   **Voies respiratoires**   **Дыхательный тракт**

       Respirationstrakt   **Vías respiratorias**   **Tractus respiratorius**   (162/163)

---

59   Hamartoma of lung   Hamartome pulmonaire   Гамартома легкого
      Chondroma of lung   Chondrome pulmonaire   Хондрома легкого

      Hamartom der Lunge   Hamartoma del pulmón   Hamartoma pulmonis
      Chondrom der Lunge   Condroma del pulmón   Chondroma pulmonis

60   Carcinoid tumor of bronchus   Carcinoïde bronchique   Карциноид бронха
      Adenoma of bronchus,   Adénome bronchique, type   Аденома бронха типа
        carcinoid type   carcinoïde   карциноида

      Bronchuscarcinoid   Carcinoide bronquial   Adenoma bronchiale
      Bronchusadenom vom   Adenoma bronquial tipo   carcinoides
        Carcinoidtyp   carcinoide   Tumor bronchialis
                                                     carcinoides

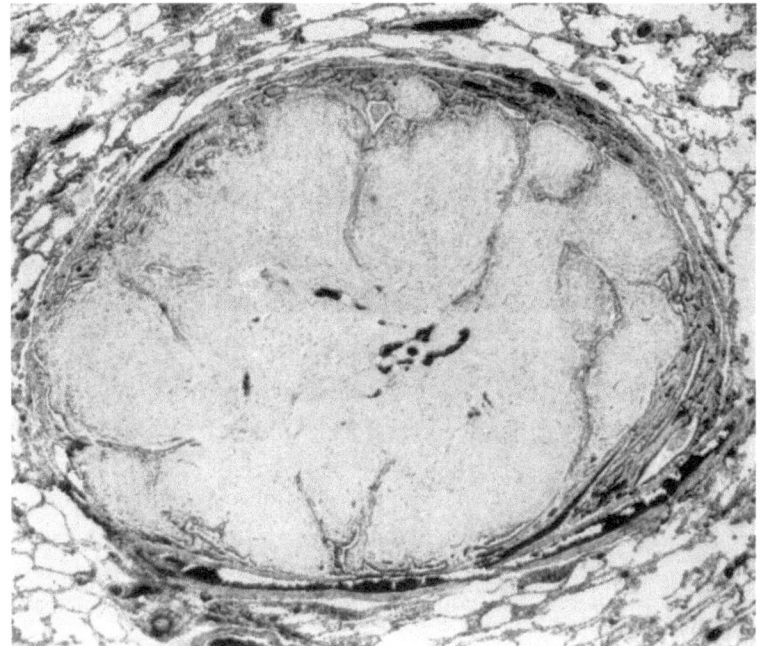

Fig. 59. × 27.   F 17 145—192

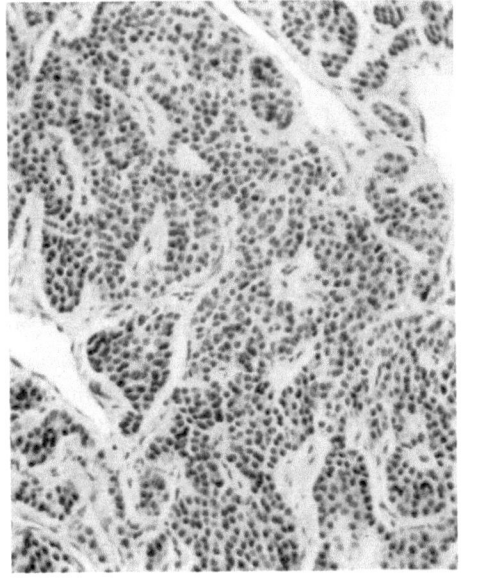
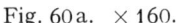
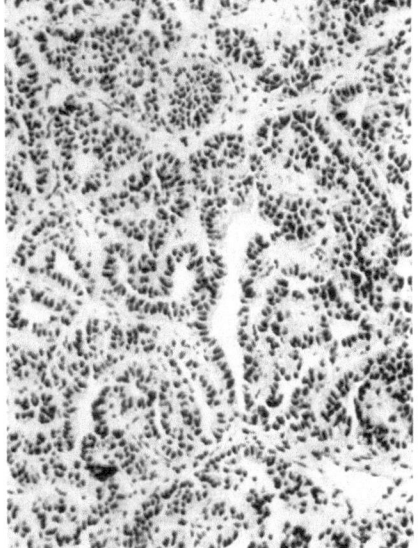

Fig. 60a. × 160.   F 17 35—30   Fig. 60b.   F 17 35—32

61 Adenoma of bronchus,
cylindromatous type
Adenocarcinoma of bron-
chus, cylindromatous
type
Cylindroma of bronchial
glands

Cylindrom des Bronchus
Bronchusadenom vom
Cylindromtyp

Epithélioma glandulaire
bronchique, type
cylindromateux
Cylindrome des glandes
bronchiques
Adénome bronchique, type
cylindromateux

Adenocarcinoma bronquial,
tipo cilindromatoso
Cilindroma de glándulas
bronquiales
Adenoma bronquial, tipo
cilindromatoso

Аденоидно-кистозная
карцинома бронха
Аденокарцинома бронха
типа цилиндромы
Цилиндрома бронхиальных
желез
Аденома бронха типа
цилиндромы

Adenocarcinoma cylindro-
matosum bronchiale
Cylindroma glandulae
bronchialis
Adenoma cylindromatosum
bronchiale

62 Alveolar cell carcinoma
Bronchiolar carcinoma

Alveolarzellcarcinom
Bronchiolarcarcinom

Epithélioma à cellules
alvéolaires
Epithélioma bronchiolaire

Carcinoma alveolar
Carcinoma bronquiolar

Альвеолярноклеточный
рак
Бронхиолярный рак

Carcinoma alveolo-cellulare
Carcinoma bronchiolare

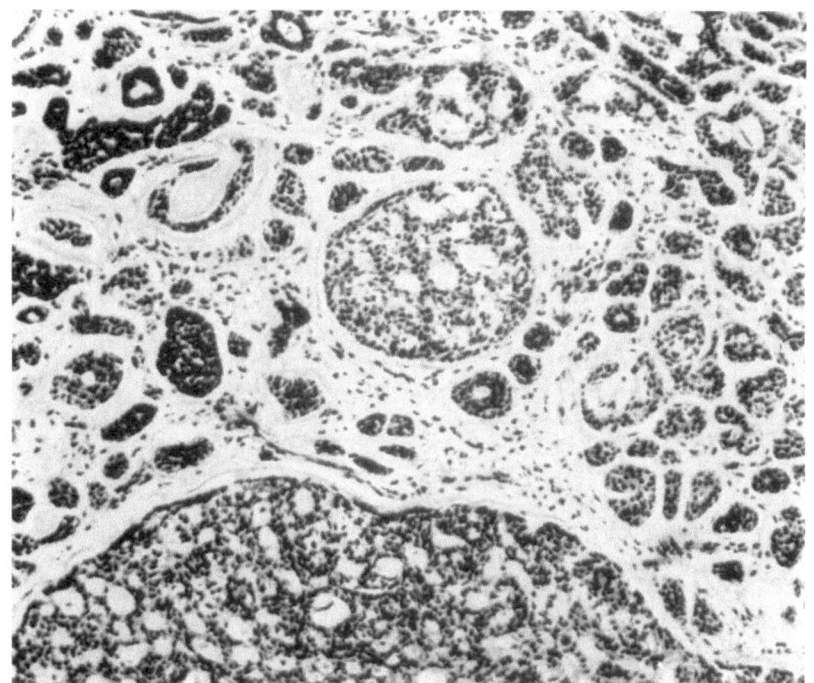

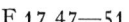

Fig. 61. × 105.   F 17 47—51

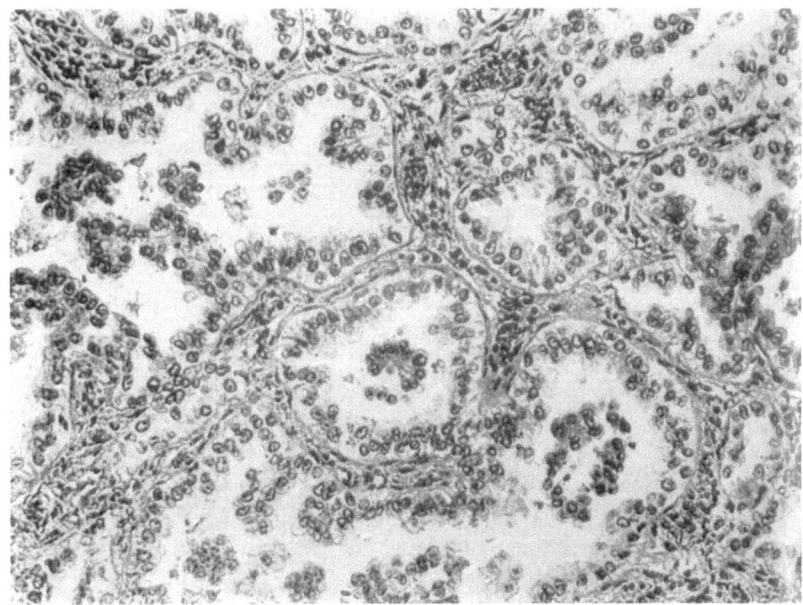

Fig. 62.   M 416

63   Carcinoma of Bronchus   Carcinome bronchique   Карцинома бронха
    a) small cell type   a) à petites cellules   а) мелкоклеточный тип
    b) big cell type   b) à grandes cellules   б) крупноклеточный тип
    c) giant cell type   c) à cellules géantes   в) гигантоклеточный тип

    Bronchuscarcinom   Carcinoma bronquial   Carcinoma bronchiale
    a) kleinzellig   a) de células pequenas   a) parvocellulare
    b) großzellig   b) de células redondas   b) magnocellulare
    c) riesenzellig   c) de células gigantes   c) gigantocellulare

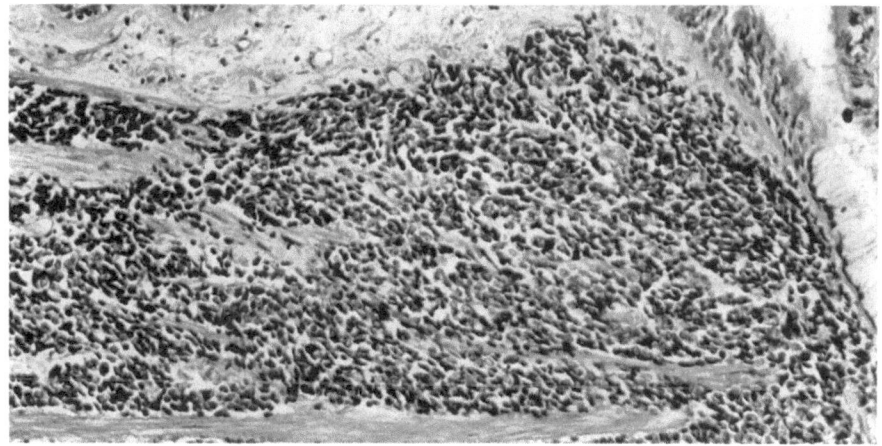

Fig. 63a. × 150.

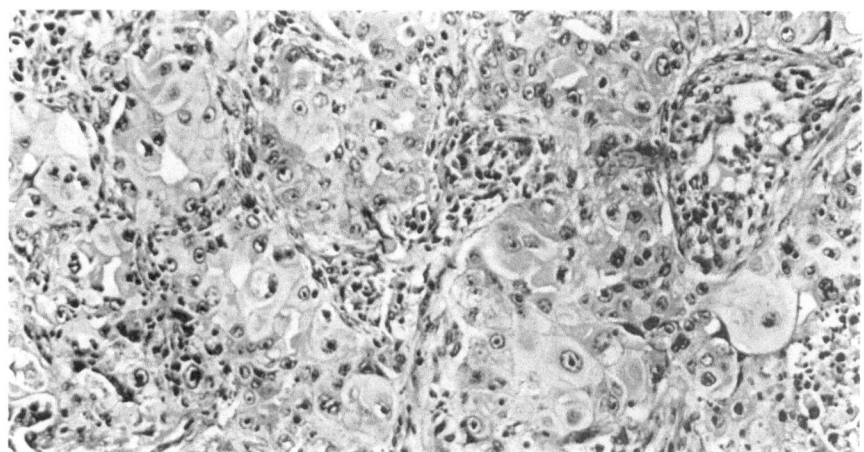

Fig. 63b. × 150.

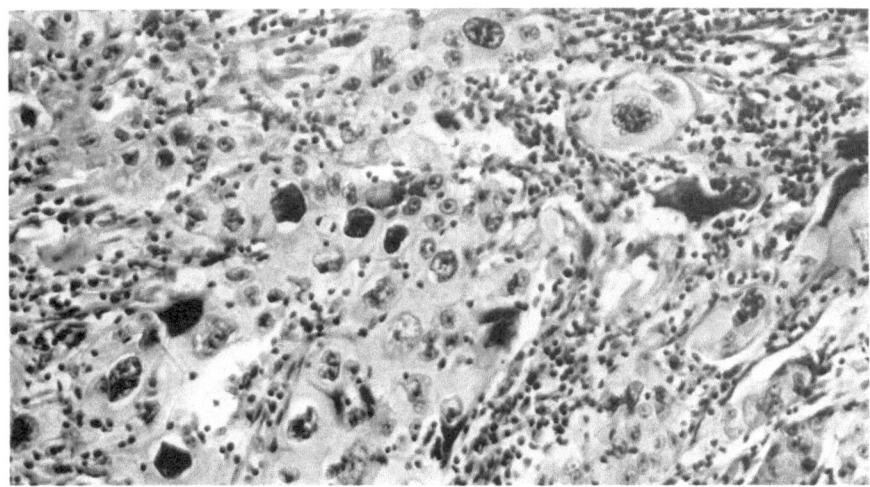

Fig. 63c. × 190.

7. **Breast**   Glande mammaire   Молочная железа

     Brustdrüse   Mama   Mamma   (174)

---

64   Pericanalicular fibro-adenoma   Fibro-adénome péri-canaliculaire   Периканаликулярная фиброаденома

     Pericanaliculäres Fibro-adenom   Fibroadenoma pericanalicu-lar   Fibroadenoma peri-canaliculare

65   Intracanalicular fibro-adenoma   Fibro-adénome intra-canaliculaire   Интраканаликулярная фиброаденома

     Intracanaliculäres Fibro-adenom   Fibroadenoma intra-canalicular   Fibroadenoma intra-canaliculare

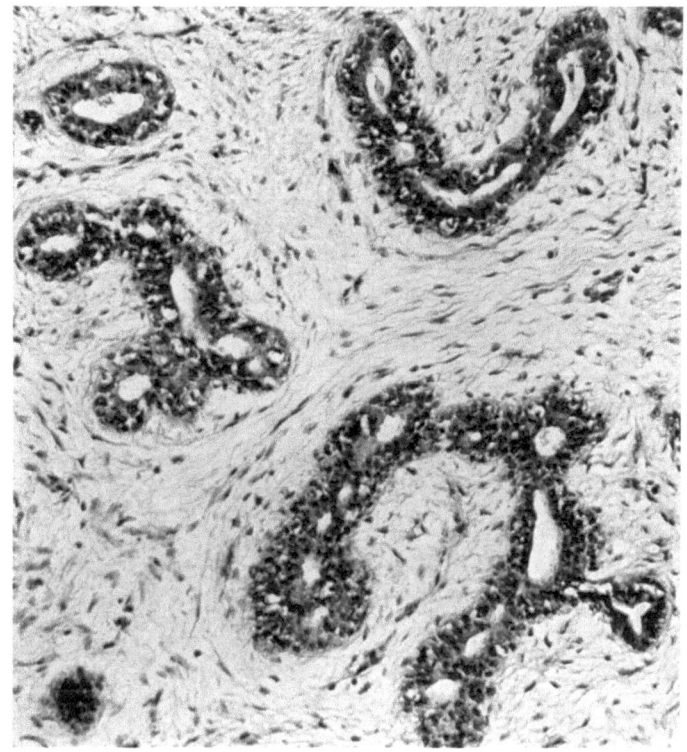

Fig. 64. × 150.

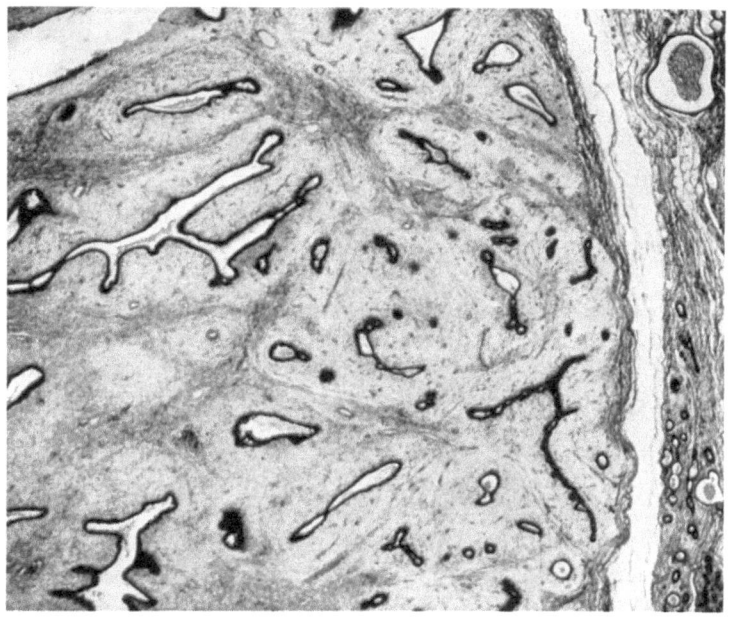

Fig. 65. × 15.

5*

66 Tubular adenoma   Adénome tubuleux   Тубулярная аденома

     Tubuläres Adenom   Adenoma tubular   Adenoma tubulare

67 Fibroadenoma phyllodes   Fibro-adénome phyllode   Филлоидная фибро аденома

     Giant fibroadenoma   Fibro-adénome géant   Гигантская фиброаденома

     Fibroadenoma phyllodes   Fibroadenoma filodes   Fibroadenoma phyllodes

     Riesen-Fibroadenom   Fibroadenoma gigante   Fibroadenoma gigantosum

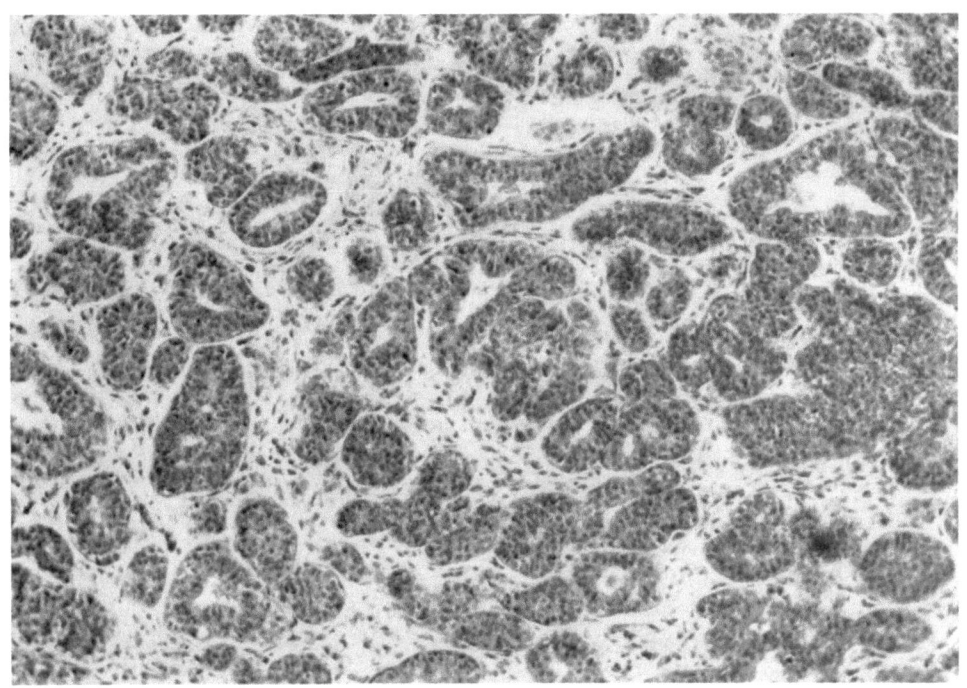

Fig. 66. × 54.

v. A. 257—290

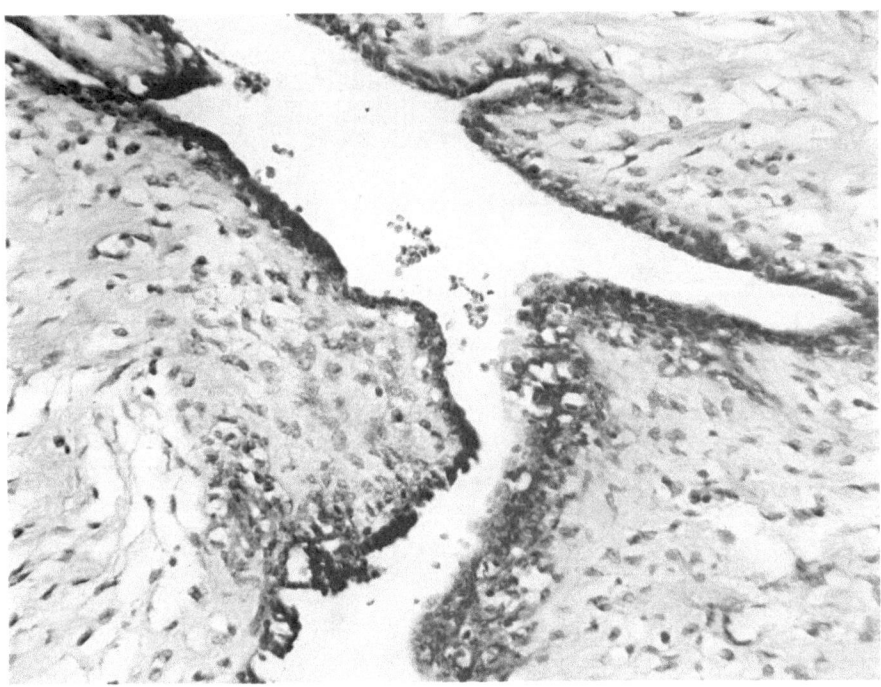

Fig. 67. × 275.

68 Intraductal papilloma   Papillome intra-canalicu-   Интрадуктальная
    Duct papilloma   laire (Tumeur dendri-   папиллома
                                    tique)   Папиллома молочных
                                    Papillome canaliculaire   протоков

    Intracanaliculäres Papillom   Papiloma intracanalicular   Papilloma intraductale
    Milchgangspapillom   Papiloma de los conductos   Papilloma ductale

69 Lobular carcinoma   Epithélioma lobulaire   Лобулярная карцинома

    Lobuläres Carcinom   Carcinoma lobular   Carcinoma lobulare

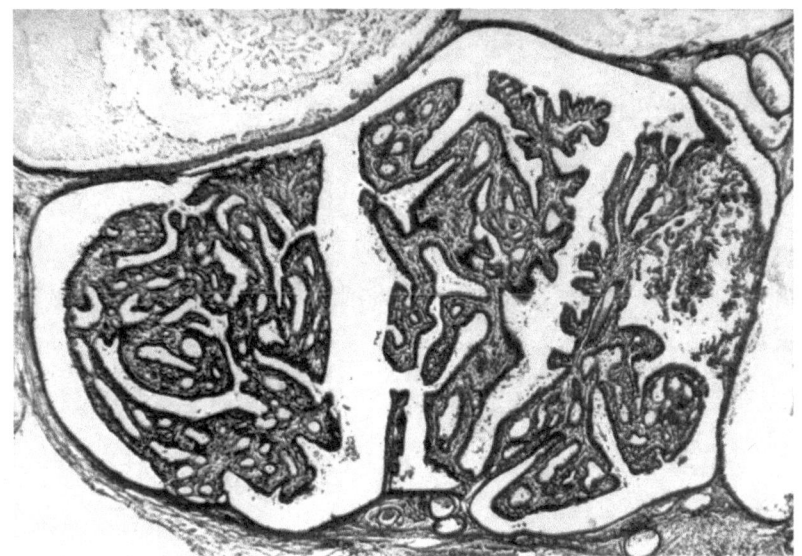

Fig. 68.   H 756—659

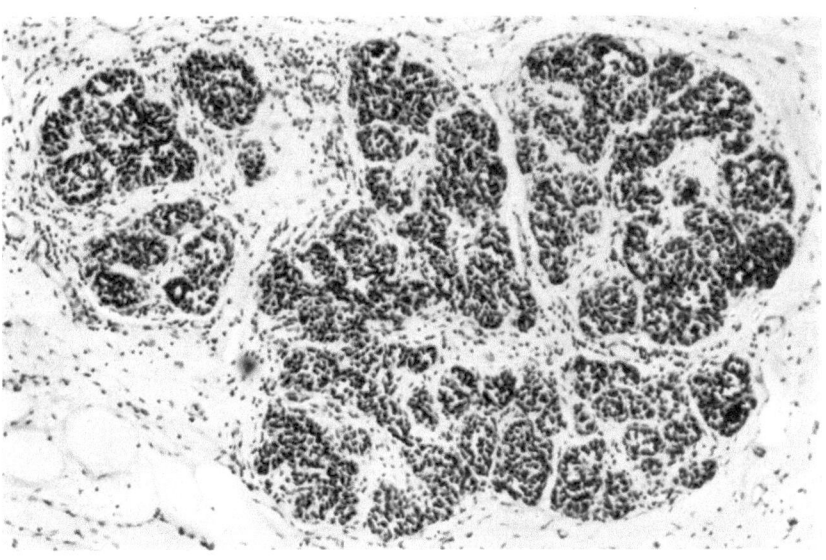

Fig. 69.   × 75.

70 Adenoma of nipple   Adenome mamelonnaire   Аденома соска молочной железы

   Adenom der Brustwarze   Adenoma pezón   Adenoma mammillae

71 Cribriform carcinoma   Epithélioma cribriforme   Криброзная карцинома
    (épithélioma en rognons
    ou à rosettes, selon Del-
    bet-Herrenschmidt)

   Cribriformes Carcinom   Carcinoma cribiforme   Carcinoma cribriforme

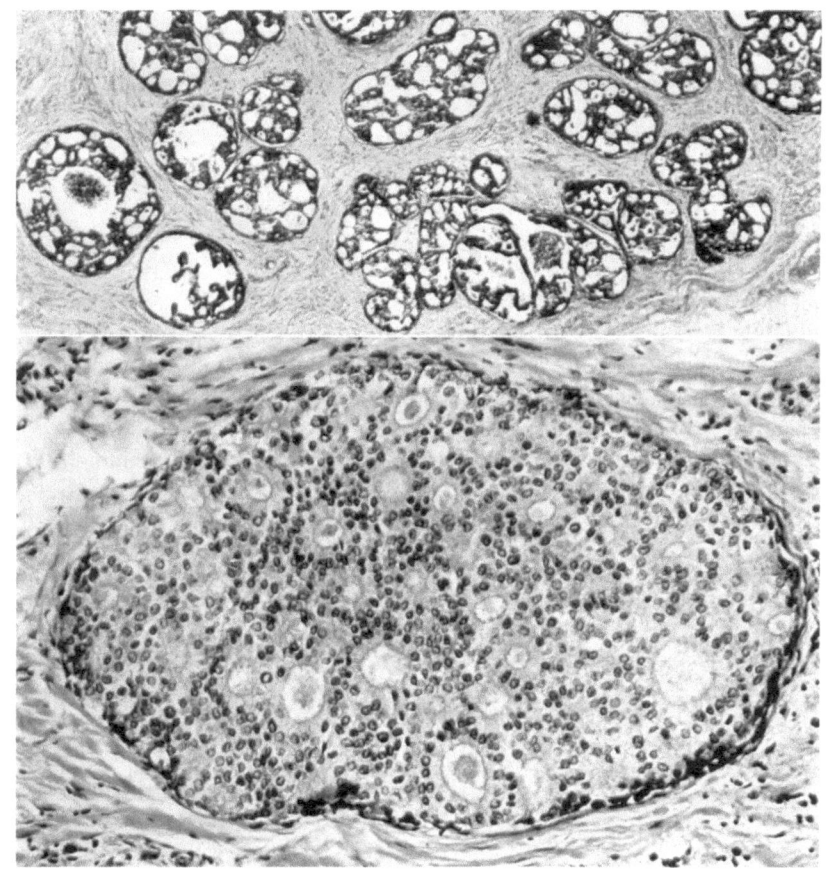

Fig. 70. × 30. × 150.

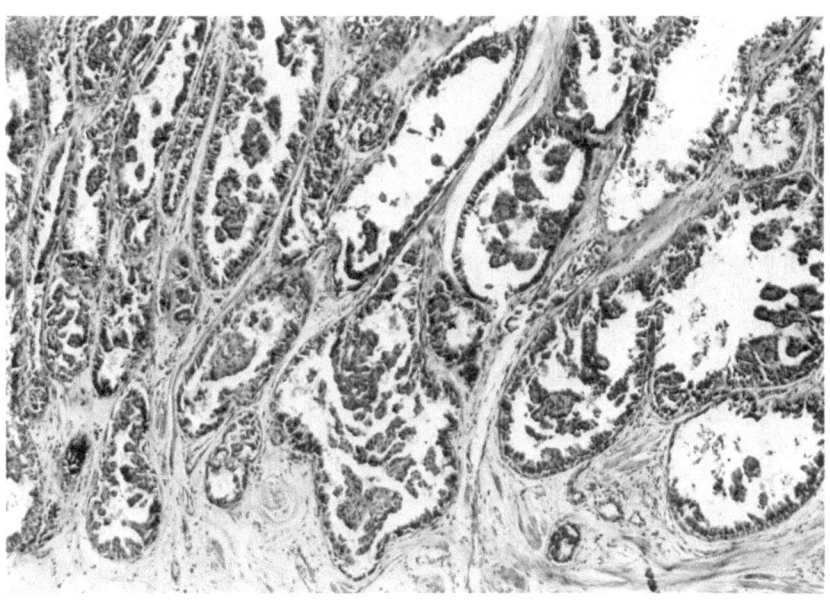

Fig. 71. × 60.

72 Intraductal carcinoma
Comedocarcinoma

Epithélioma intra-
canaliculaire
Comedocarcinome

Интрадуктальная
карцинома
Комедокарцинома

Intracanaliculäres Carcinom
Comedocarcinom

Carcinoma intracanalicular
Comedocarcinoma

Carcinoma intraductale
Comedocarcinoma

73 Intraepidermal carcinoma
of the nipple (Paget's
disease of the breast)

Epithélioma intra-épider-
mique du mamelon (Ma-
ladie de Paget de la glande mammaire)

Интраэпителиальный рак
соска (болезнь Пэджета)

Intraepidermales Carcinom
der Mamille (Morbus
Paget)

Carcinoma intraepidérmico
del pezón (Enfermedad
de Paget de la mama)

Carcinoma intradermale
mamillae (Morbus Paget
mammae)

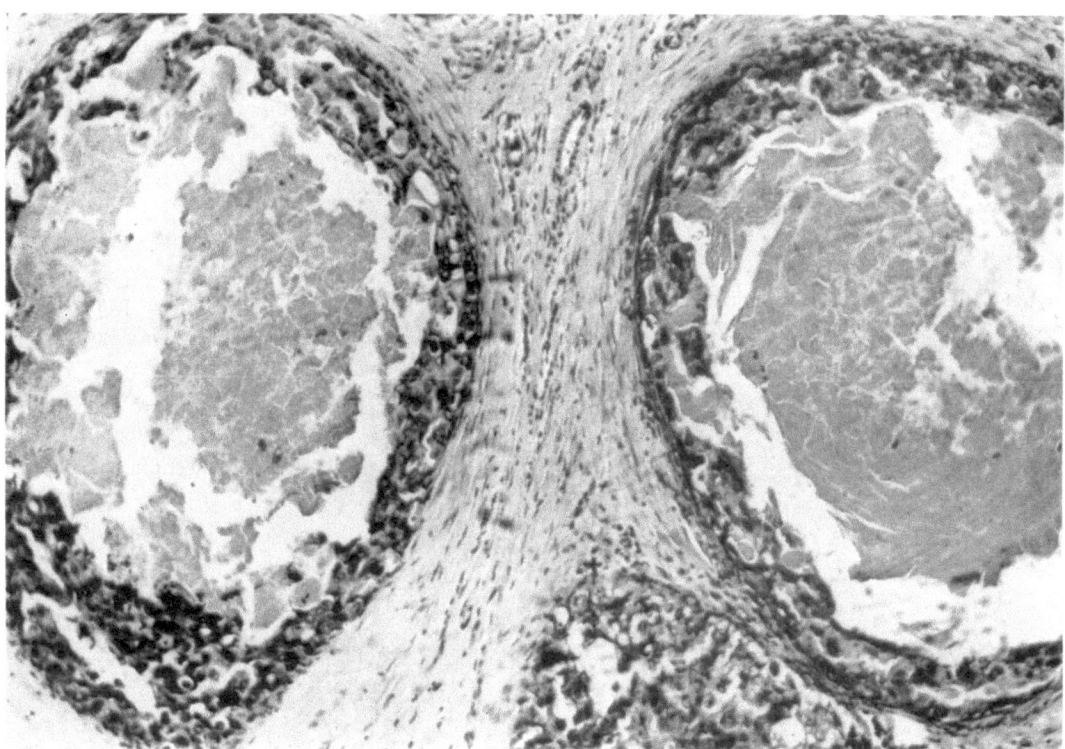

Fig. 72. F 34 33—15

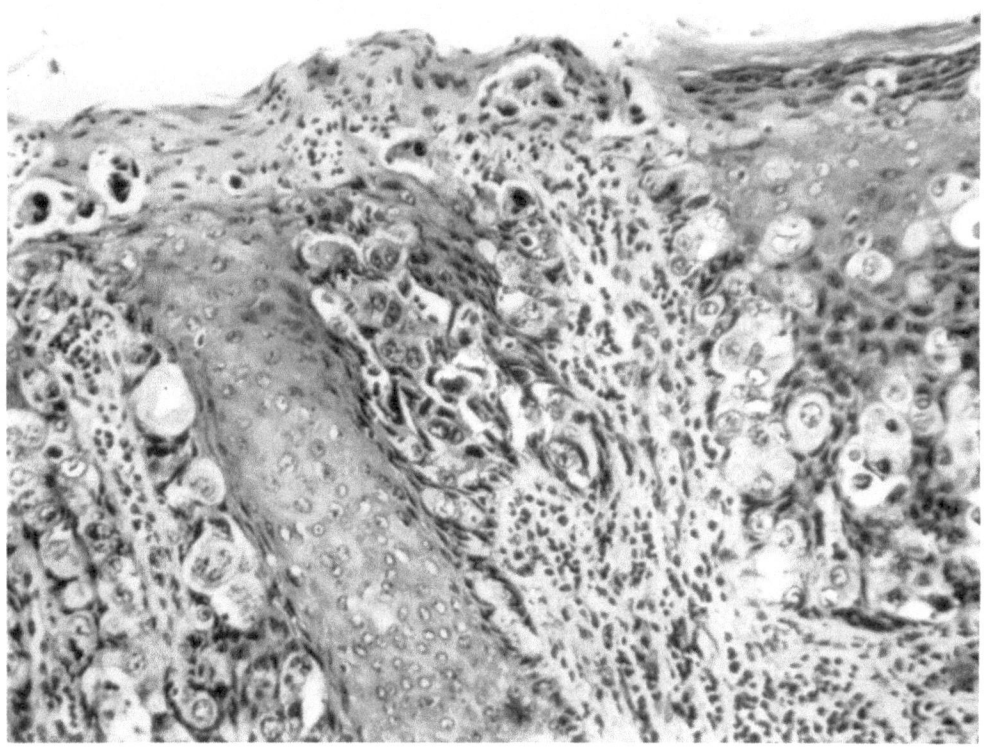

Fig. 73. F 34 17—1

74 Carcinoma — spindle cell type
Carcinosarcoma

Spindelzellcarcinom
Carcinosarkom

Epithélioma à cellules fusiformes
Epithélio-sarcome

Carcinoma fusocelular
Carcinosarcoma

Веретеноклеточный рак
Карциносаркома

Carcinoma fusicellulare
Carcinosarcoma

75 Cystosarcoma phyllodes

Cystosarcoma phyllodes

Cystosarcome phyllode

Cistosarcoma filodes

Филлоидная цистосаркома

Cystosarcoma phyllodes

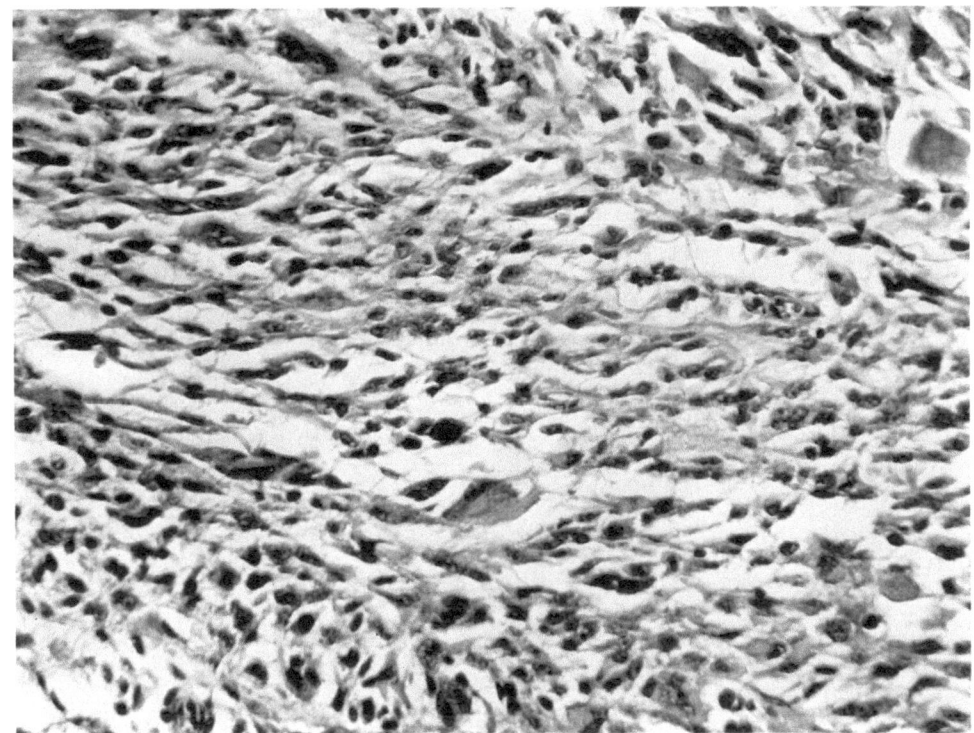

Fig. 74. × 300.

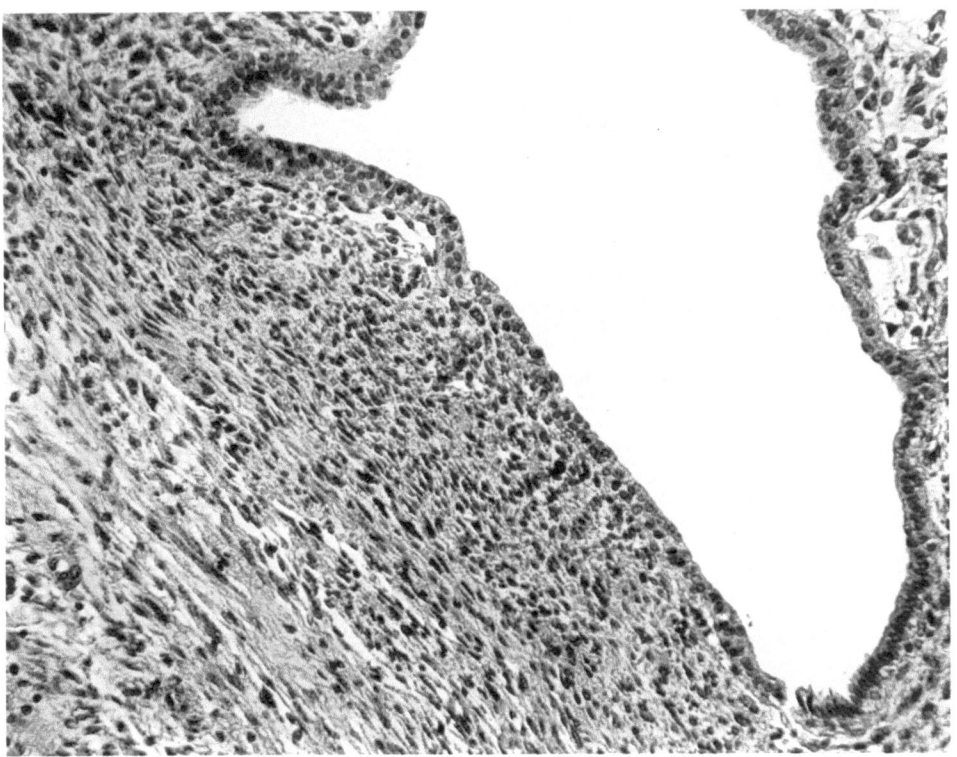

Fig. 75. × 250.

76 Adenoid cystic carcinoma

    Adenocystisches Carcinom
    Cylindromatöses Carcinom

Epithélioma adénoïde cystique (cylindromateux)

Carcinoma adenoide quístico

Аденоидо-кистозная
карцинома

Carcinoma adenoides cysticum

77 Medullary carcinoma with
    lymphoid stroma

    Medulläres Carcinom mit
    lymphoidem Stroma

Epithélioma encéphaloïde à
stroma lymphoïde

Carcinoma medular con
estroma linfoide

Медуллярный рак с
лимфоидной стромой

Carcinoma medullare cum
stromate lymphoide

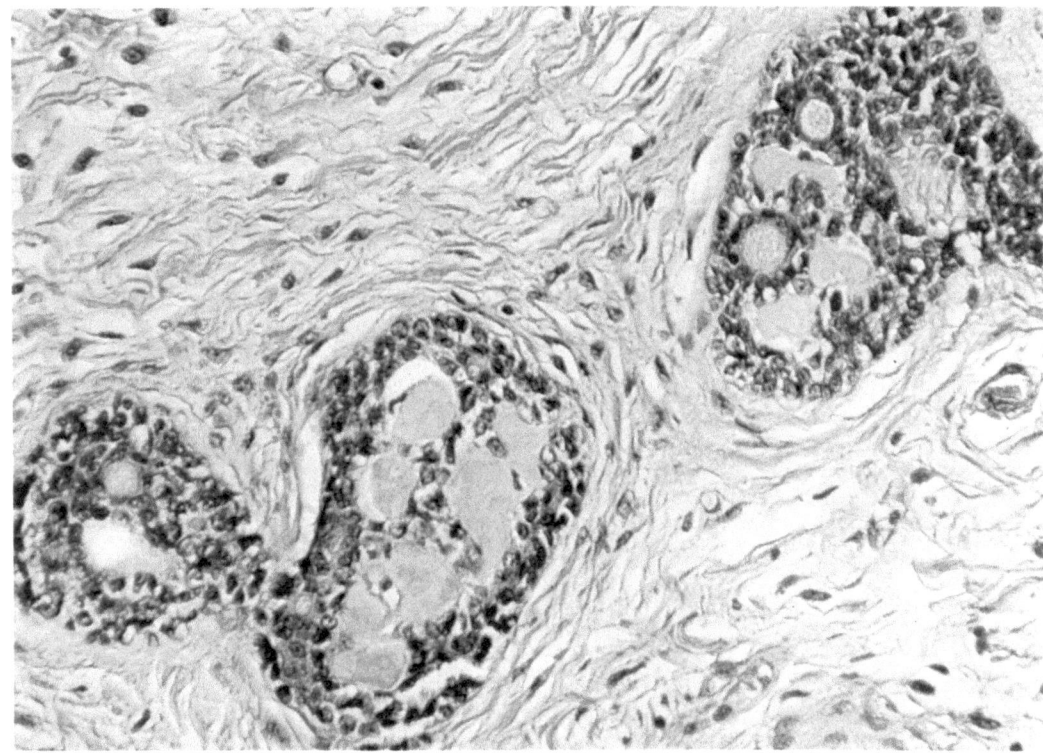

Fig. 76. × 300.

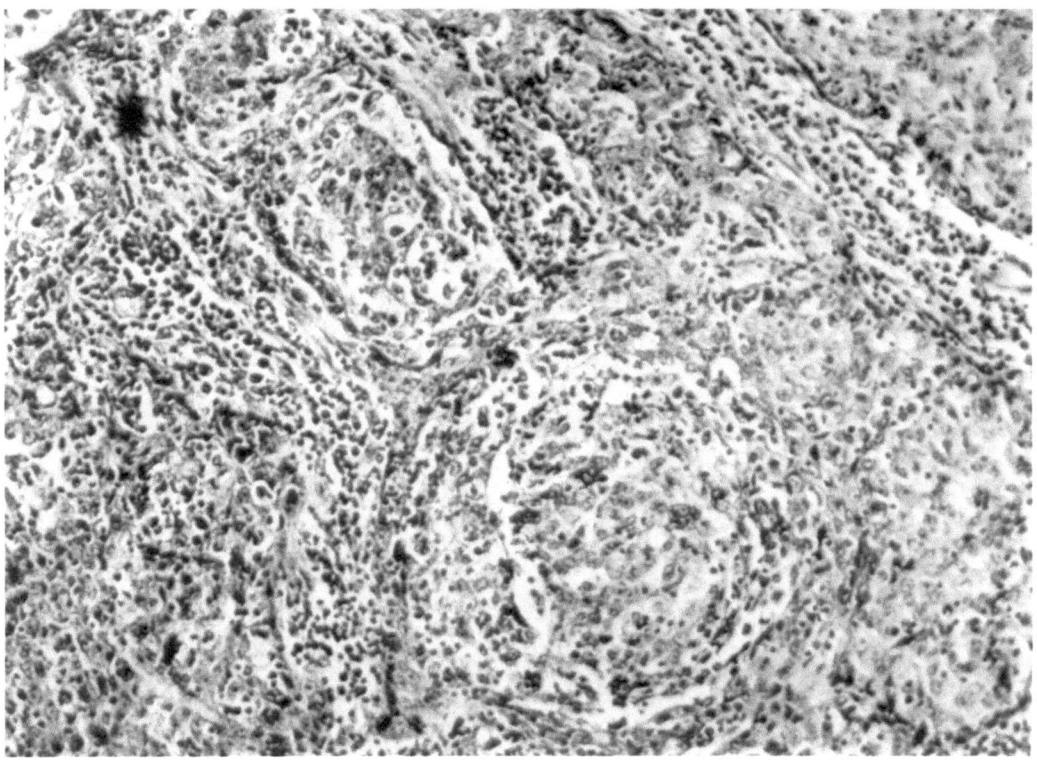

Fig. 77.

8. Uterus   Utérus   **Матка**

Gebärmutter   Utero   **Uterus**   (180—182)

78	Polyp of cervix	Polype cervical	Полип шейки
	Cervixpolyp	Pólipo cervical	Polypus cervicis uteri

79	Polyp of corpus	Polype corporéal	Полип тела
	Polyp of endometrium	Polype endométrial	Полип эндометрия
	Corpuspolyp	Pólipo del endometrio	Polypus corporis uteri
			Polypus endometrii

80	Hydatidiform mole	Môle hydatiforme	Пузырный занос
	Blasenmole	Mola hidatidiforme	Mola hydatidosa

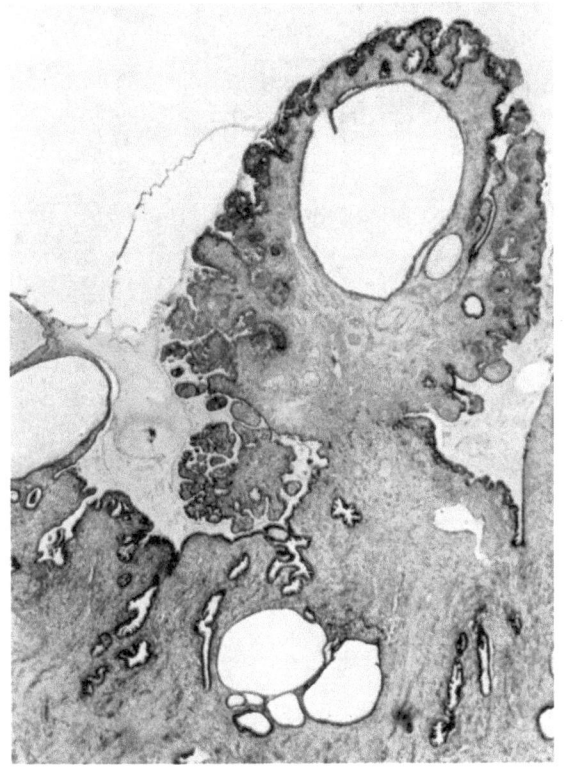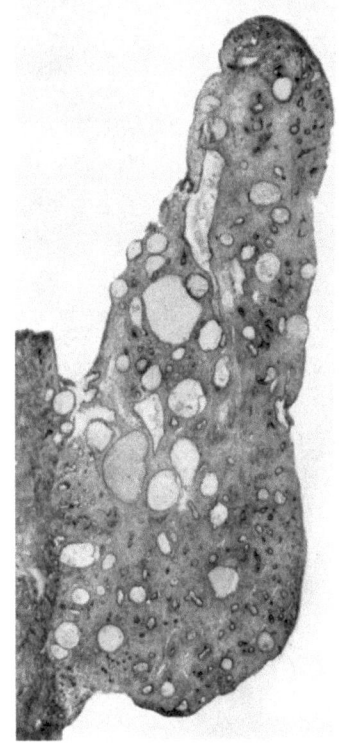

Fig. 78. × 8.   F 33/2 89—62   Fig. 79. × 5. F 33/2 179—151

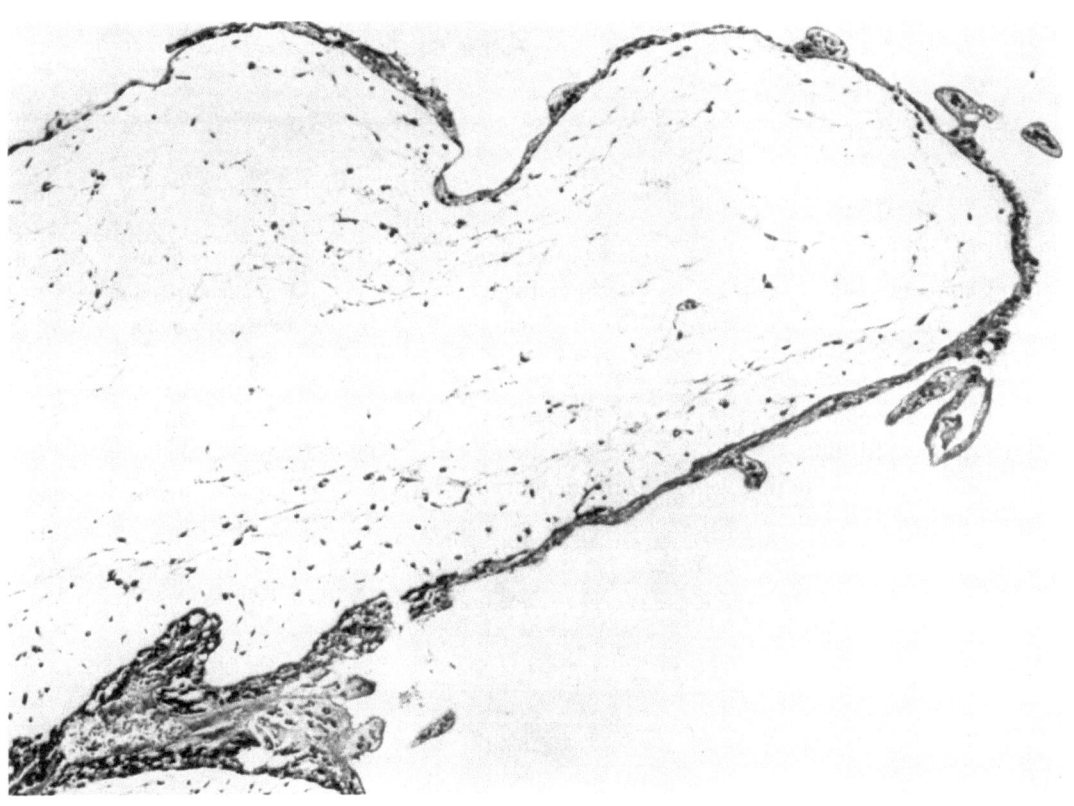

Fig. 80. × 100.   F 33/1 39—20

81 Invasive hydatidiform mole   Môle hydatiforme   Деструирующий пузырный
                                       envahissante   занос

    Destruierende Blasenmole   Mola hidatidiforme invasiva Mola hydatidosa invasiva

82 Choriocarcinoma   Choriocarcinome   Хориокарцинома
    Chorioepithelioma   Chorio-épithéliome   Хорионэпителиома
    Destructive chorioadenoma   Môle disséquante   Деструирующая
                                                                  хорионаденома

    Choriocarcinom   Coriocarcinoma   Choriocarcinoma
    Chorionepitheliom   Corioepitelioma   Chorioepithelioma
    Destruierendes Chorio-   Corioadenoma destructivo   Chorioadenoma destruens
      adenom

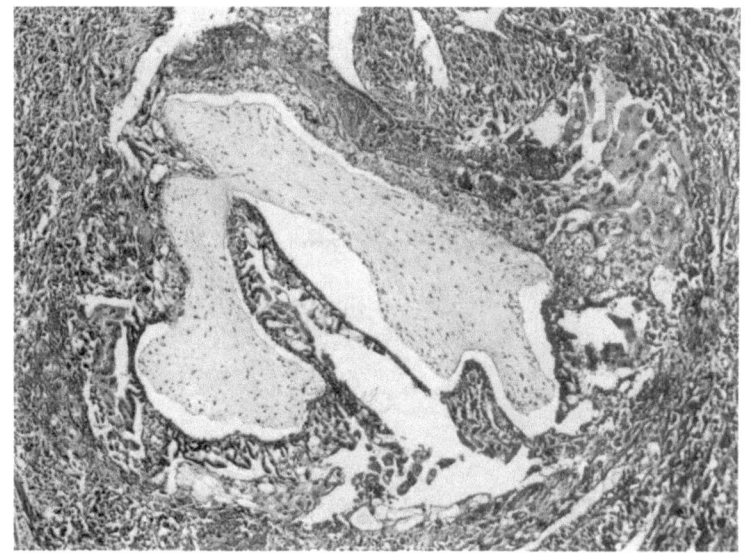

Fig. 81. ×48.   F 33/1 55—53

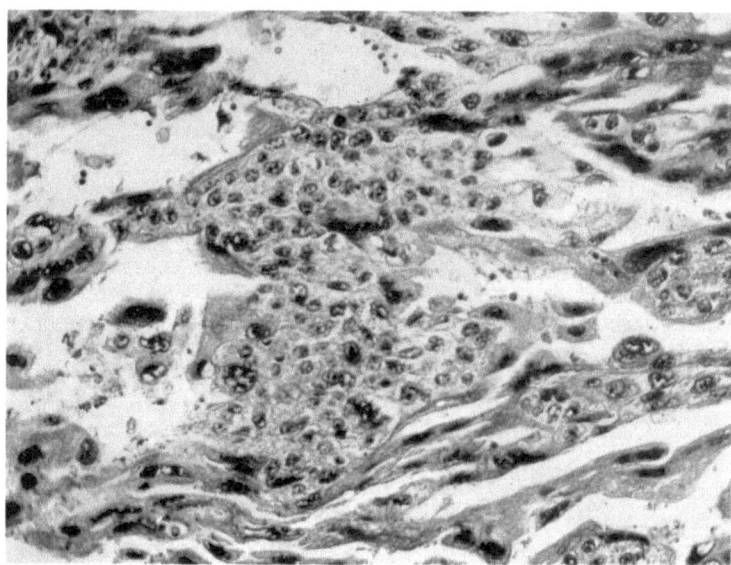

Fig. 82. ×185.   F 33/1 57—57

83 Endometrial carcinoma   Epithélioma corporéal   Эндометриальный рак

    Endometriales Carcinom   Carcinoma endometrial   Carcinoma endometriale

84 Endometrial sarcoma   Sarcome du chorion   Эндометриальная саркома
                                 cytogène

    Endometriales Sarkom   Sarcoma endometrial   Sarcoma endometriale

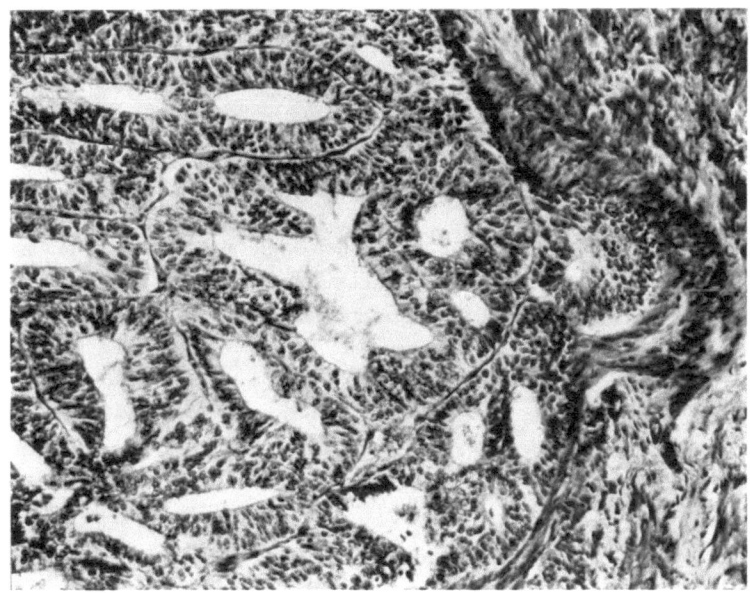

Fig. 83. × 120.

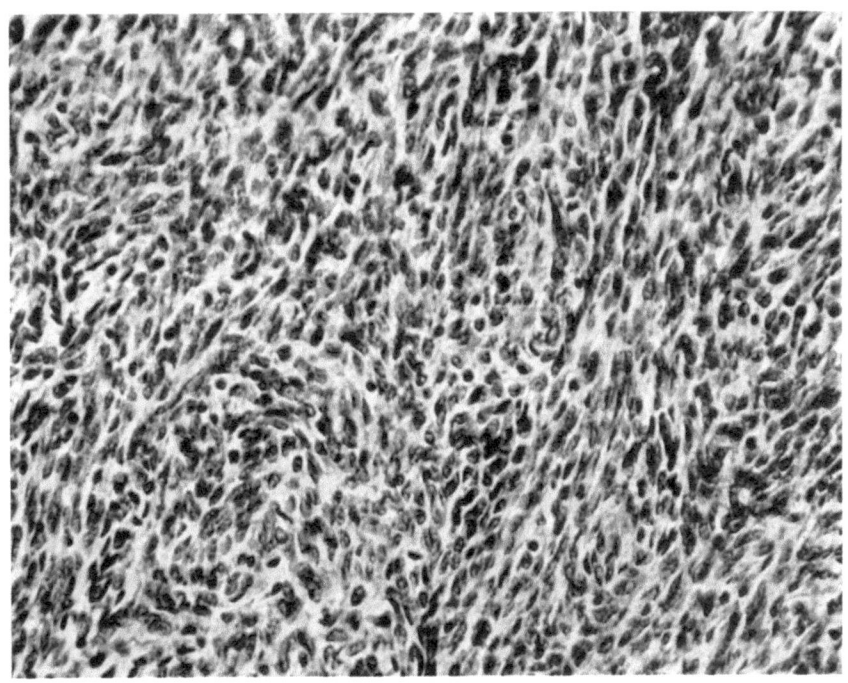

Fig. 84. × 250.

85	Mesodermal mixed tumor Sarcoma botryoides	Tumeur mésodermique à structure complexe Sarcome botryoïde	Мезодермальная смешанная опухоль Ботриоидная саркома
	Mesodermaler Mischtumor Botryoides Sarkom	Tumor mixto mesodérmico Sarcoma botrioides	Tumor mixtus meso- dermalis Sarcoma botryoides
86	Carcinosarcoma of uterus	Epithélio-sarcome	Карциносаркома
	Carcinosarkom	Carcinosarcoma del útero	Carcinosarcoma

The histological picture of adenomatoid tumor of tube is considered as identical with adenomatoid tumor of testis; the mesonephroma of cervix as identical with mesonephroma of ovary — see these.

L'aspect histologique des tumeurs adénomateuses de la trompe est identique à celui des tumeurs adénomateuses du testicule; le mésonéphrome du col est analogue à celui de l'ovaire — se reporter à ces organes.

Гистологическое строение аденоматоидной опухоли трубы рассматривается как идентичное адено- матоидной опухоли яичка; мезонефрома шейки матки идентична мезонефроме яичника - см. 9.

Das histologische Bild der adenomatösen Tumoren der Tube wird als identisch mit dem der adeno- matösen Tumoren des Hodens, das der Mesonephrome der Cervix als identisch mit dem der Meso- nephrome des Ovariums angesehen — siehe jeweils dort.

El cuadro histológico del tumor adenomatoide de la trompa se considera idéntico con el tumor adeno- matoide del testículo; el mesonefroma cervical como idéntico con el mesonefroma del ovario: ver éstos.

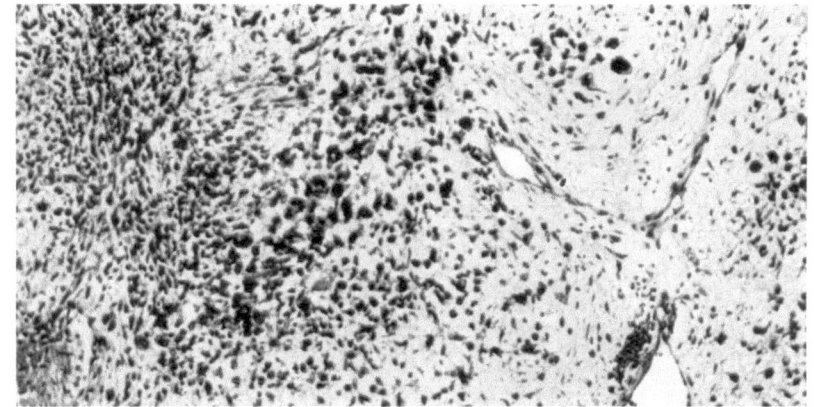

Fig. 85a. ×125. F 33/2 163—139

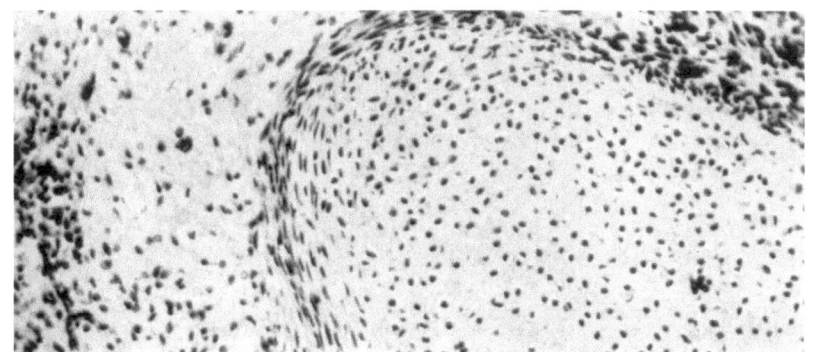

Fig. 85b. ×145. F 33/2 163—140

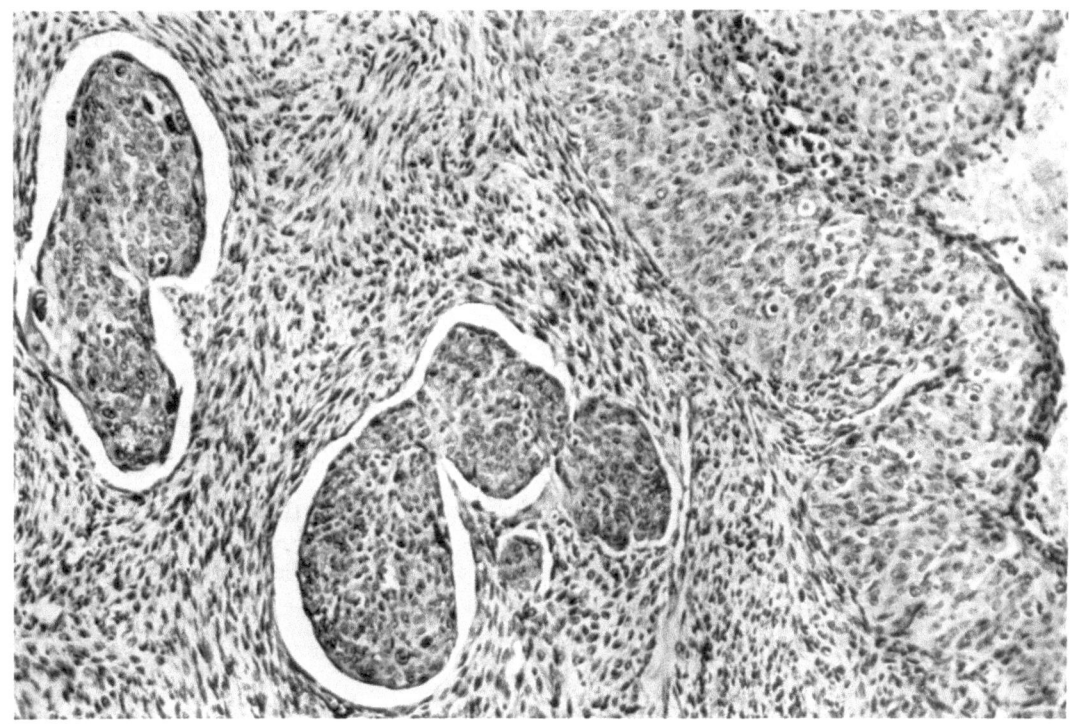

Fig. 86. ×114. F 33/2 165—141

---

9. Ovary　　　Ovaire　　　**Яичник**

Eierstock　　Ovario　　　Ovariae　　(183)

87　Thecoma　　　　　　　Thécome　　　　　　　　Текома
　　Theca cell tumor　　　Tumeur à cellules thécales　Текаклеточная опухоль

　　Thekom　　　　　　　Tecoma　　　　　　　　　Thecoma
　　Thecazelltumor　　　　Tumor de células de la teca　Tumor thecocellularis

88　Serous papillary cyst-　Kyste germinatif végétant　Серозная папиллярная
　　　adenoma　　　　　　Kyste séreux papillaire　　　кистаденома
　　Serous papillary cystoma　Kyste à épithélium cilié　Серозная папиллярная
　　Cilioepithelial cystoma　　　　　　　　　　　　кистома
　　　　　　　　　　　　　　　　　　　　　　　Кистома из мерцательного
　　　　　　　　　　　　　　　　　　　　　　　　эпителия

　　Seröses papilläres Cyst-　Cistoadenoma papilífero　Cystadenoma papilliferum
　　　adenom　　　　　　　seroso　　　　　　　　　serosum
　　Seröses papilläres Cystom　Cistoma papilífero seroso　Cystoma papilliferum
　　Flimmerepithel-Cystom　Cistoma de células epite-　　serosum
　　　　　　　　　　　　　liales ciliadas　　　　　Cystoma cilioepitheliale

89　Surface papilloma　　　Papillome de surface　　　Поверхностная папиллома

　　Oberflächenpapillom　　Papiloma de superficie　　Papilloma superficiale

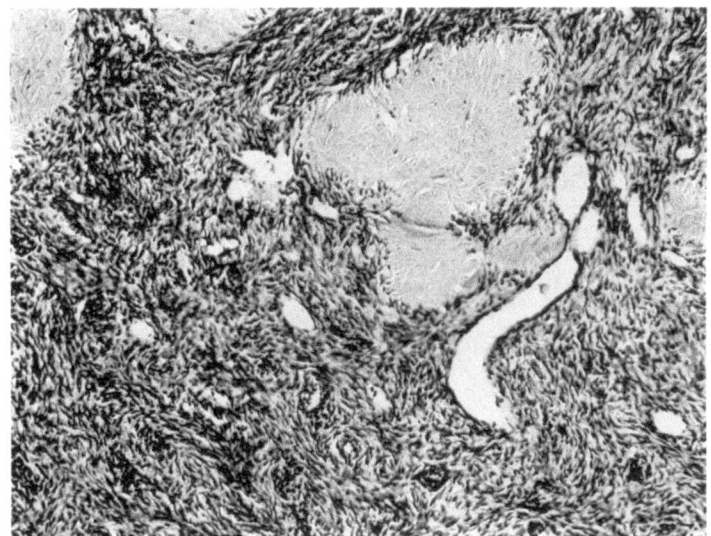

Fig. 87. × 85.

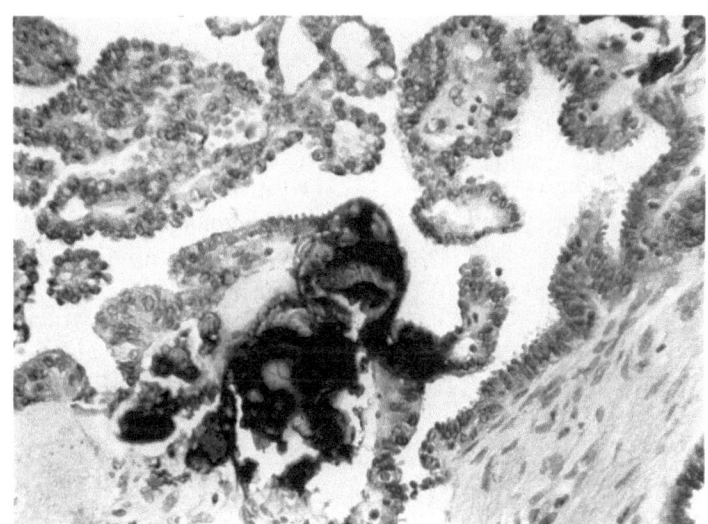

Fig. 88. × 200.

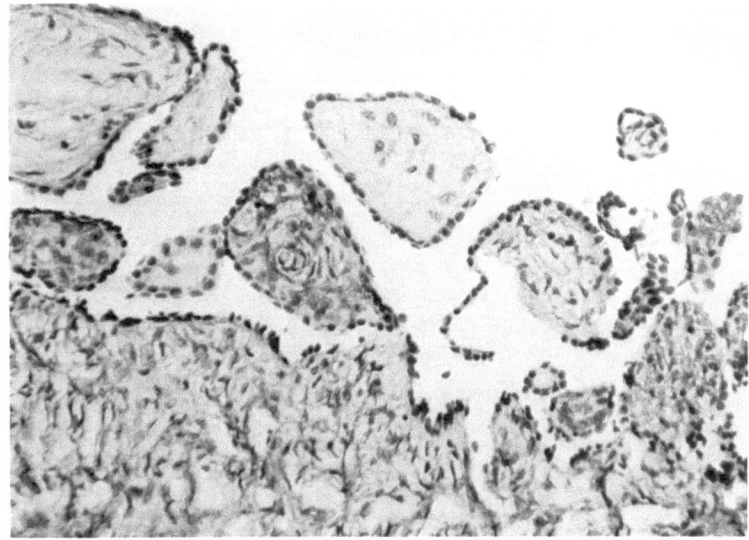

Fig. 89. × 150.

90	Mucinous cystadenoma Mucinous cystoma	Kyste mucineux (entéroïde) Kyste uni- ou multi-loculé mucineux	Муцинозная кистаденома Муцинозная кистома
	Mucinöses Cystadenom Mucincystom	Cistoadenoma mucinoso Cistoma mucinoso	Cystadenoma mucinosum Cystoma mucinosum

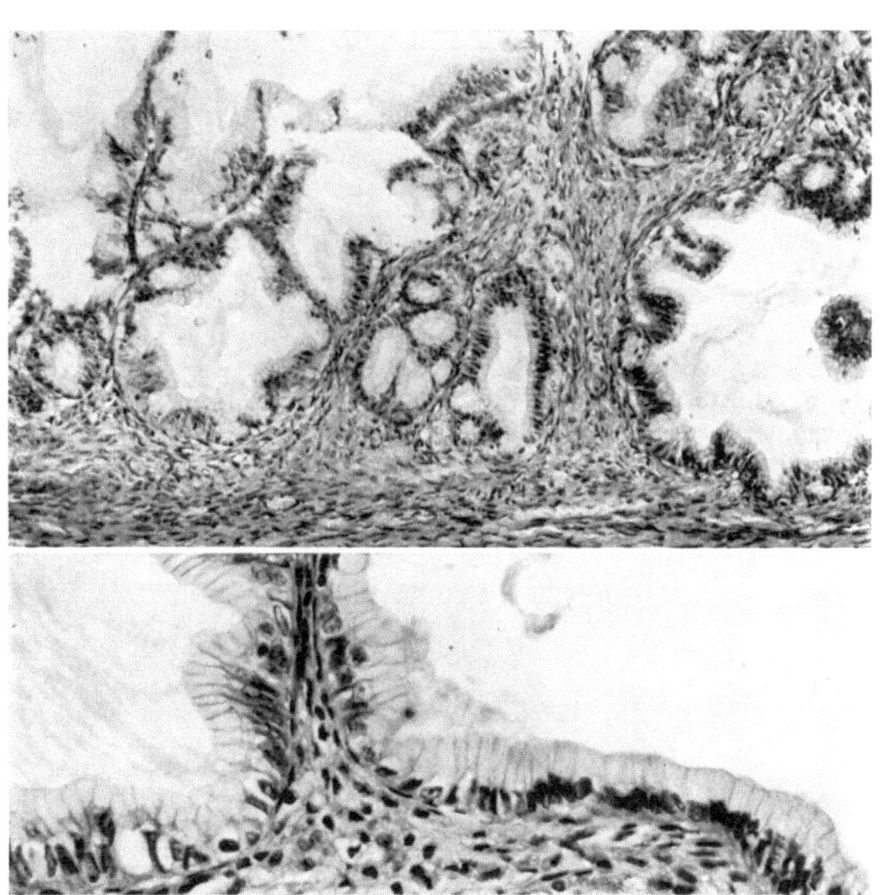

Fig. 90. × 120. × 300.

91   Teratoma   Tératome   Тератома

     Teratom   Teratoma   Teratoma

92   Adenofibroma   Adénofibrome   Аденофиброма

     Adenofibrom   Adenofibroma   Adenofibroma

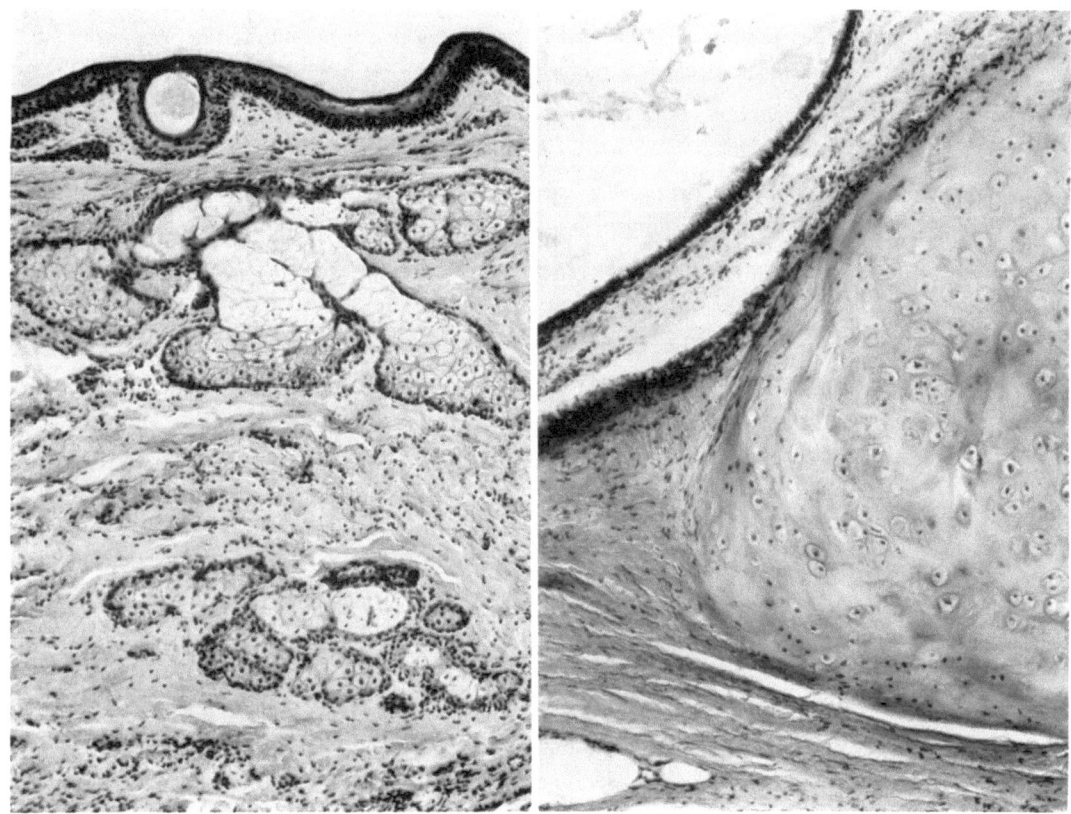

Fig. 91. × 90.

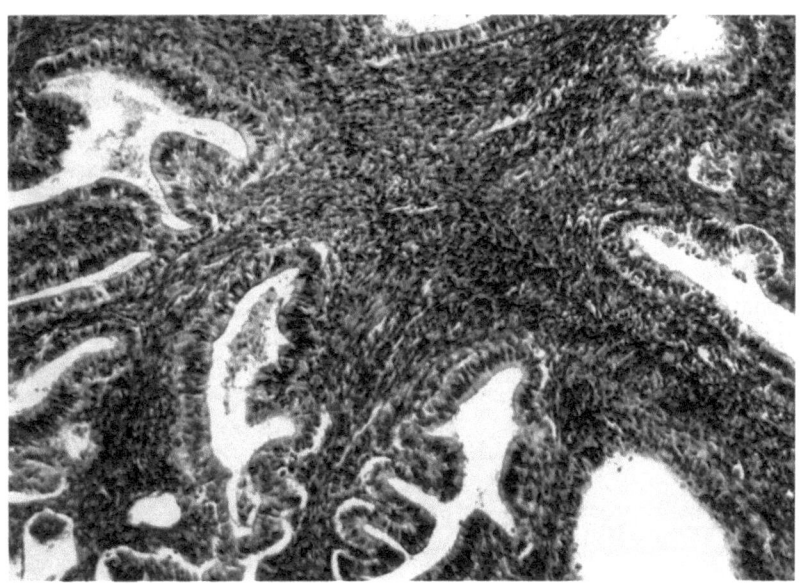

Fig. 92. ×115.   Glaz. 80—47

Arrhenoblastoma — *designation for some tumors with hormonal masculinizing properties but of variable histological patterns*, (91—94):

Arrhénoblastome — *désignation de certaines tumeurs ayant des propriétés hormonales masculinisantes, mais de structures histologiques variables*, (91—94):

Арренобластома — *название для опухолей различного гистологического строения, обладающих гормональными маскулинизирующими свойствами* (91—94):

Arrhenoblastom — *Bezeichnung für Tumoren mit maskulinisierenden hormonellen Eigenschaften verschiedenen histologischen Baues*, (91—94):

Arrenoblastoma — *designación para tumores con efecto hormonal masculinizante y cuadro histológico variable*, (91—94):

93 Arrhenoblastoma
   a) testicular (tubular)
      adenoma
   b) Sertoli cell tumor
   c) intermediate type
   d) sarcomatoid type
   e) Sertoli-Leydig-
      cell tumor

Arrhénoblastome
   a) adénome testiculaire
      (tubuleux)
   b) tumeur à cellules
      de Sertoli
   c) type intermediaire
   d) type sarcomatoíde
   e) tumeur à cellules
      type Sertoli-Leydig

Арренобластома
   а) тестикулярная аденома
      (тубулярная)
   б) опухоль из
      сертолиевых клеток
   в) промежуточный тип
   г) саркоматозный тип
   е) опухоль из клеток
      Сертоли-Лейдига

Arrhenoblastom
   a) testiculäres (tubuläres)
      Adenom
   b) Sertolizell-Tumor
   c) intermediärer Typ
   d) sarcomatoider Typ
   e) Sertoli-Leydig-Zell-
      Tumor

Arrenoblastoma
   a) adenoma testicular
      (tubular)
   b) tumor de células
      de Sertoli
   c) de tipo intermedio
   d) de tipo sarcomatoso
   e) tumor de células
      de Sertoli y de Leydig

Arrhenoblastoma
   a) Adenoma testiculare
      (tubulare)
   b) Adenoma
      Sertoli-cellulare
   c) Typus intermedius
   d) Typus sarcomatodes
   e) Tumor Sertoli-Leydig
      cellularis

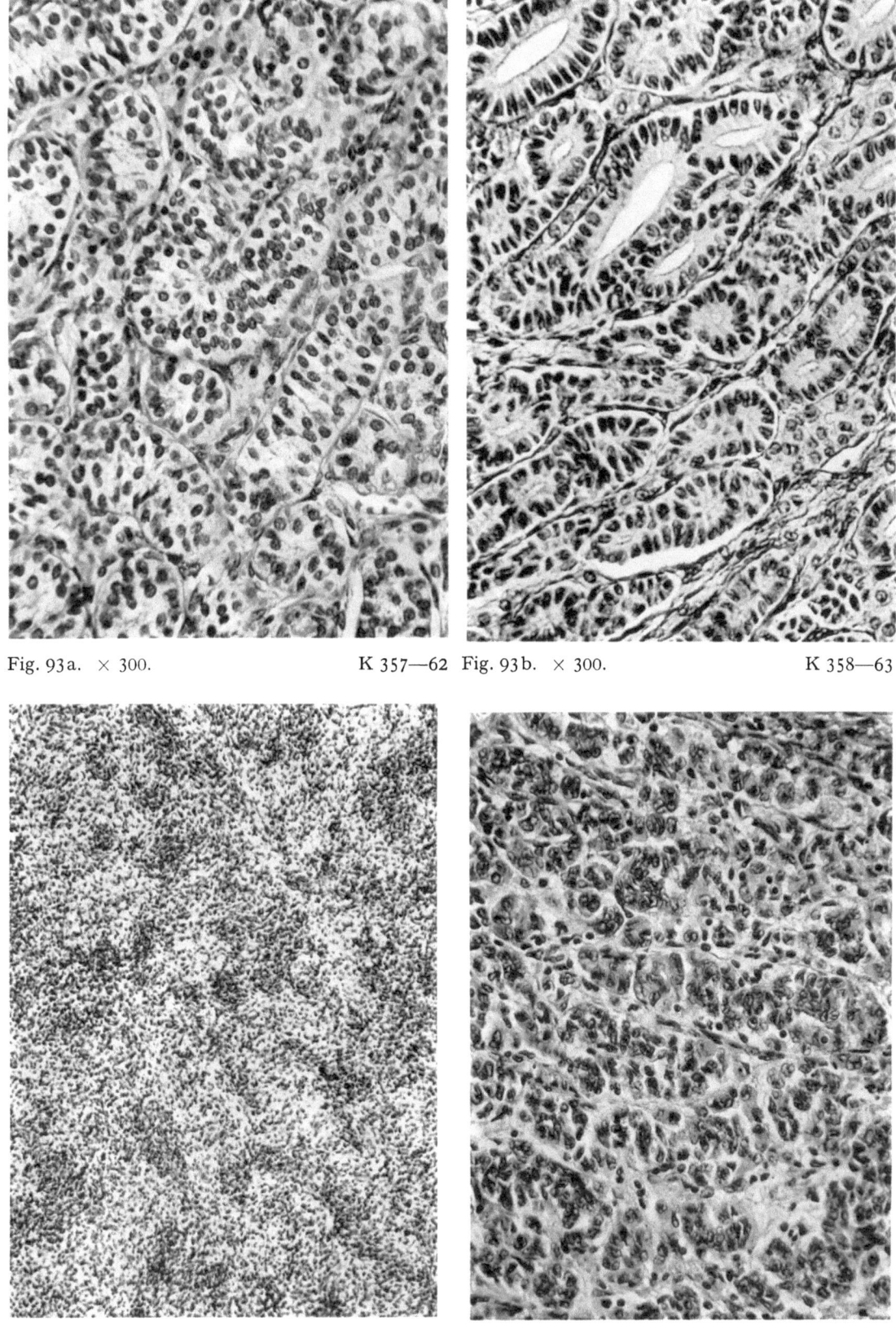

Fig. 93a. × 300.   K 357—62   Fig. 93b. × 300.   K 358—63

Fig. 93c. × 85.   K 359—65.   Fig. 93d. × 300.   K 360—66

| 94 | Leydig cell tumor
Hilus cell tumor
Interstitial cell tumor | Tumeur à cellules de Leydig
Tumeur à cellules hilaires
Tumeur à cellules inter-
    stitielles | Опухоль из клеток Лейдига
Опухоль из хилюсных
    клеток
Опухоль из
    интерстициальных клеток |
| | Leydigzell-Tumor
Hiluszell-Tumor
Tumor der interstitiellen
    Zellen | Tumor de células de Leydig
Tumor de células hiliares
Tumor de células inters-
    ticiales | Tumor Leydigcellularis
Tumor hilocelluare
Tumor interstitio-cellularis |

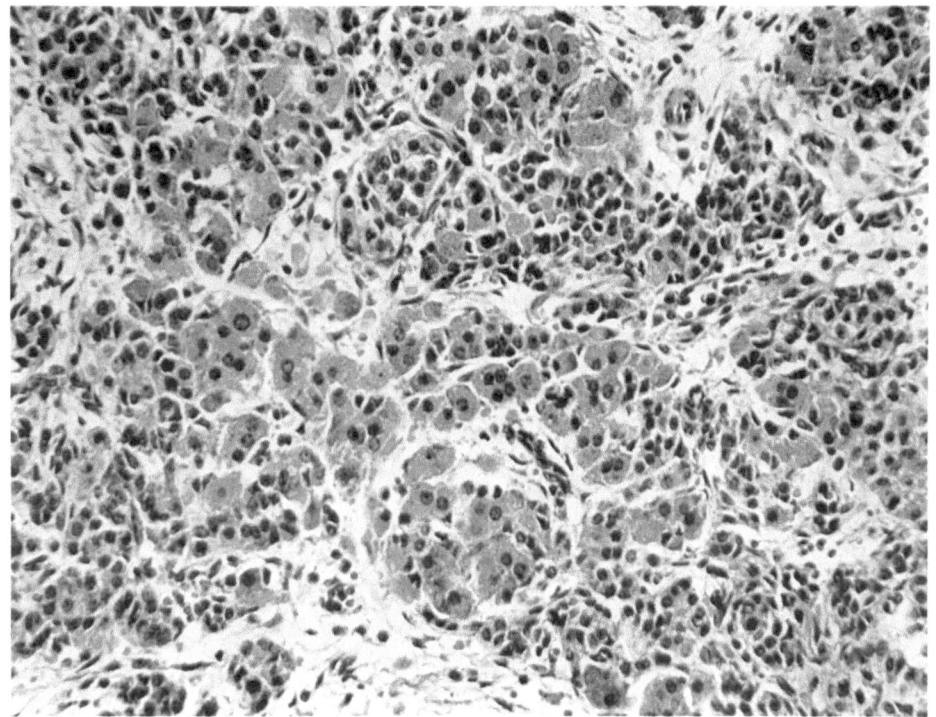

Fig. 93e. × 275. K 358—64

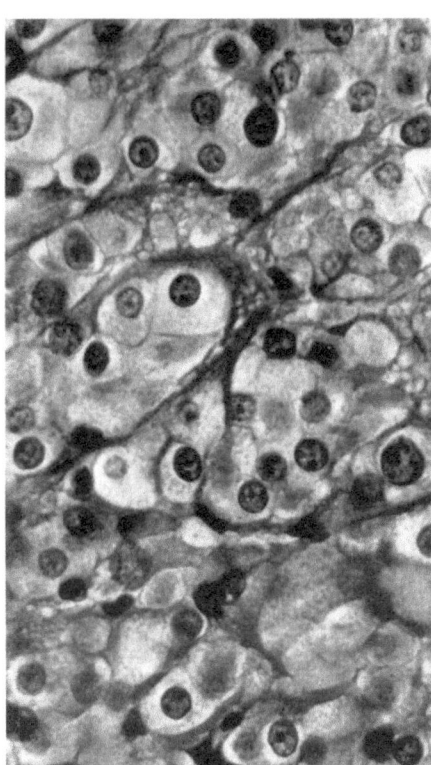

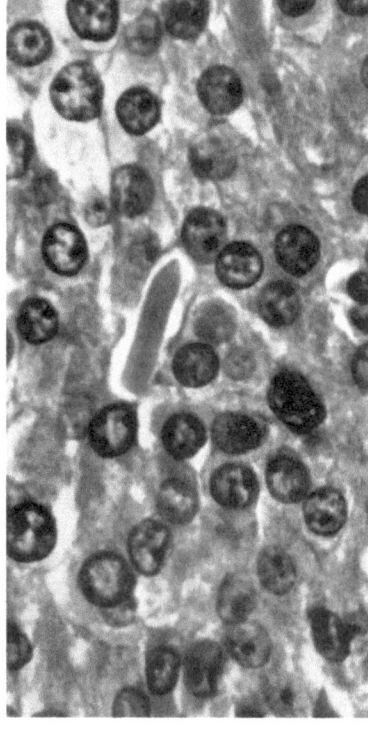

Fig. 94a. ×400. F 33/3 135—128   Fig. 94b. ×670. F 33/3 135—129

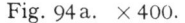

7 Nomenclature, 2. Edit.

95 Brenner tumor	Tumeur de Brenner	Опухоль Бреннера
Brenner-Tumor	Tumor de Brenner	Tumor Brenner

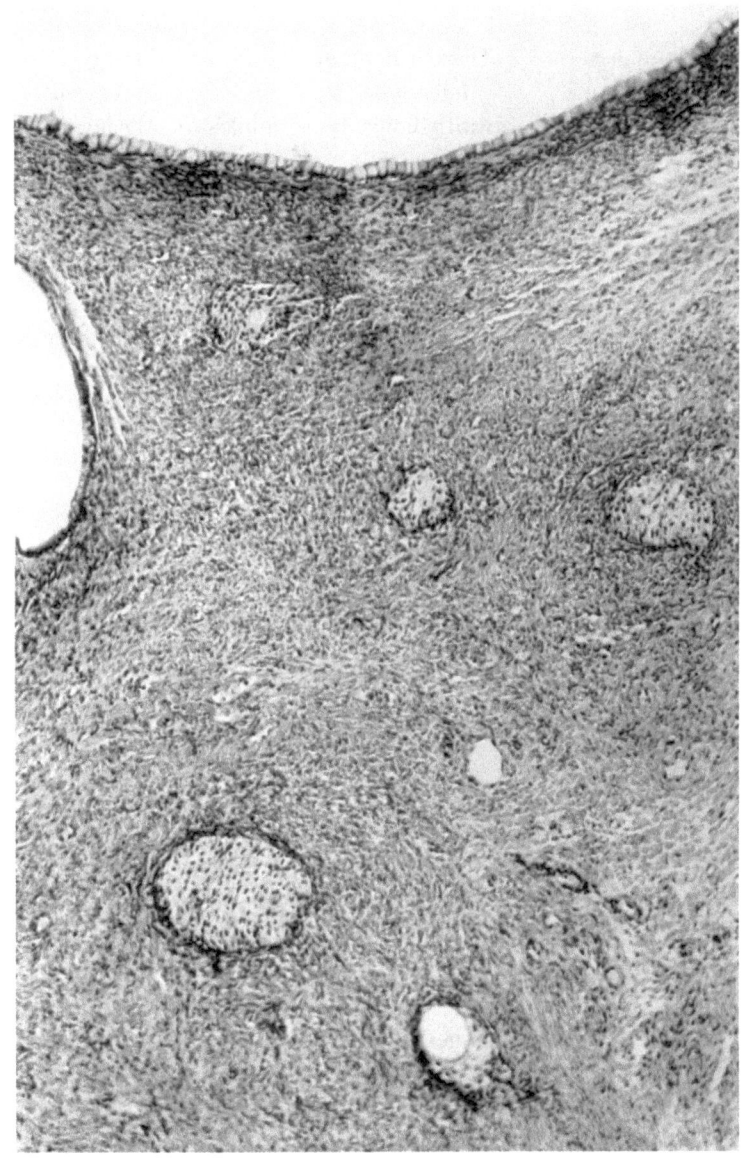

Fig. 95. × 100.   F 33/3 129—115

96	Granulosa cell tumor Granulosa cell carcinoma	Tumeur de la granulosa ou folliculome Epithélioma de la granulosa	Гранулезоклеточная опухоль Гранулезоклеточный рак
	Granulosazelltumor Granulosazellcarcinom	Tumor de células de la granulosa Carcinoma de células de la granulosa	Tumor granulosocellulare Carcinoma granulosocellu- lare
97	Dysgerminoma Dysgerminom	Dysgerminome Disgerminoma	Дисгерминома Dysgerminoma

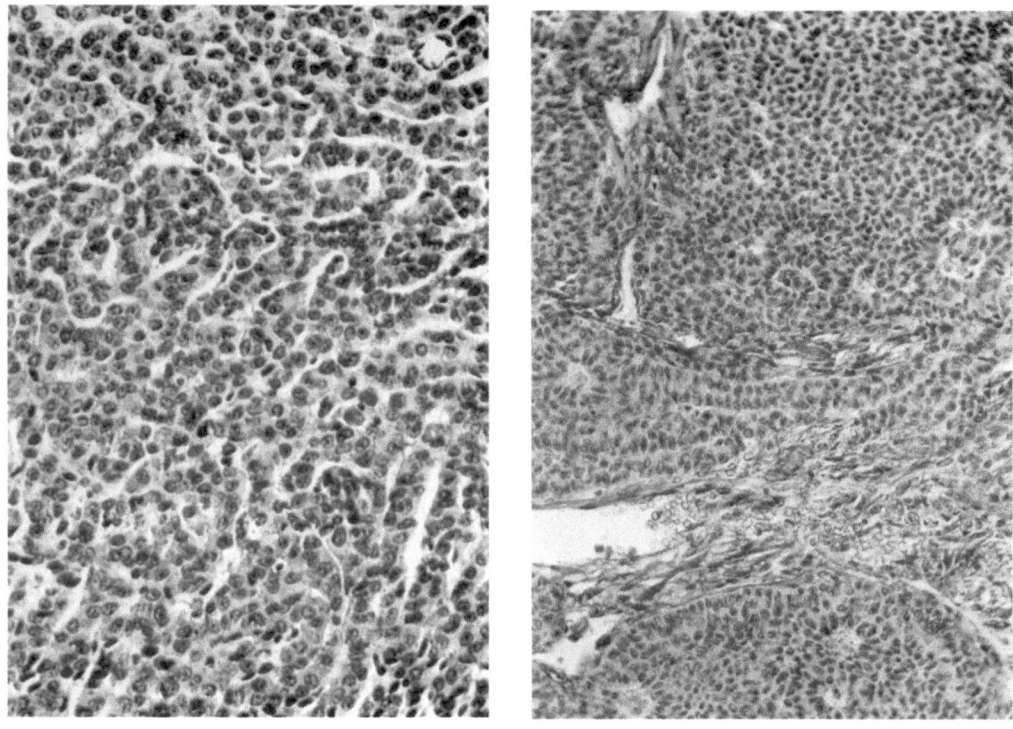

Fig. 96a. × 200.   F 33/3 27—13   Fig. 96b. × 160.   F 33/3 25—11

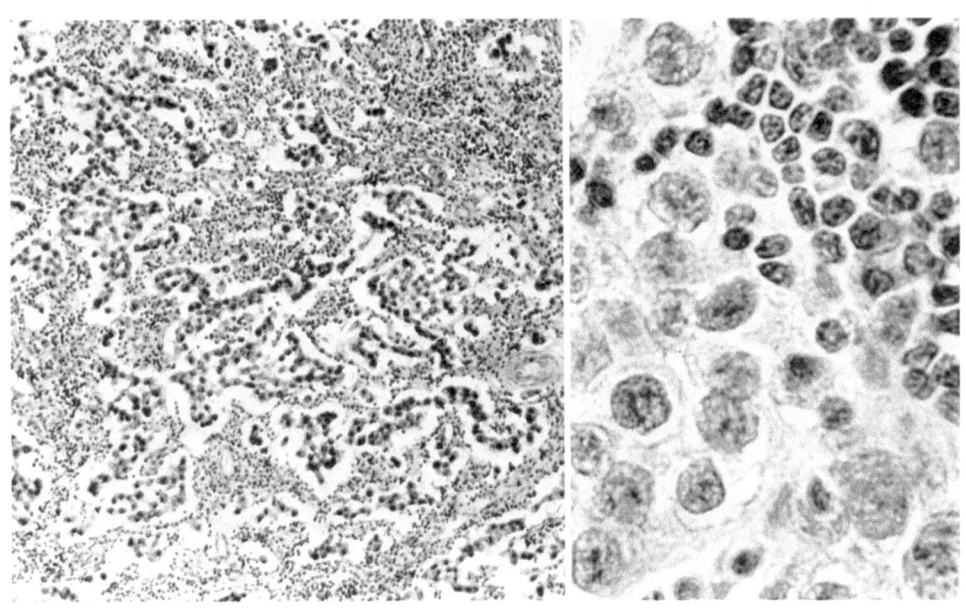

Fig. 97. × 75. × 720.

| 98 | Mucinous cystadeno-carcinoma | Epithélioma mucineux (entéroïde) | Муцинозная кистаденокарцинома |
| | Mucinöses Cystadeno-carcinom | Cistoadenocarcinoma mucinoso | Cystadenocarcinoma muci-nosum carcinomatosum |

| 99 | Serous papillary cystadeno-carcinoma | Epithélioma germinatif végétant | Серозная папиллярная кистаденокарцинома |
| | Seröses papilläres Cyst-adenocarcinom | Cistoadenocarcinoma papilífero seroso | Cystadenocarcinoma papil-liferum serosum |

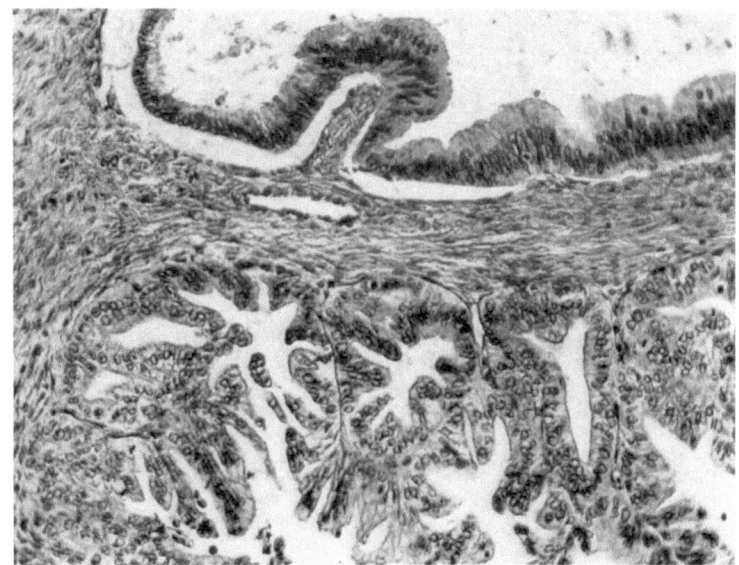

Fig. 98. × 160.   F 33/3 101—95

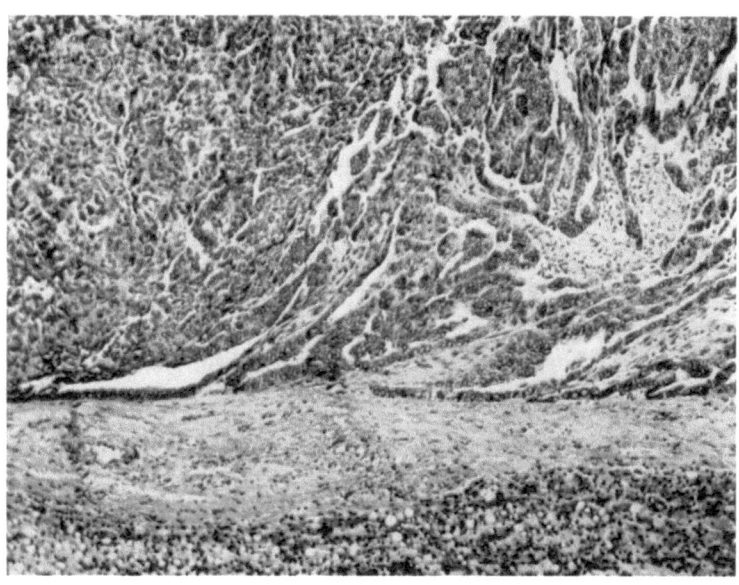

Fig. 99. × 75.   F 33/3 93—81

| 100 | Psammocarcinoma | Psammo-épithélioma papillaire | Псаммокарцинома |
| | Psammocarcinom | Psamocarcinoma | Psammocarcinoma |

| 101 | Mesonephroma | Mesonéphrome | Мезонефрома |
| | Mesonephrom | Mesonefroma | Mesonephroma |

This list does not include secondary tumors such as Krukenberg tumor.

La liste ne contient pas de tumeurs secondaires comme par exemple la tumeur de Krukenberg.

Этот перечень не содержит метастатических опухолей, как напр. опухоли Крукенберга.

Diese Aufzählung enthält keine sekundären Tumoren, wie z. B. den sog. Krukenberg-Tumor.

La lista no incluye tumores metastásicos como el tumor de Krukenberg.

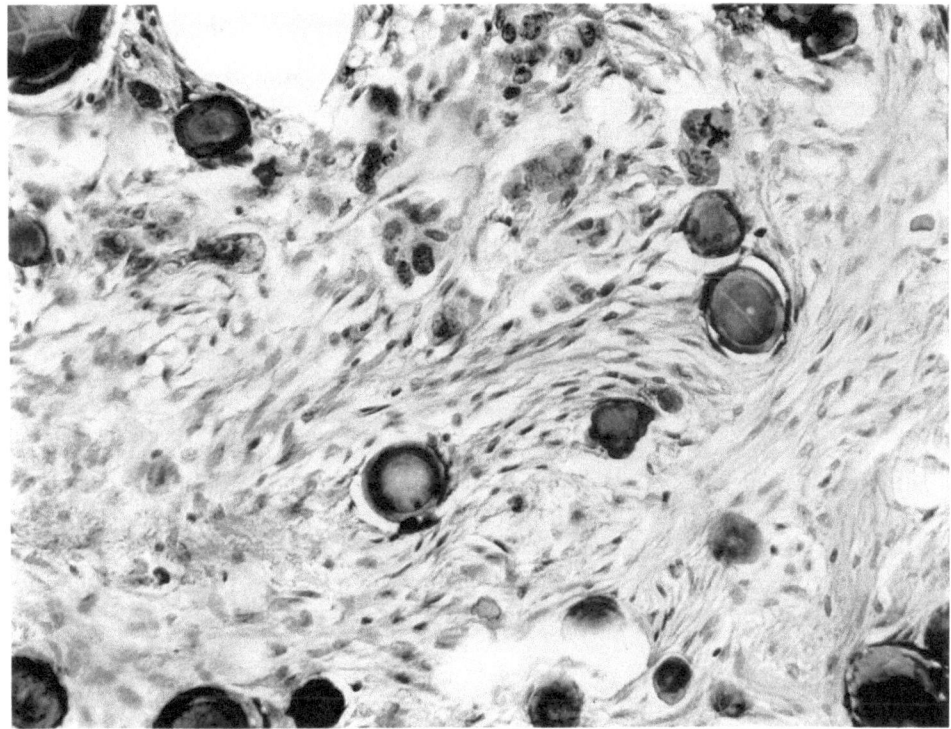

Fig. 100. × 300.

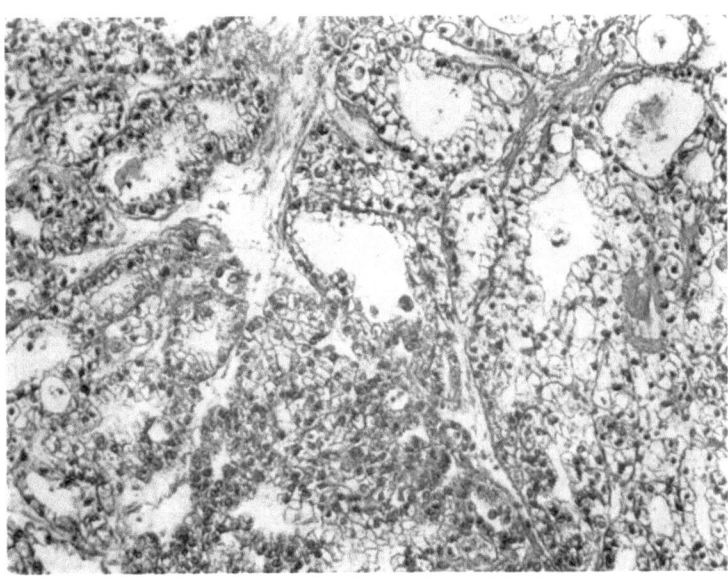

Fig. 101. × 125.   F 33/3 127—113

106

10. Prostate Prostate Предстательная железа

Vorsteherdrüse Próstata Prostata (185)

---

102 Differentiated adenocarcinoma

Epithélioma glandulaire
différencié

Дифференцированная
аденокарцинома

Differenziertes Adeno-
carcinom

Adenocarcinoma diferen-
ciado

Adenocarcinoma maturum

103 Anaplastic adenocarcinoma
Anaplastic small cell
carcinoma

Epithélioma glandulaire
anaplasique
Epithélioma anaplasique à
petites cellules

Анапластическая
аденокарцинома
Анапластическая
мелкоклеточная карци-
нома

Anaplastisches Adeno-
carcinom
Anaplastisches kleinzelliges
Carcinom

Adenocarcinoma ana-
plásico
Adenocarcinoma anaplásico
de células pequeñas

Adenocarcinoma ana-
plasticum
Carcinoma parvocellulare
anaplasticum

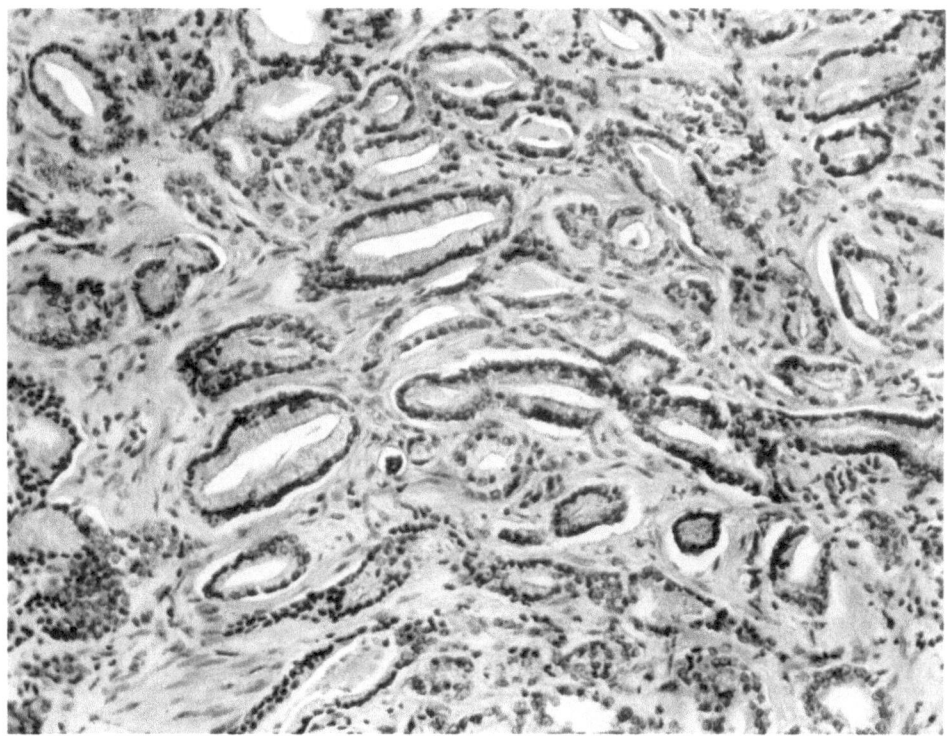

Fig. 102. × 185. F 32 23—8

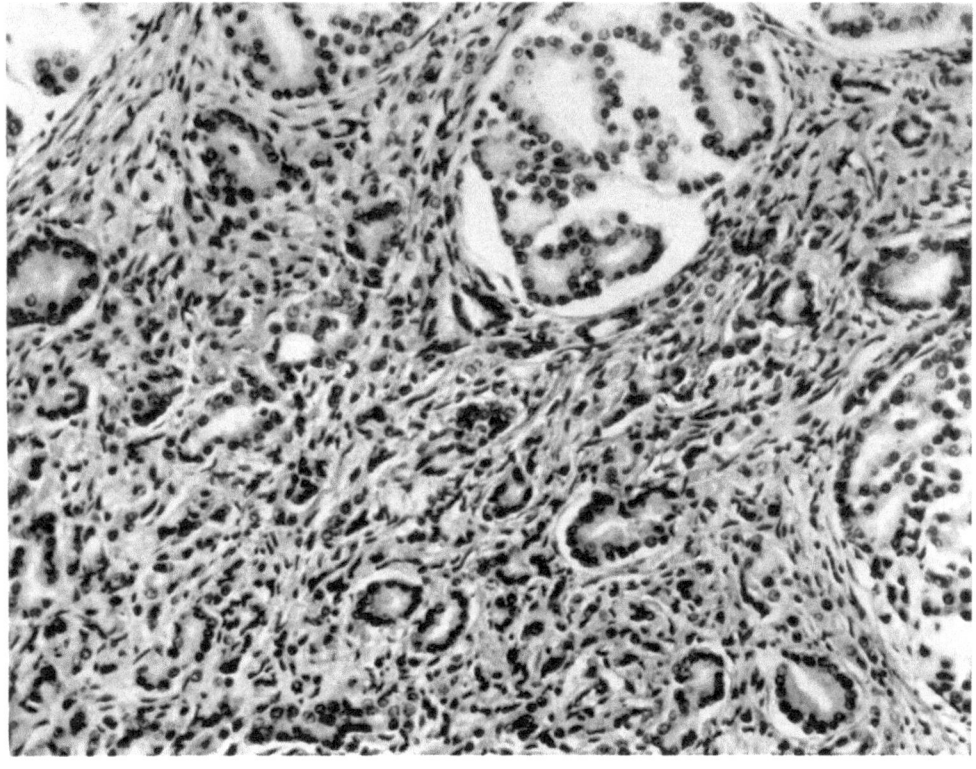

Fig. 103. × 185. F 32 25—10

104 Cribriform carcinoma   Epithélioma cribriforme   Крибрознаяя карцинома

Cribriformes Carcinom   Carcinoma cribiforme   Carcinoma cribriforme

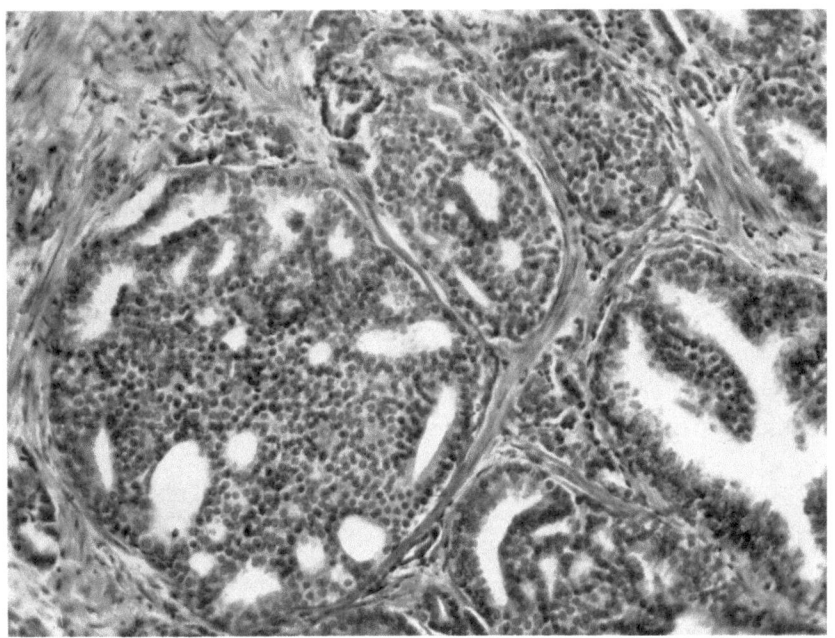

Fig. 104. × 158.   v. A. 311—363

110

11. Testis   Testicule   Яичко   (186)
    Hoden   Testículo   Testis

105	Tubular adenoma Sertoli cell tumor	Adénome tubuleux Tumeur à cellules de Sertoli	Тубулярная аденома Опухоль из клеток Сертоли
	Tubuläres Adenom Sertolizell-Tumor	Adenoma tubular Tumor de células de Sertoli	Adenoma tubulare Tumor Sertoli-cellularis

106	Interstitial cell tumor Leydig cell tumor	Tumeur à cellules inter- stitielles Tumeur à cellules de Leydig	Опухоль из интерстициальных клеток Опухоль из клеток Лейдига
	Tumor der interstitiellen Zellen Leydigzell-Tumor	Tumor de células inters- ticiales Tumor de células de Leydig	Tumor interstitio-cellularis Tumor Leydig-cellularis

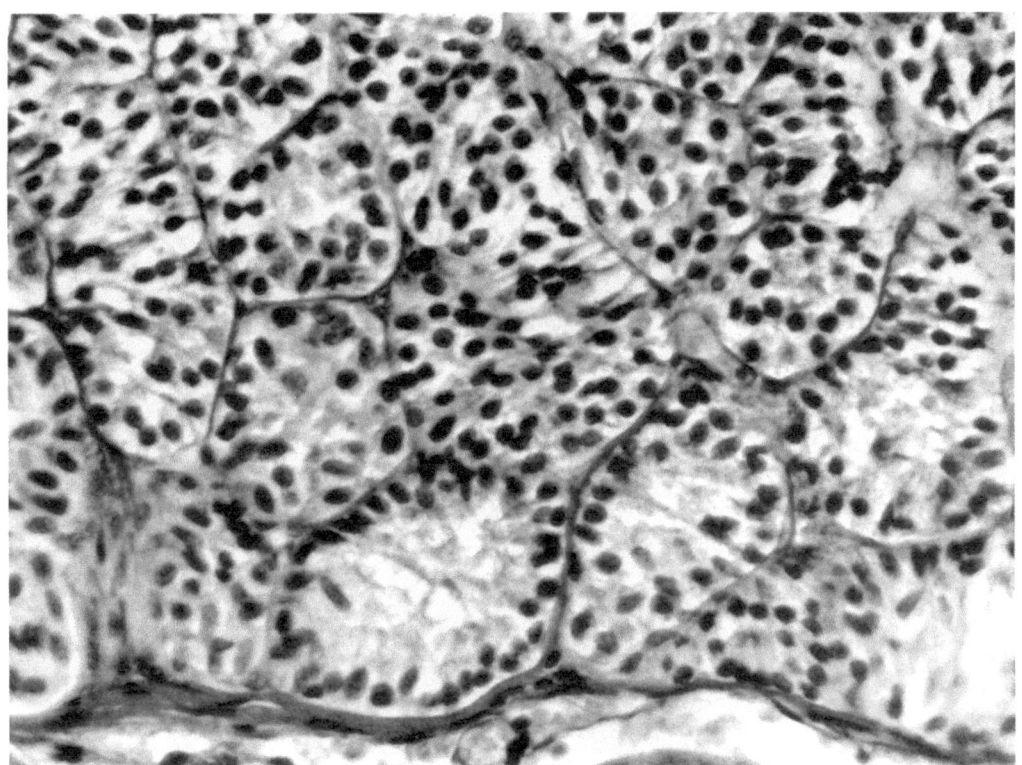

Fig. 105. × 400.   F 32 123—85

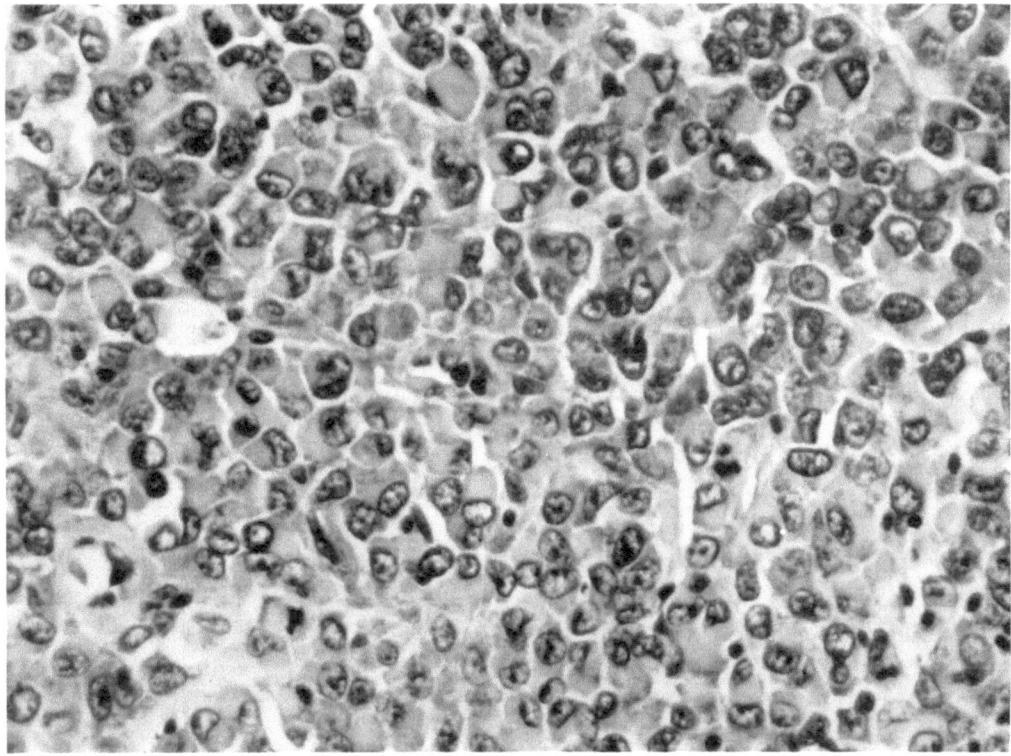

Fig. 106. × 400.   F 32 117—81

107   Adenomatoid tumor   Tumeur adenomatoide   Аденоматоидная опухоль

Adenomatoider Tumor   Tumor adenomatoide   Tumor adenomatoides

108   Seminoma   Séminome   Семинома

Seminom   Seminoma   Seminoma

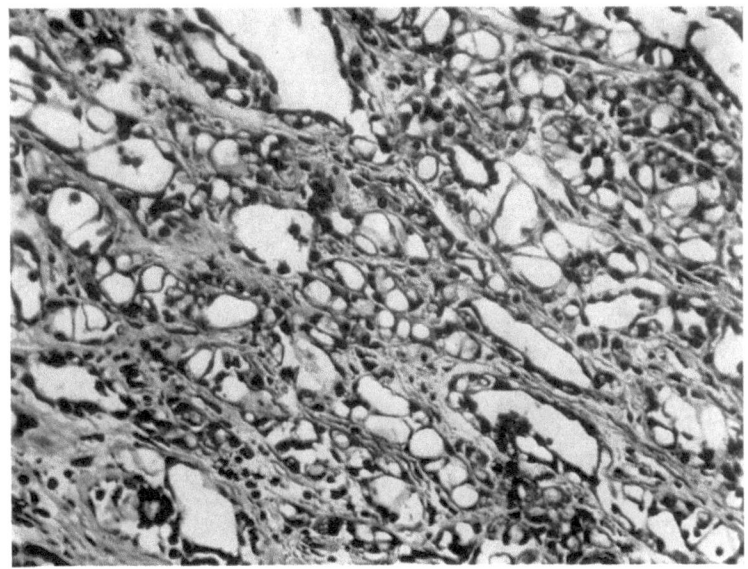

Fig. 107. × 165.   F 32 133—95

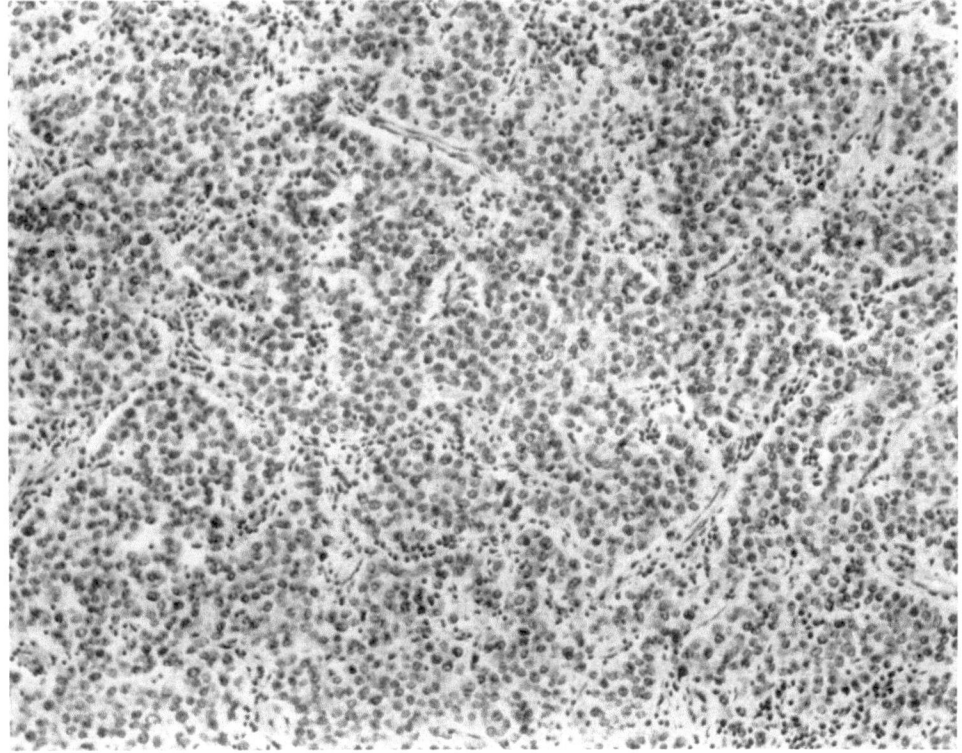

Fig. 108. × 155.   F 32 63—34

109 Spermatocytoma	Spermatocytome	Сперматоцитома
Spermatocytom	Espermatocitoma	Spermatocytoma

110 Teratoma	Tératome	Тератома
Teratom	Teratoma	Teratoma

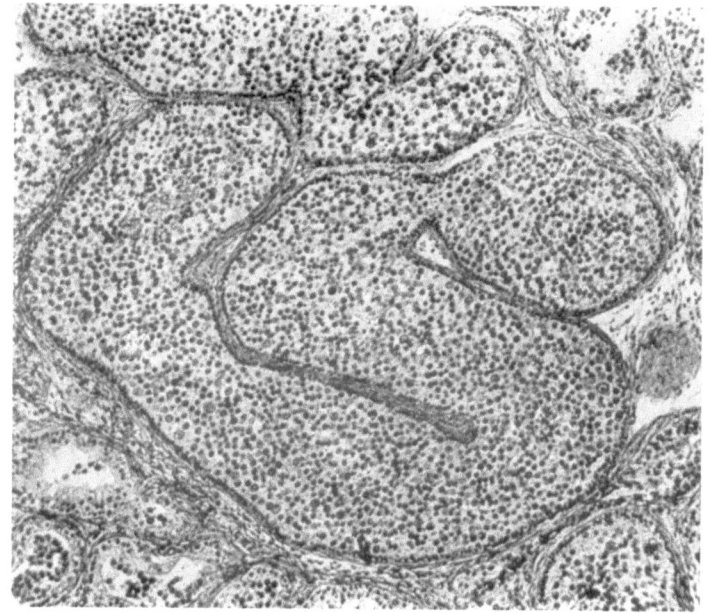

Fig. 109.   M 671—609

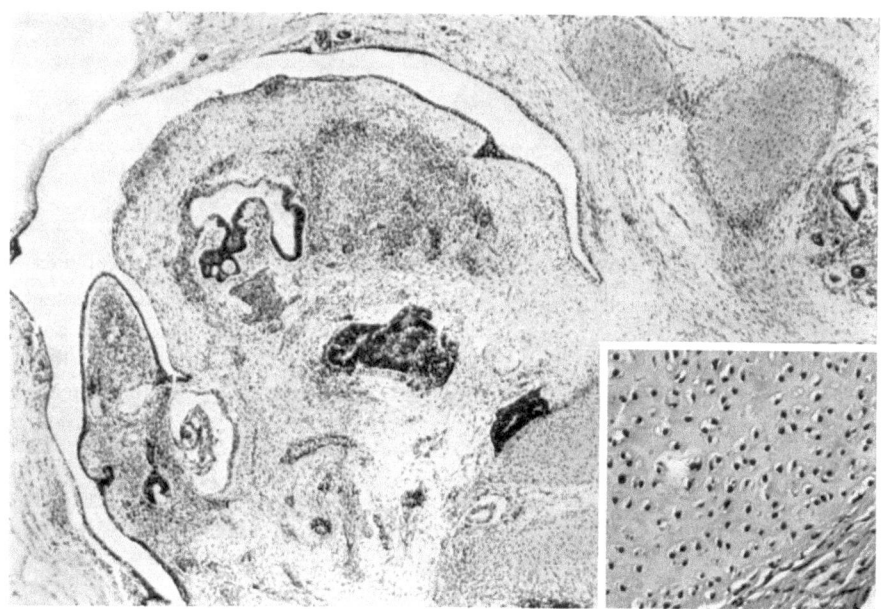

Fig. 110. × 38, × 150.

116

111 Embryonal carcinoma   Epithéolima embryonnaire   Эмбриональная карцинома
Malignant teratoblastoma   Tératoblastome malin   Злокачественная
Malignant mixed tumor   Tumeur maligne à structure   тератобластома
Malignant teratoma   complexe   Злокачественная
    Tératome malin   смешанная опухоль
    Злокачественная тератома

Embryonales Carcinom   Carcinoma embrionario   Carcinoma embryonale
Bösartiges Teratoblastom   Teratoblastoma maligno   Teratoblastoma malignum
Bösartiger Mischtumor   Tumor mixto maligno   Tumor mixtus malignus
Bösartiges Teratom   Teratoma maligno   Teratoma malignum

112 Choriocarcinoma   Choriocarcinome   Хориокарцинома
Chorioepithelioma   Chorio-épithéliome   Хориоэпителиома

Choriocarcinom   Coriocarcinoma   Choriocarcinoma
Chorionepitheliom   Corioepitelioma   Chorioepithelioma

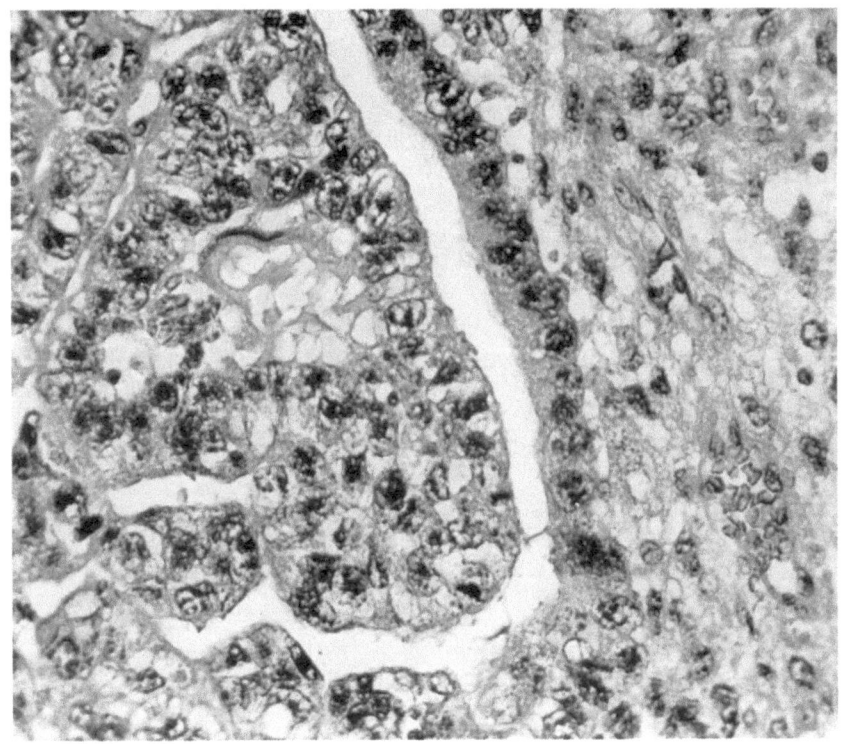

Fig. 111. × 280. F 32 83—52

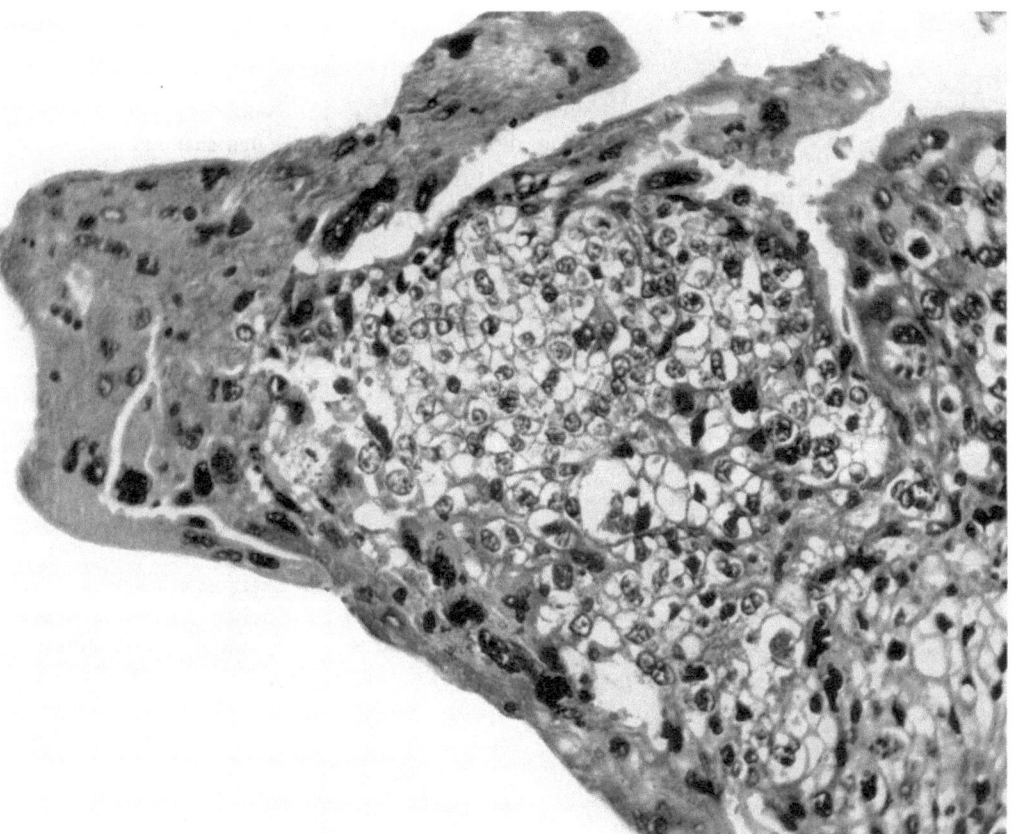

Fig. 112. × 235. F 32 103—70

12. **Kidney**   **Rein**   **Почка**   (189)

  Niere   **Riñón**   **Renes**

113   Tubular adenoma   Adénome tubuleux   Тубулярная аденома

  Tubuläres Adenom   Adenoma tubular   Adenoma tubulare

114   Basophilic papillary
adenoma   Adénome papillaire
basophile   Базофильная папилларная аденома

  Basophiles papilläres
Adenom   Adenoma papilífero
basófilo   Adenoma papilliferum
basophile

115   Acidophilic papillary
adenoma   Adénome papillaire
acidophile   Ацидофильная папилларная аденома

  Acidophiles papilläres
Adenom   Adenoma papilífero
acidófilo   Adenoma papilliferum
acidophile

116   Clear cell adenoma   Adénome à cellules claires   Светлоклеточная аденома

  Klarzell-Adenom (Adenom
von wasserklaren Zellen)   Adenoma de células claras   Adenoma clarocellulare

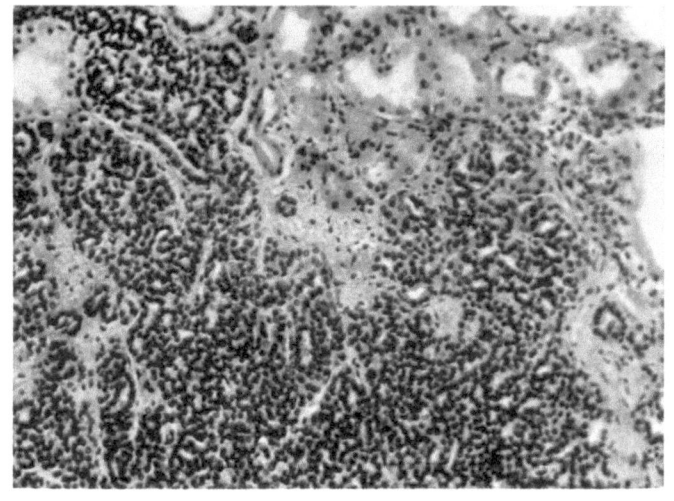

Fig. 113. × 125.   F 30 33—11

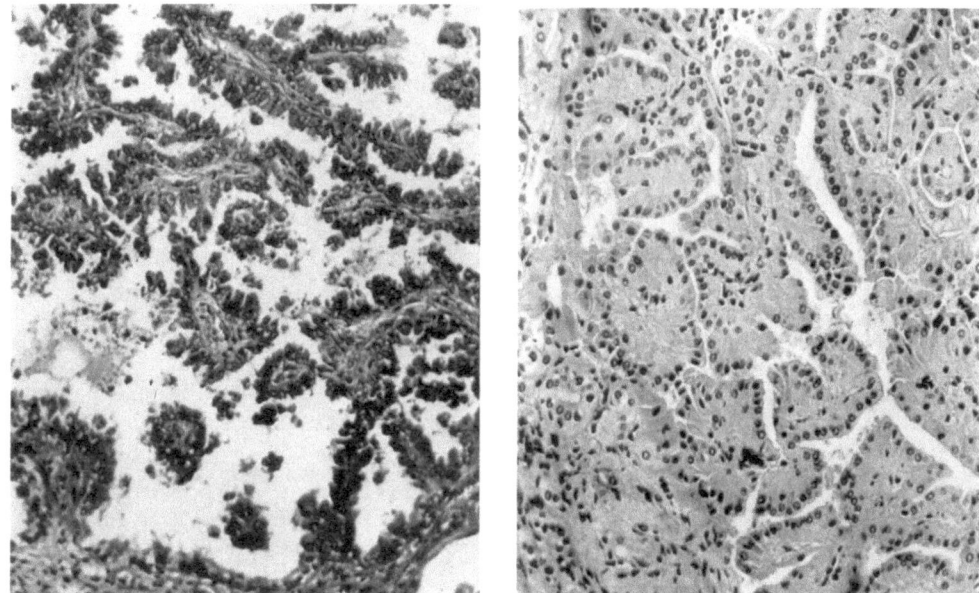

Fig. 114. × 125.   F 30 33—9   Fig. 115. × 145.   F 30 39—17

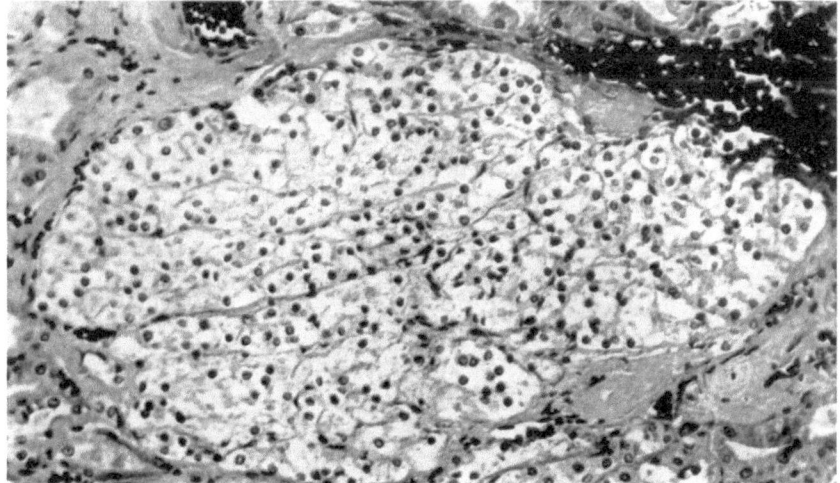

Fig. 116. × 185.   F 30 39—18

117   Papillary adenocarcinoma   Epithélioma glandulaire   Папилларная аденокарци-
                                        papillaire   нома

      Papilläres Adenocarcinom   Adenocarcinoma papilífero   Adenocarcinoma papillife-
                                                                    rum

118   Tubular adenocarcinoma   Epithélioma glandulaire   Тубулярная аденокарци-
                                        tubuleux   нома

      Tubuläres Adenocarcinom   Adenocarcinoma tubular   Adenocarcinoma tubulare

119   Clear cell carcinoma   Epithélioma à cellules claires   Светлоклеточный рак
      Hypernephroma   Hypernéphrome   Гипернефроидный рак

      Hellzelliges Carcinom   Carcinoma de células claras   Carcinoma clarocellulare
      Hypernephrom   Hipernefroma   Hypernephroma

121

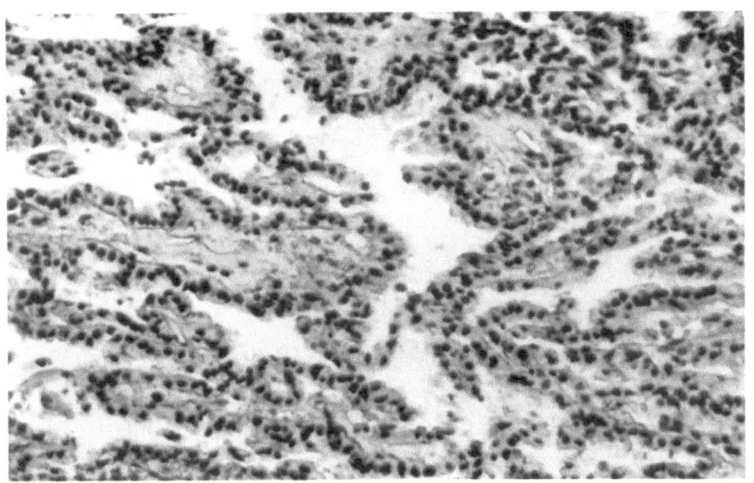

Fig. 117. × 175.   F 30 67—51

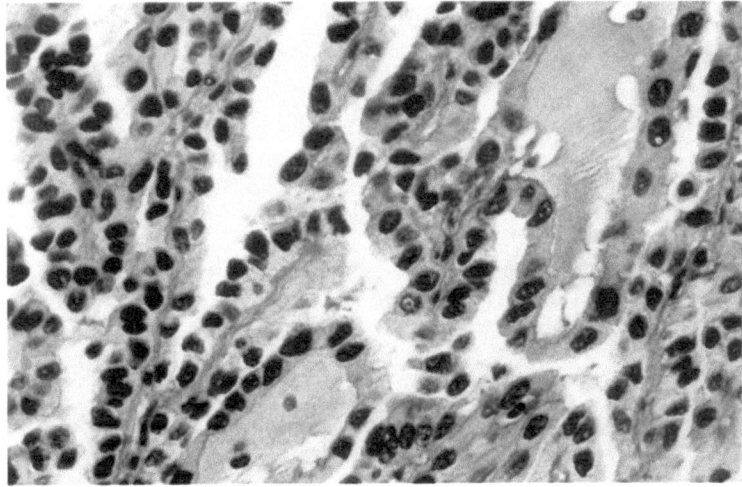

Fig. 118. × 360.   F 30 67—50

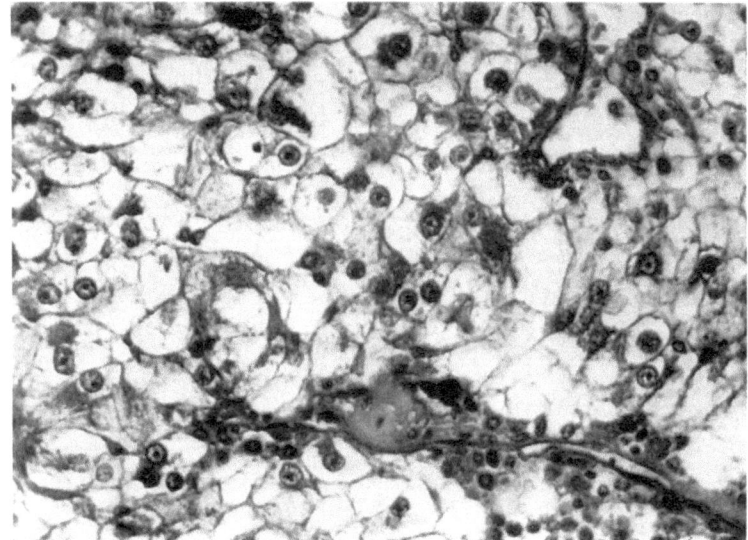

Fig. 119. × 310.   F 30 61—39

| 120 | Granular cell carcinoma | Epithélioma à cellules granuleuses | Гранулярноклеточный рах |
| | Gekörntzelliges Carcinom | Carcinoma de células granulosas | Carcinoma granulocellulare |

121	Embryonic nephroma (Wilms)	Tumeur de blastème rénal (Wilms)	Эмбриональная нефрома (Вильмс)
	Adenosarcoma	Adénosarcome	Аденосаркома
	Nephroblastoma	Néphroblastome	Нефробластома
	Wilms tumor	Tumeur de Wilms	Опухоль Вильмса

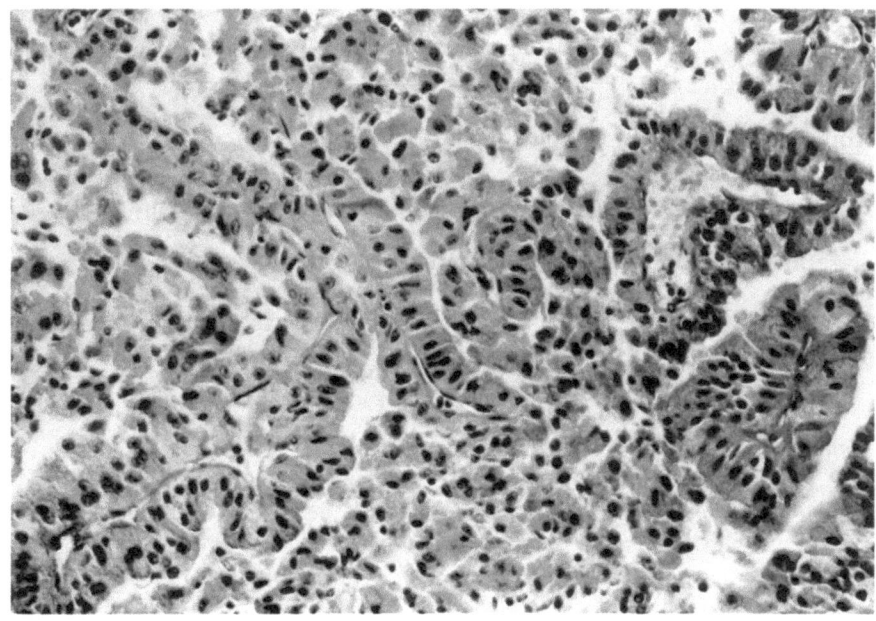

Fig. 120. × 190.

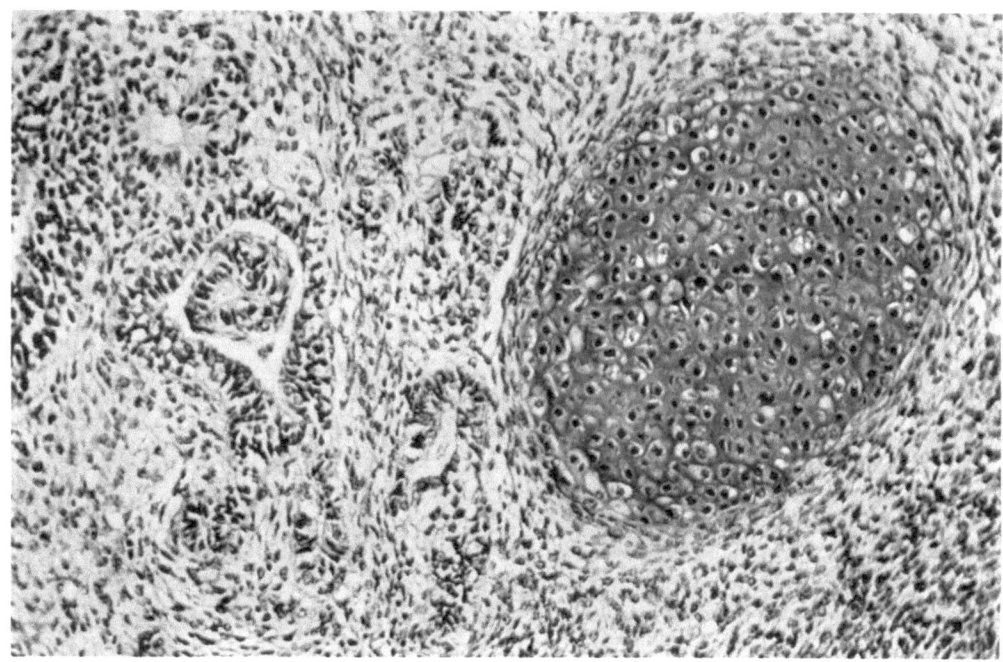

Fig. 121. × 205.

F 30 105—90

13. **Urinary duct system** **Voies urinaires extra-** **Мочевые пути**
Renal pelvis, Ureter, **rénales** Почечная лоханка,
Urinary bladder, Bassinet, uretère, vessie, мочеточник, мочевой
пузырь,

Harnwege **Vías urinarias** **Viae urinariae**
Nierenbecken, Harnleiter, **extrarrenales** Pelvis renalis, ureter
Harnblase, Pelvis renal, uréter, vesica urinaria, (188, 189)
vejiga,

---

122 Papilloma Papillome Папиллома

Papillom Papiloma Papilloma

123 Transitional cell carcinoma Epithélioma de type para- Переходноклеточный рак
malpighien

Übergangszell-Carcinom Carcinoma de células de Carcinoma transitio-
transición cellulare

Other common types of tumors see I/1;
Adenocarcinoma
Epidermoid carcinoma
Mucous carcinoma (possibly arising from urachus).

Pour les autres formes courantes des tumeurs voir I/1;
Epithélioma glandulaire
Epithélioma épidermoïde
Epithélioma muqueux (développé peut-être aux dépens de l'ouraque).

Другие, встречающиеся здесь типы опухолей (см. I/1)
Аденокарцинома
Плоскоклеточный рак
Слизеобразующий рак (возможно происходящий из урахуса).

Andere hier vorkommende Tumortypen (s. I/1) wie
Adenocarcinom
Epidermoidcarcinom
Schleimbildendes Carcinom (möglicherweise vom Urachus ausgehend).

Para otros tipos corrientes de tumores, véase I/1
Adenocarcinoma
Carcinoma epidermoide
Carcinoma mucoso (probablemente originado en el uraco).

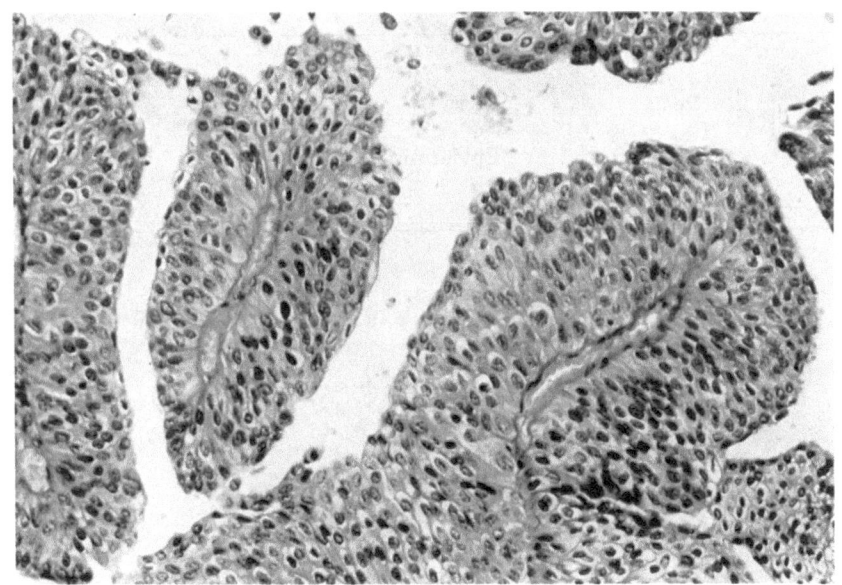

Fig. 122. × 150.

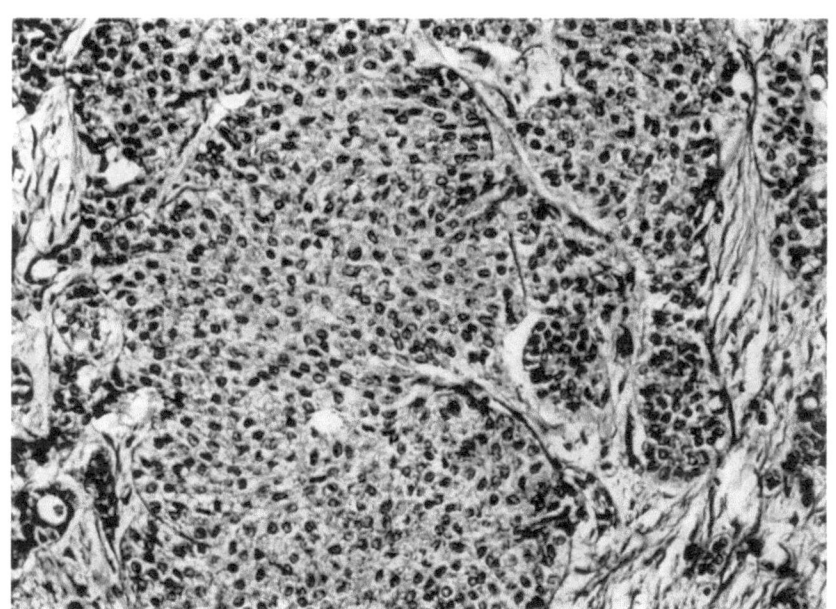

Fig. 123. × 190.

14. Skin   Peau   Кожа

Haut   Piel   Epidermis   (173)

124 Calcifying epithelioma
    (Malherbe)
    Pilomatrixoma

Verkalkendes Epitheliom
    (Malherbe)

Epithélioma calcifié
    (Malherbe)

Epitelioma calcificante
    (Malherbe)

Обизвествлевающая
    эпителиома (Мальэрб)

Epithelioma calcificans
    (Malherbe)

125 Syringoma

Syringom

Syringome

Siringoma

Сирингома

Syringoma

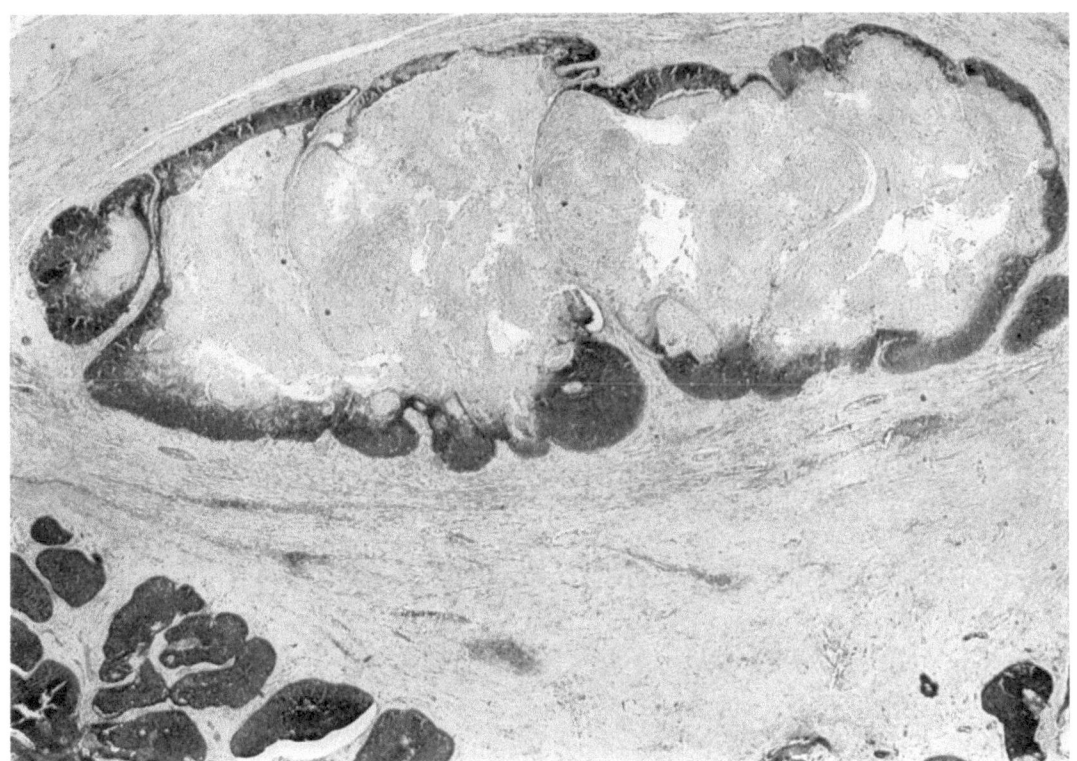

Fig. 124.   F 2 149—104

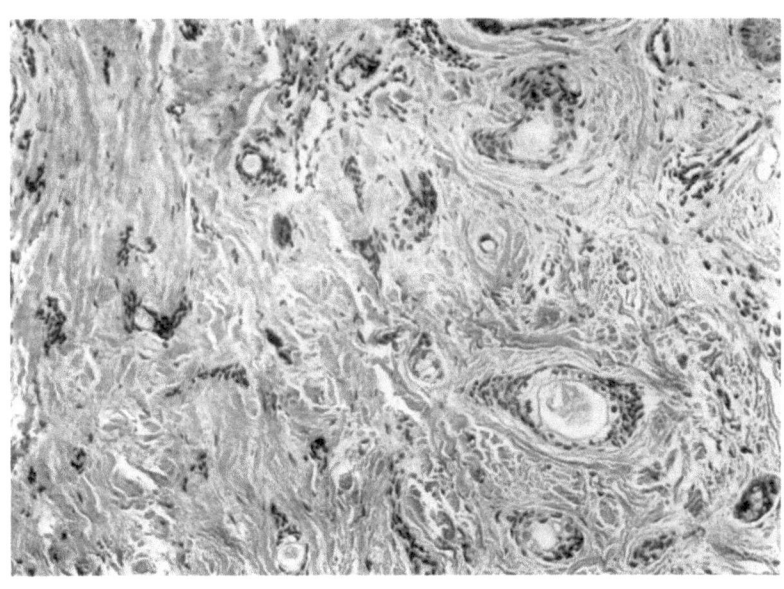

Fig. 125.   × 126.   F 2 89—51

126 Papillary syringadenoma   Syringo-cystadénome   Папиллярная
                        papillifère   сирингоаденома

Papilläres Syringadenom   Siringoadenoma papilífero   Syringadenoma papilli-
                                                             ferum

127 Papillary hidradenoma   Hydradénome papillaire   Папиллярная аденома
                                                             потовых желез

Papilläres Schweißdrüsen-   Hidroadenoma papilífero   Hidradenoma papilliferum
    adenom

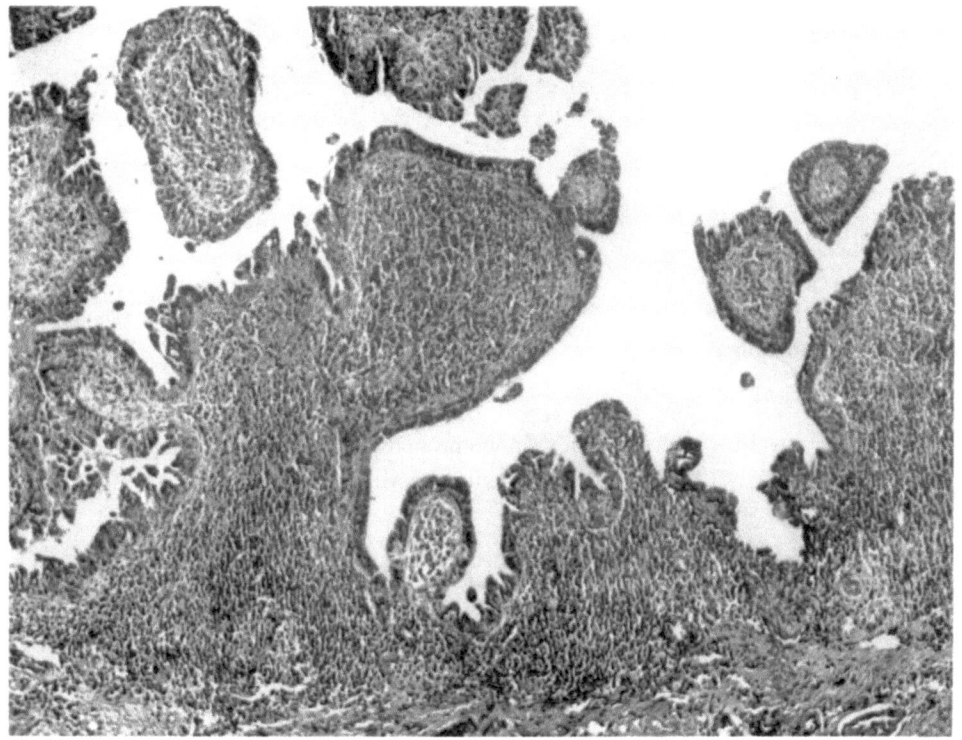

Fig. 126. ×79. F 2 91—53

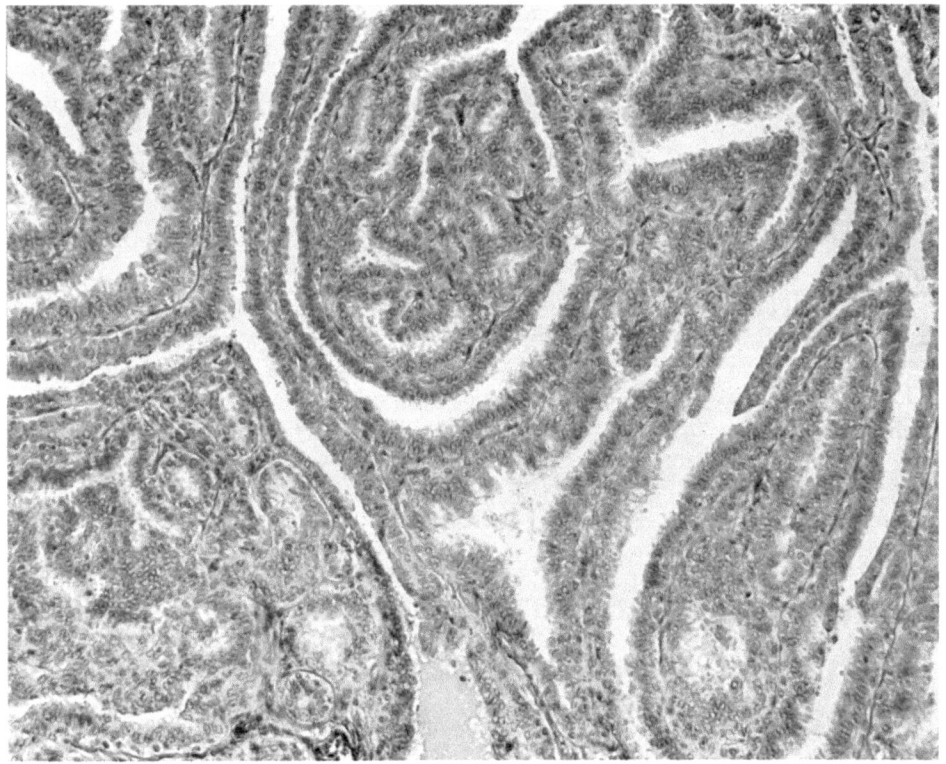

Fig. 127. ×150. K 60—2.23

128 Nodular hidradenoma   Hydradénome nodulaire   Узловатая аденома потовых
     Eccrine spiradenoma   желез
                                                       Эккринная спираденома

     Noduläres Schweiß-   Hidroadenoma nodular   Hidradenoma nodulare
       drüsenadenom   Espiroadenoma ecrino

129 Clear cell hidradenoma   Hydradénome à cellules   Светлоклеточная аденома
                             claires   потовых желез

     Klarzelliges Schweiß-   Hidroadenoma de células   Hidradenoma clarocellu-
       drüsenadenom   claras   lare

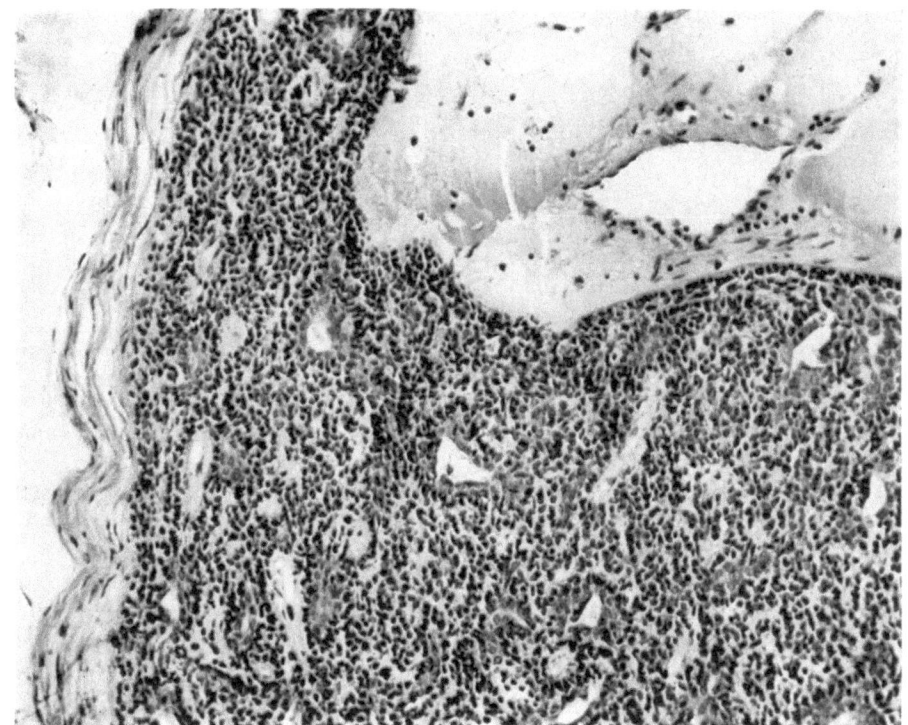

Fig. 128. × 205.   F 2 107—70

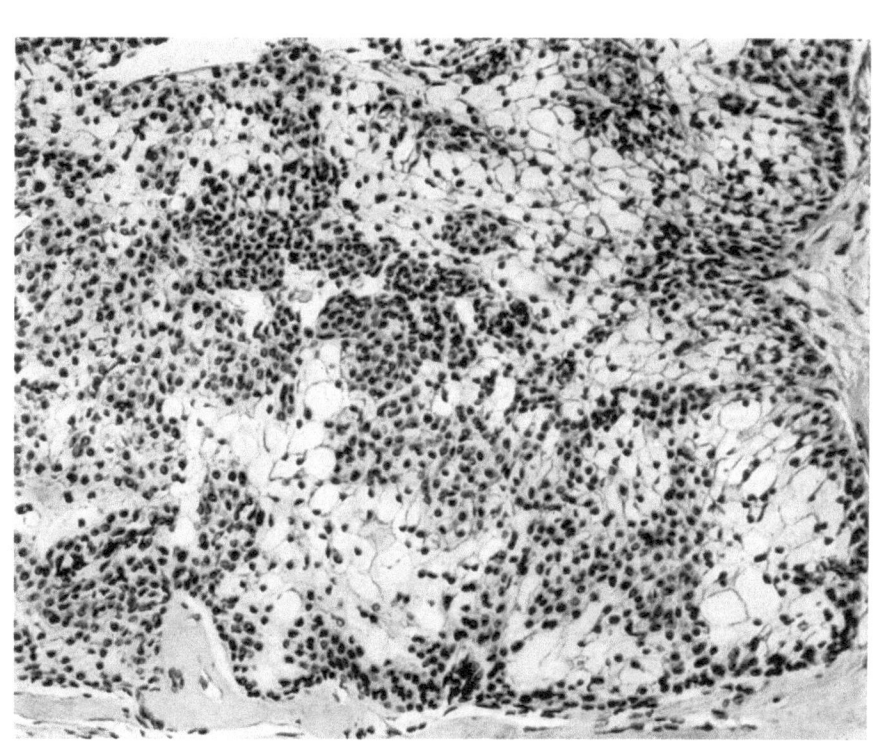

Fig. 129. × 165.   F 2 111—75

9*

130 Mixed tumor of skin (salivary gland type)
Chondroid syringoma

Mischtumor der Haut vom Speicheldrüsentyp
Chondroides Syringom

Tumeur mixte de la peau (de type salivaire)
Syringome chondroïde

Tumor mixto de la piel (tipo glándula salivar)
Siringoma condroide

Смешанная опухоль кожи (типа слюнной железы)
Хондроидная сирингома

Tumor mixtus sialoides
Syringoma chondroides

131 Cylindroma (dermal) including Turban tumor

Cylindrom — einschließlich des besonders lokalisierten Turbantumors (Spiegler)

Cylindrome — comprenant, la tumeur en turban

Cilindroma (dérmico), inclusive Tumor en turbante

Цилиндрома — включая Тюрбанную опухоль Шпиглера

Cylindroma (cutaneum)
Tumor Turbani

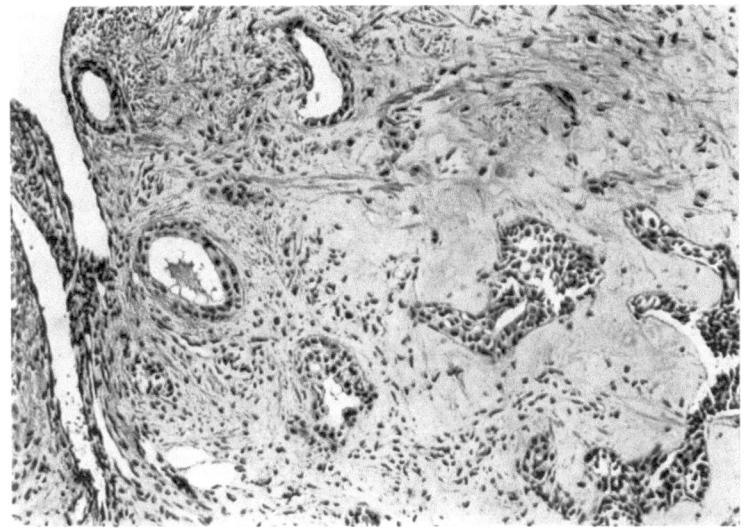

Fig. 130.   × 117.   F 2 109—73

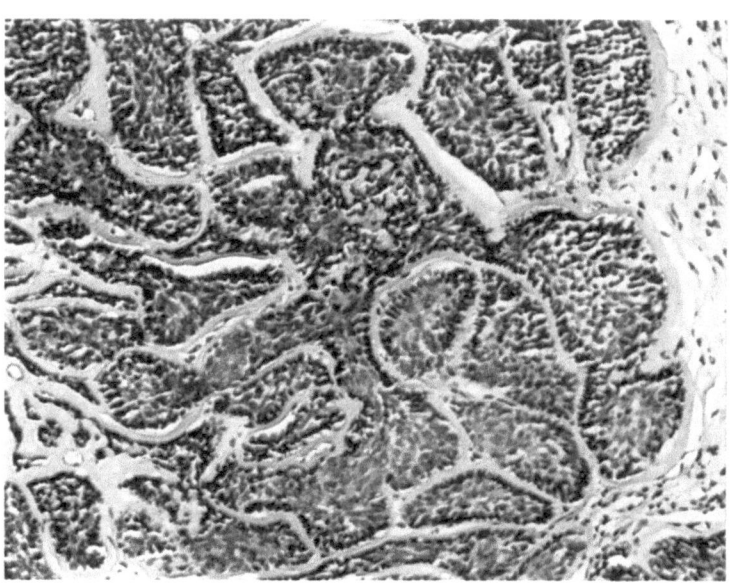

Fig. 131.   × 142.   F 2 93—57

134

132 Sebaceous adenoma   Adénome sébacé   Аденома из сальных желез

Talgdrüsenadenom   Adenoma sebáceo   Adenoma sebaceum

133 Trichoepithelioma   Tricho-épithélioma   Трихоэпителиома
      Benign adenoid cystic epi-   Epithélioma adénoïde   Доброкачественная
      thelioma (Brooke)   cystique bénin (Brooke)   аденокистозная
              эпителиома (Брук)

Trichoepitheliom   Tricoepitelioma   Trichoepithelioma
Gutartiges adenoid-cysti-   Epitelioma adenoide quís-   Epithelioma adenoides
   sches Epitheliom   tico benigno (Brooke)   cysticum benignum
   (Brooke)   (Brooke)

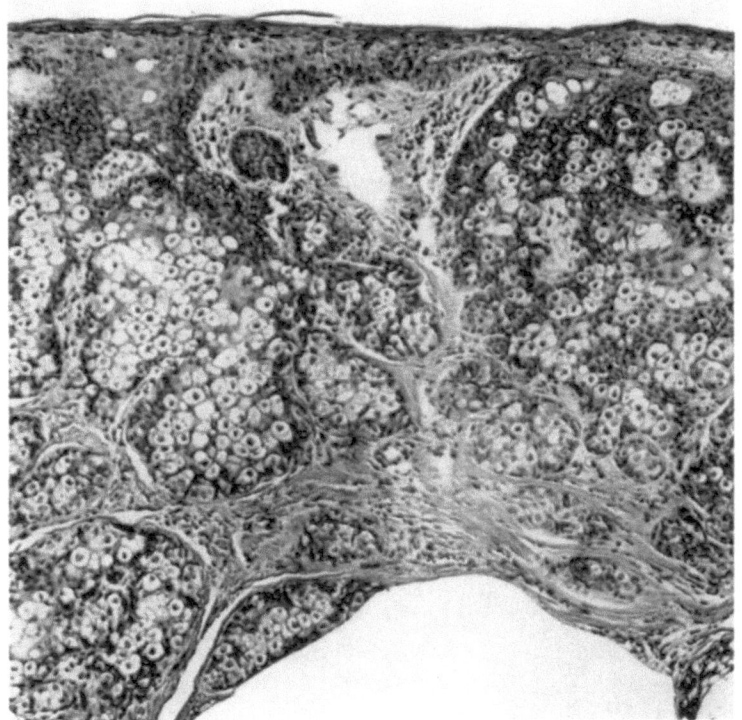

Fig. 132. × 102.   F 2 129—90

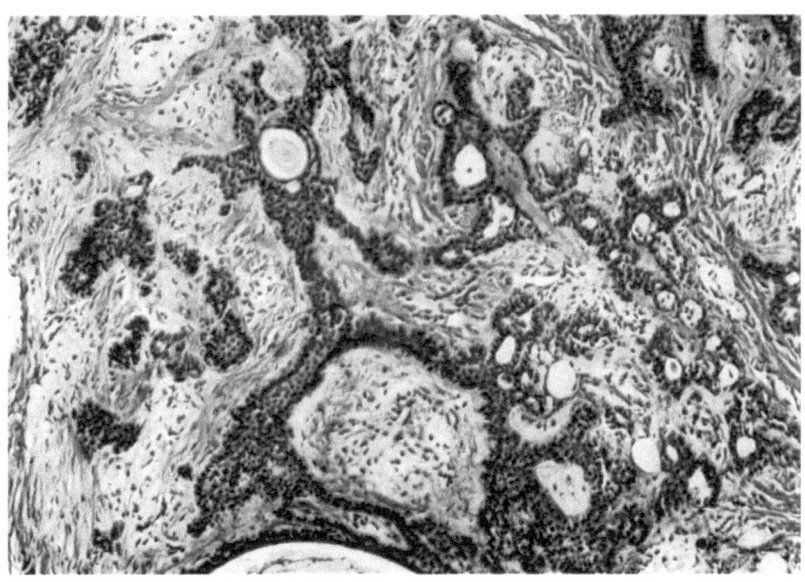

Fig. 133. × 79.   F 2 85—49

134 Squamous cell papilloma | Papillome kératinisant | Плоскоклеточная папиллома

Hyperkeratotisches Papillom | Papiloma escamoso o espinocelular | Papilloma spinocellulare

135 Fibroepithelial papilloma | Papillome fibro-épithélial | Фиброэпителиальная папиллома

Fibroepitheliales Papillom | Papiloma fibroepitelial | Papilloma fibroepitheliale

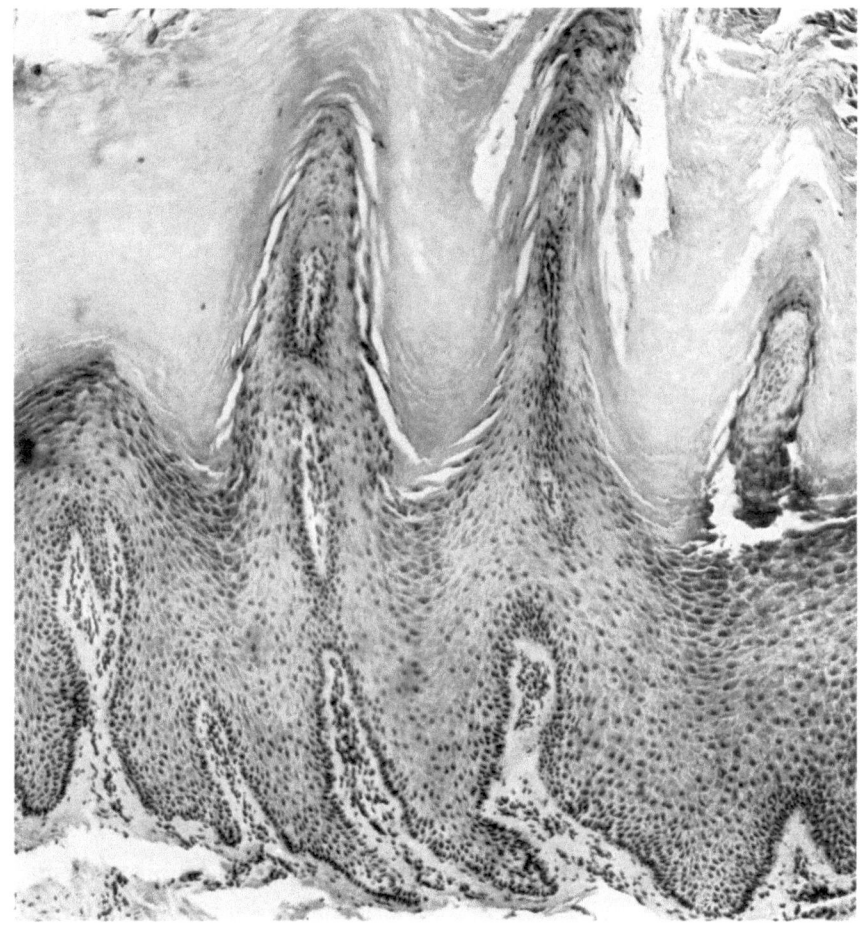

Fig. 134. × 100.   F 2 31—3

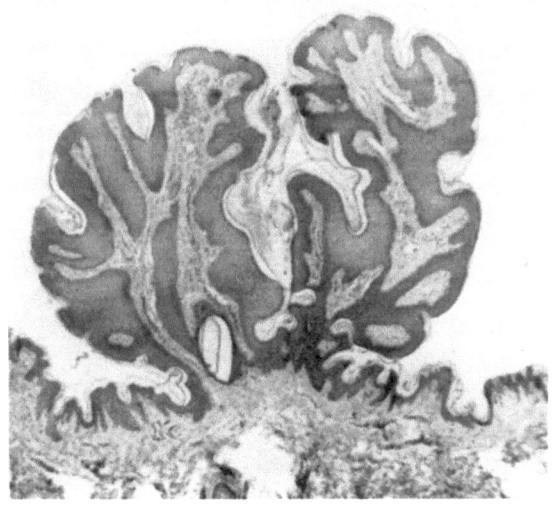

Fig. 135. × 15.   F 2 61—29

136 Keratoacanthoma   Kérato-acanthome   Кератоакантома
     Molluscum sebaceum   Molluscum sébacé   Сальный моллюск

     Keratoakanthom   Queratoacantoma   Keratoacanthoma
     Molluscum sebaceum   Molusco sebáceo   Molluscum sebaceum

137 Basal cell papilloma   Papillome basocellulaire   Базальноклеточная
     Seborrheic keratosis   Kératose séborrhéique   папиллома
                                                      Себорройный кератоз

     Seborrhoische Keratose   Papiloma basocelular   Papilloma basocellulare
                                            Queratosis seborreica   Keratosis seborrhoica

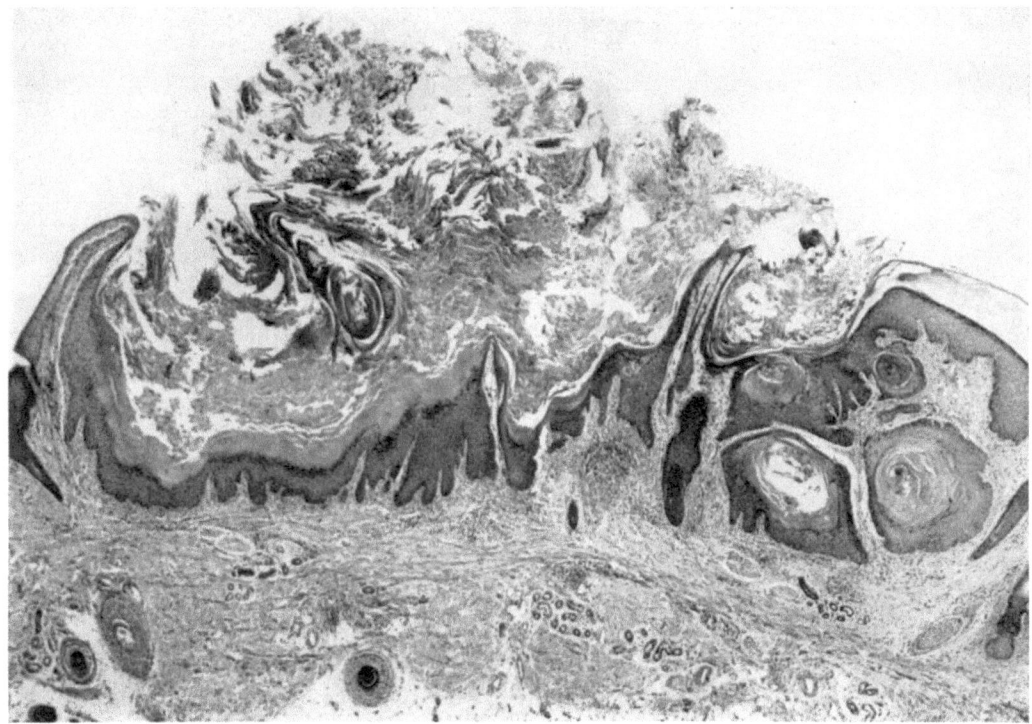

Fig. 136.   F 2 73—40

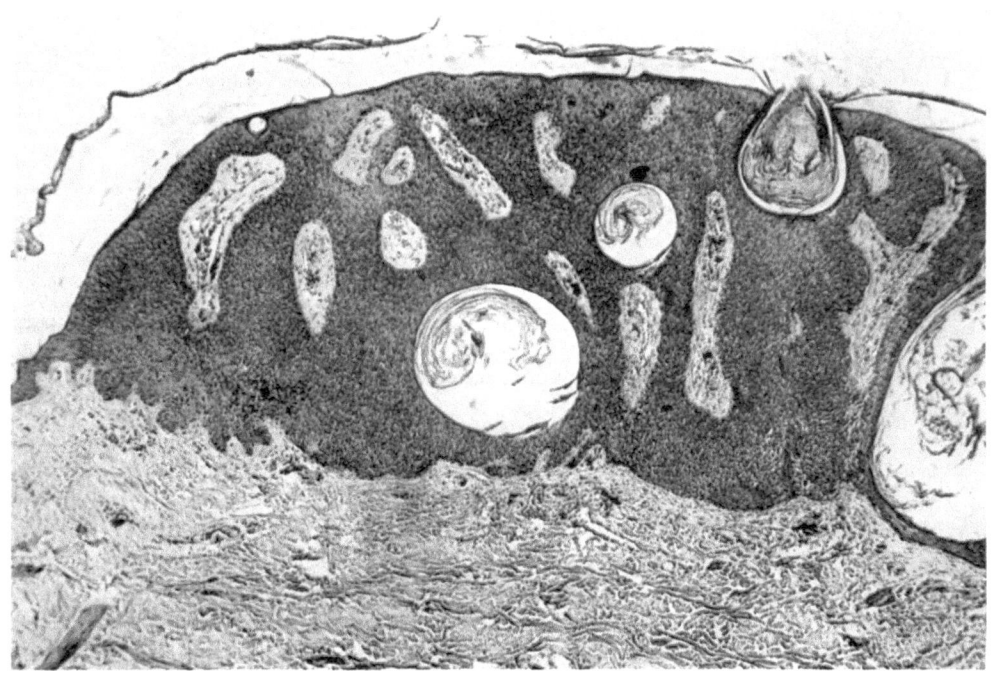

Fig. 137. ×48.   F 2 47—15

138 Intraepidermal (basal cell) epithelioma (Jadassohn)

Epithélioma basocellulaire intra-dermique (Jadassohn)

Интраэпидермальная (базальноклеточная) эпителиома (Ядассон)

Intradermales Basaliom (Jadassohn)

Epitelioma (basocelular) intraepidérmico (Jadassohn)

Epithelioma intradermale basocellulare (Jadassohn)

139 Basal cell carcinoma

Epithélioma basocellulaire

Базальноклеточный рак

Basalzellcarcinom
Basaliom

Carcinoma basocelular

Carcinoma basocellulare

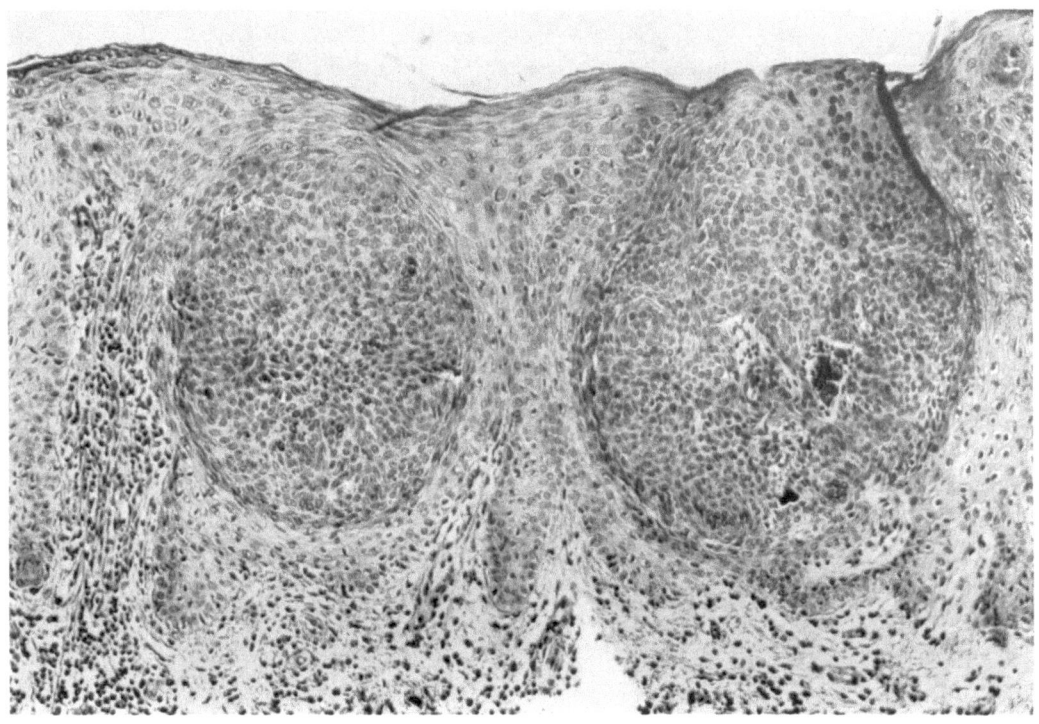

Fig. 138. × 117.   F 2 53—23

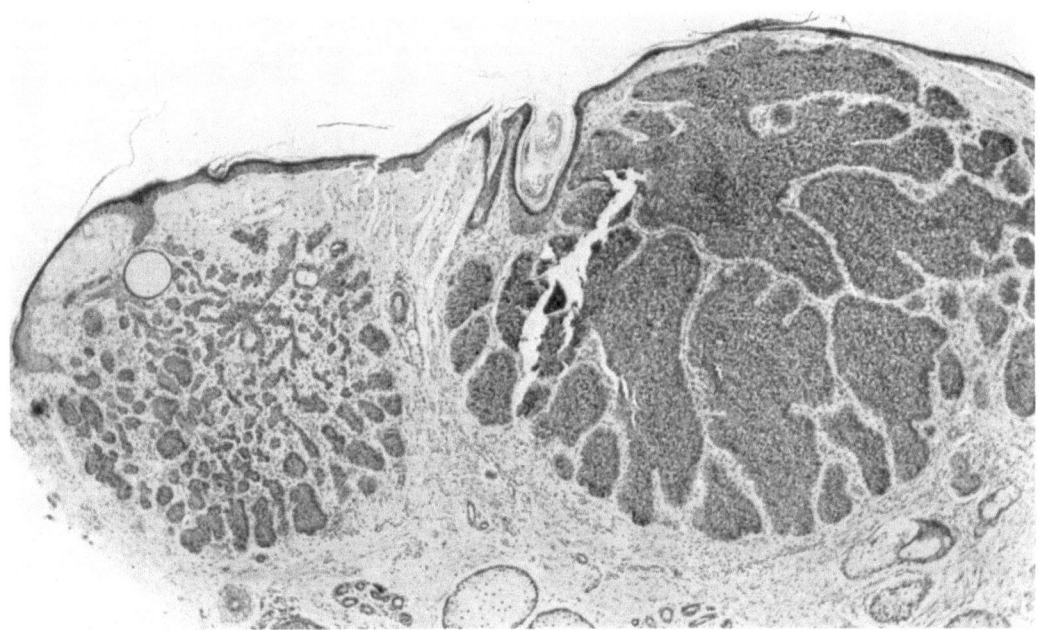

Fig. 139. × 109.   F 2 211—149

140 Basoquamous cell carcinoma with foci of keratinisation

    Spino-basocelluläres Carcinom mit herdförmiger Verhornung

Epithélioma spino-basocellulaire avec kératinisation focale

    Carcinoma espino-basocelular con focos de queratinisación

Базо-спиноцеллюлярный рак с очагами кератинизаций

    Carcinoma baso- et spinocellulare mixtum

141 Sweat gland carcinoma
Syringocarcinoma
Hidradenocarcinoma

    Schweißdrüsencarcinom
Syringocarcinom
Hydradenocarcinom

Epithélioma sudoripare
Syringoépithélioma
Hidradénocarcinome

    Carcinoma de glándulas sudoríparas
Siringocarcinoma
Hidradenocarcinoma

Рак потовых желез
Сирингокарцинома
Гидраденокарцинома

    Carcinoma hidroglandulare
Syringocarcinoma
Hidradenocarcinoma

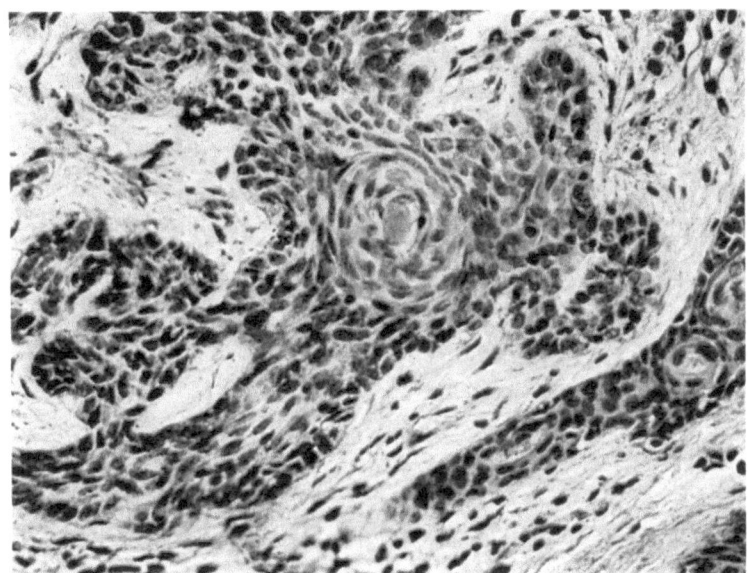

Fig. 140.   F 2 239—181

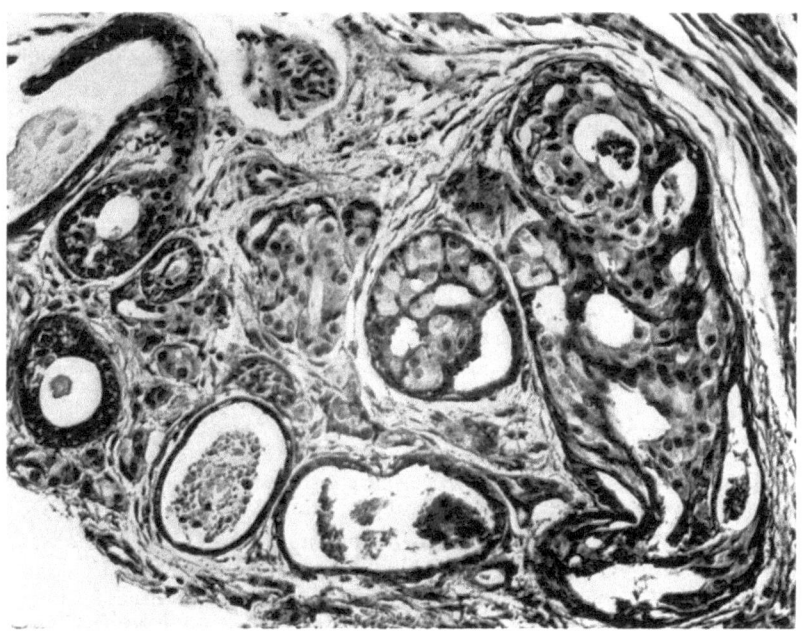

Fig. 141.   F 2 119—84

142 Sebaceous gland carcinoma   Epithélioma sébacé   Рак сальных желез

Talgdrüsencarcinom   Carcinoma de glándulas sebáceas   Carcinoma sebaceum

143 Intraepidermal carcinoma*   Epithélioma intra-épidermique*   Интраэпидермальный рак (Пэджет)*

Paget disease of breast   Maladie de Paget du sein   Болезнь Пэджета молочной железы

Intradermales Carcinom (Paget)*   Carcinoma intraepi-dérmico*   Carcino ma intradermale

Extramammärer Morbus Paget   Enfermedad de Paget extramamaria

---

* Similar lesions (extramammary Paget's disease) may occur outside the breast particularly in the ano-genital area but having different histochemical and clinical behaviour.

* Des lésions similaires (Maladie de Paget extra-mammaire) peuvent exister dans la sphère ano-génitale, mais elles ont un comportement histo-chimique et clinique différent.

* Такие же изменения (экстрамаммарная болезнь Пэджета) могут встретиться в коже других частей тела, в особенности в ано-генитальной области, имея однако другие гистохимические и клинические особенности.

* Ähnliche Veränderungen können auch außerhalb der Mamma (extramammäre Pagetsche Erkrankung), besonders in der Anogenitalregion vorkommen, doch zeigen sie hier ein anderes histochemisches und klinisches Verhalten.

* Lesiones similares (Enfermedad de Paget extramamaria) pueden ocurrir fuera de la mama, particularmente en el área ano-genital, pero teniendo diferente comportamiento clínico e histoquímico.

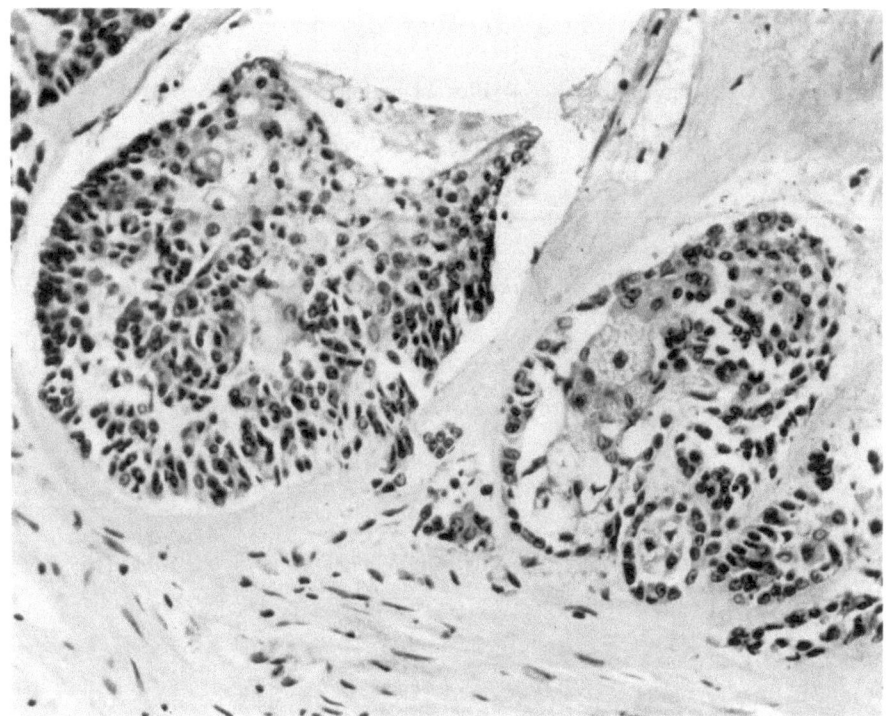

Fig. 142.   × 228.   F 2 131—94

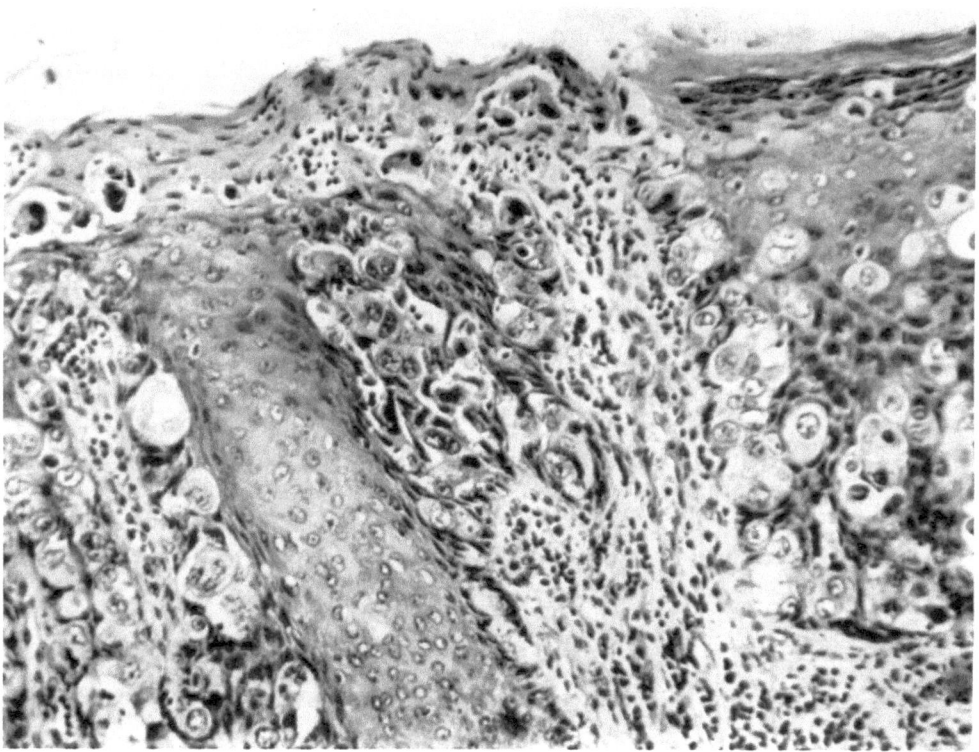

Fig. 143.   F 34 17—1

15. Thyroid   Thyroïde   Щитовидная железа

Schilddrüse   **Tiroides**   Glandula thyreoidea   (193)

Adenoma — *may be further classified on the basis of predominant histological pattern into* (145—149):

Adénome — *selon le type histologique prédominant ils peuvent être classés en* (145—149):

Аденома — *подразделяется на основании преобладающих гистологических особенностей на* (145—149):

Adenom — *weiterhin auf Grund der vorwiegenden histologischen Eigenschaft zu unterscheiden in* (145—149):

Adenoma — *según el cuadro histológico predominante, puede clasificarse como* (145—149):

144	Trabecular adenoma	Adénome trabéculaire	Трабекулярная Аденома
	Embryonal adenoma	Adénome embryonnaire	Эмбриональная Аденома
	Trabeculäres Adenom	Adenoma trabecular	Adenoma trabeculare
	Embryonales Adenom	Adenoma embrionario	Adenoma embryonale

145	Microfollicular adenoma	Adénome microfolliculaire	Микрофолликулярная Аденома
	Fetal adenoma	Adénome foetal	Фетальная Аденома
	Mikrofollikuläres Adenom	Adenoma microfolicular	Adenoma microfolliculare
	Fetales Adenom	Adenoma fetal	Adenoma foetale

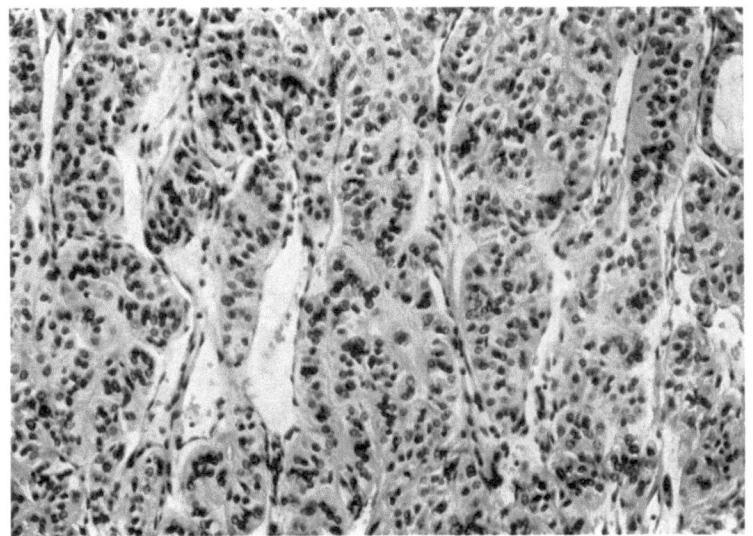

Fig. 144. × 150.

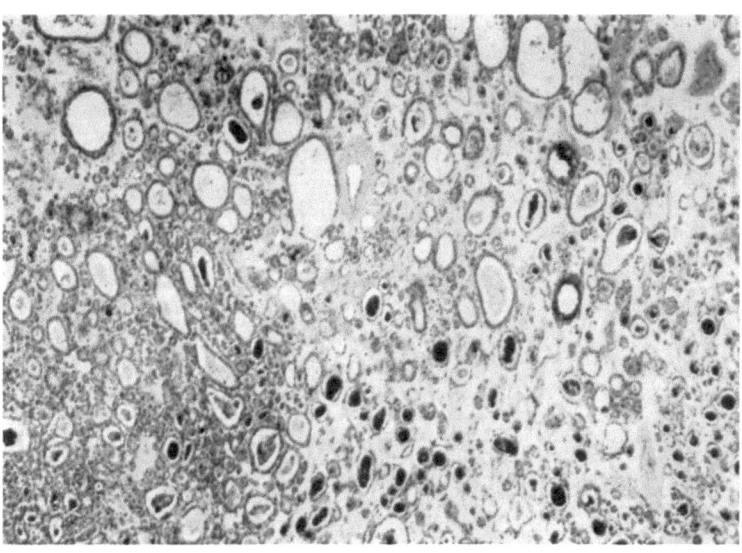

Fig. 145. ×48.   F 14 31—20

146   Macrofollicular adenoma   Adénome macrofolliculaire   Макрофолликулярная
      Colloid adenoma   Adénome colloïde   Аденома
                                                                    Коллоидная Аденома

      Makrofollikuläres Adenom   Adenoma macrofolicular   Adenoma macrofolliculare
      Kolloides Adenom   Adenoma coloide   Adenoma colloides

147   Oncocytic adenoma   Adénome oncocytaire   Онкоцитарная Аденома
      Hürthle cell adenoma   Adénome à cellules de   Аденома из клеток Гюртля
                                     Hürthle

      Onkocytäres Adenom   Adenoma oncocítico   Adenoma oncocyticum
      Hürthlezell-Adenom   Adenoma de células de   Adenoma Hürthle-cellu-
                                     Hürthle   lare

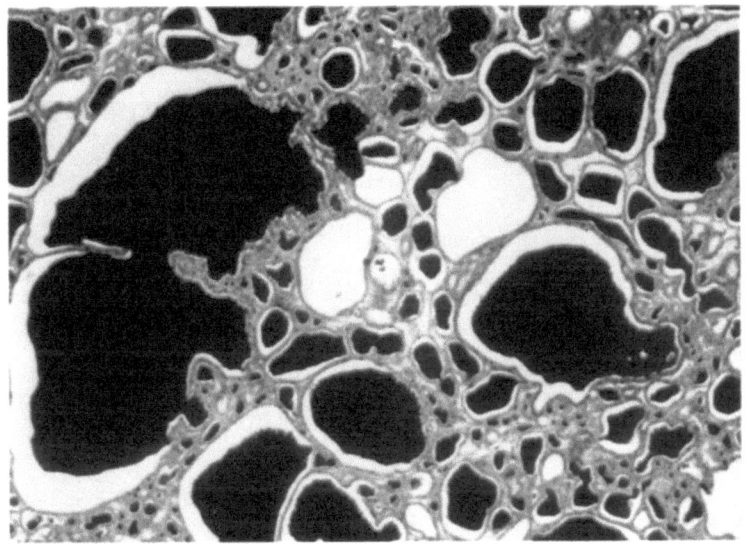

Fig. 146. × 48.   F 14 31—22

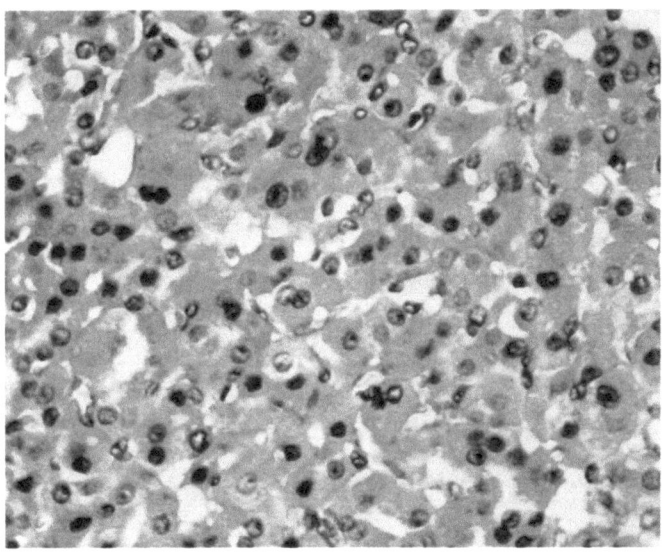

Fig. 147. × 400.   F 14 33—23

148 Alveolar adenocarcinoma Epithélioma alvéolaire Альвеолярная аденокарци-
Follicular adenocarcinoma Epithélioma folliculaire нома
                                                      Фолликулярная адено-
                                                      карцинома

Alveoläres Adenocarcinom Adenocarcinoma alveolar Adenocarcinoma alveolare
Follikuläres Adenocarci- Adenocarcinoma folicular Adenocarcinoma folliculare
nom

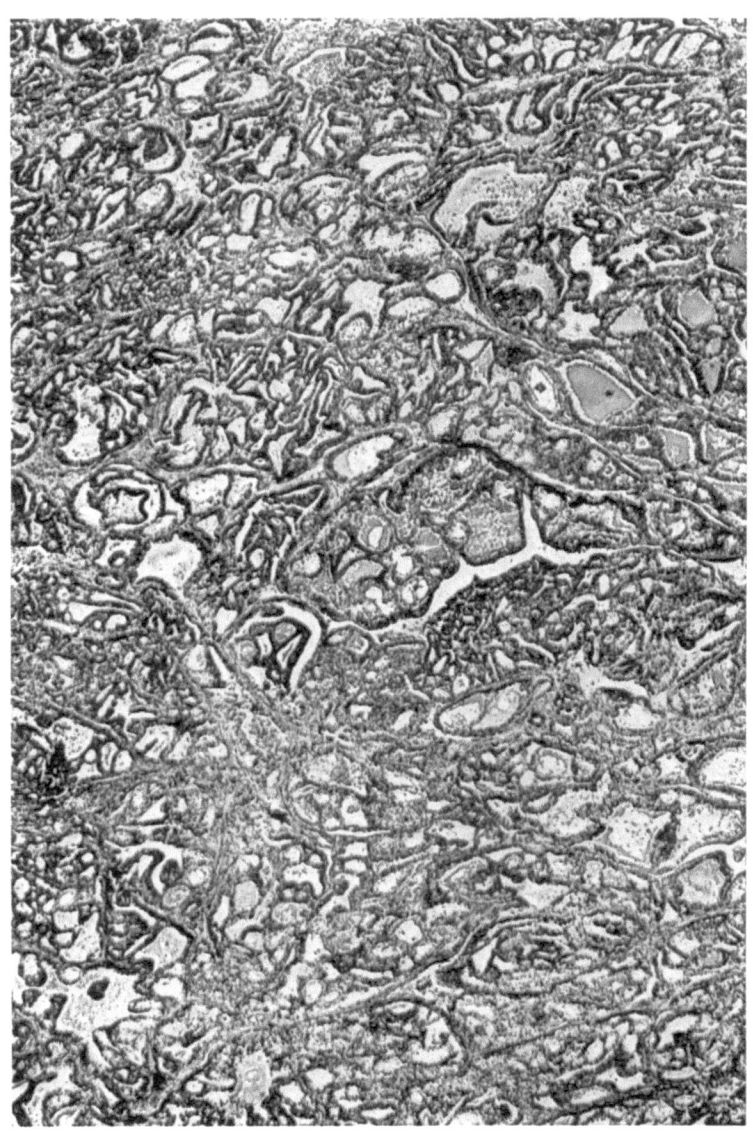

Fig. 148. × 50.

F 14 61—43

149	Alveolar adenocarcinoma Follicular adenocarcinoma (Langhans)	Epithélioma alvéolaire Epithélioma folliculaire (Langhans)	Альвеолярная адено- карцинома Фолликулярная адено- карцинома Растущая струма (Лангханса)
	Alveoläres Adenocarcinom Follikuläres Adenocarci- nom Wuchernde Struma (Lang- hans)	Adenocarcinoma alveolar Adenocarcinoma folicular Struma proliferante (Langhans)	Adenocarcinoma alveolare Adenocarcinoma folliculare Struma proliferans (Lang- hans)
150	Sclerosing adenocarcinoma	Epithélioma glandulaire sclérosant	Склерозирующая аденокарцинома
	Sklerosierendes Adeno- carcinom	Adenocarcinoma esclero- sante	Adenocarcinoma sclerosans

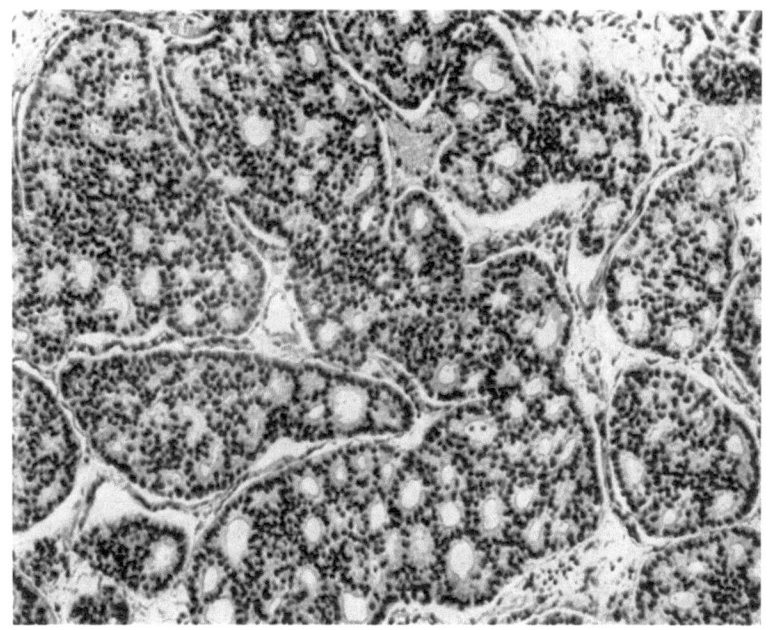

Fig. 149.   M 495—338

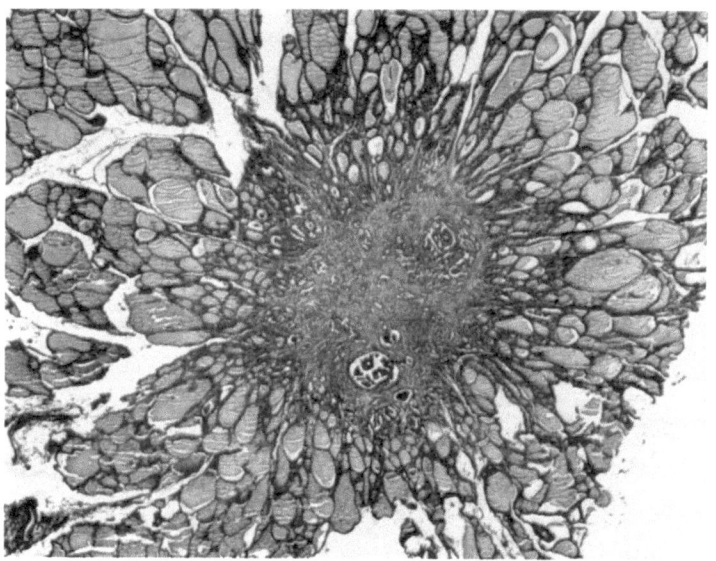

Fig. 150. × 15.   F 14 67—50

151 Papillary adenocarcinoma   Epithélioma glandulaire   Папиллярная
                                            papillaire   аденокарцинома

Papilläres Adenocarcinom   Adenocarcinoma papilífero   Adenocarcinoma papilli-
                                                                                ferum

152 Giant cell carcinoma   Epithélioma à cellules   Гигантоклеточная
                                            géantes   карцинома

Riesenzellcarcinom   Carcinoma de células   Carcinoma gigantocellulare
                                     gigantes

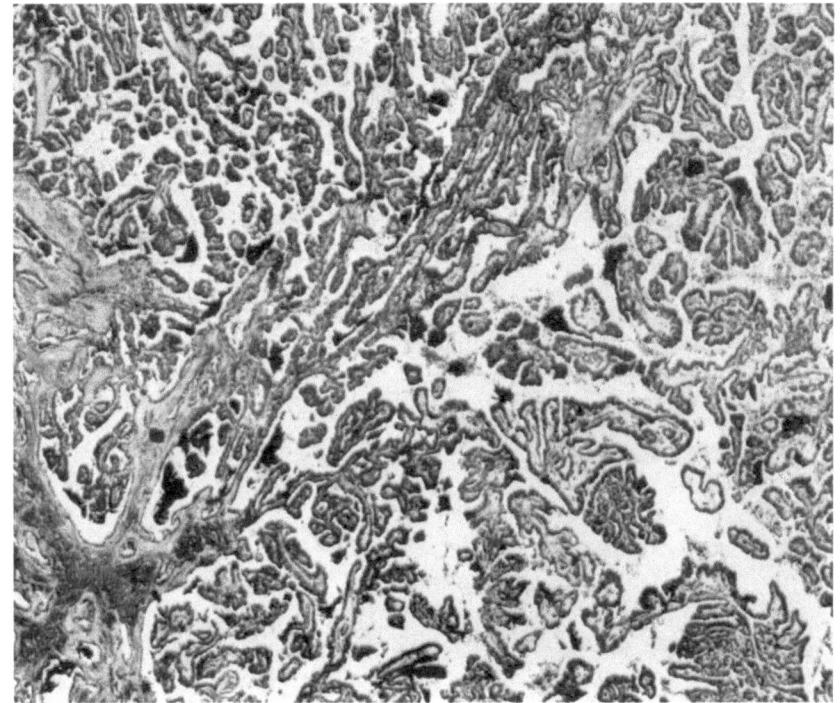

Fig. 151. × 50.   F 14 73—54

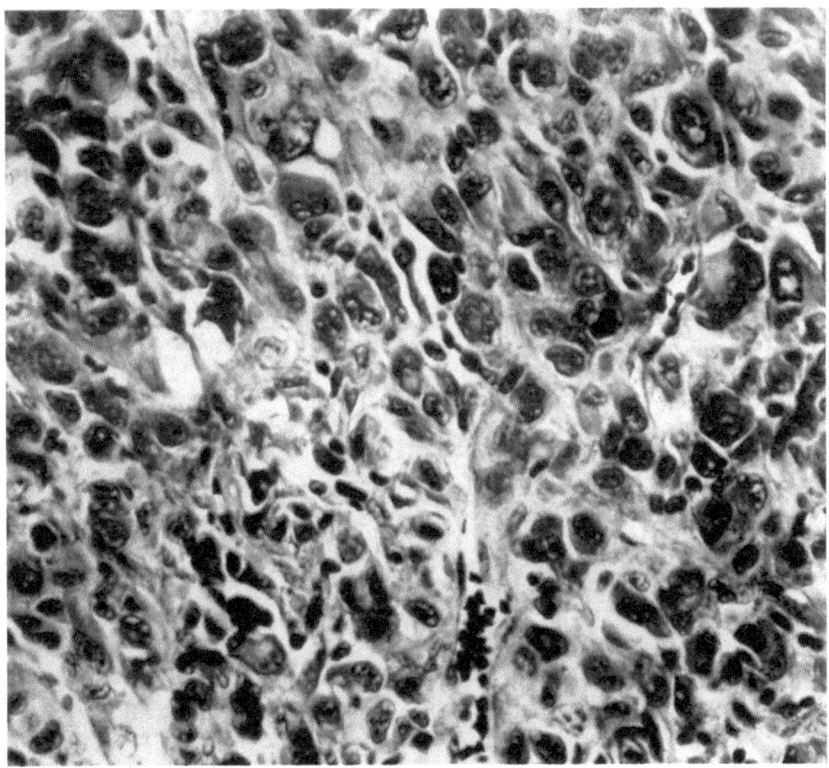

Fig. 152. × 400.   F 14 85—71

153   Small cell carcinoma   Epithélioma à petites   Мелкоклеточная карцинома
cellules

      Kleinzelliges Carcinom   Carcinoma de células   Carcinoma parvocellulare
pequeñas

154   Oncocytic carcinoma   Epithélioma oncocytaire   Онкоцитарная карцинома
      Hürthle cell carcinoma   Epithélioma à cellules de   Рак из клеток Гюртля
Hürthle

      Onkocytäres Carcinom   Carcinoma oncocítico   Carcinoma oncocyticum
      Hürthlezell-Carcinom   Carcinoma de células de   Carcinoma Hürthle-cellu-
Hürthle   lare

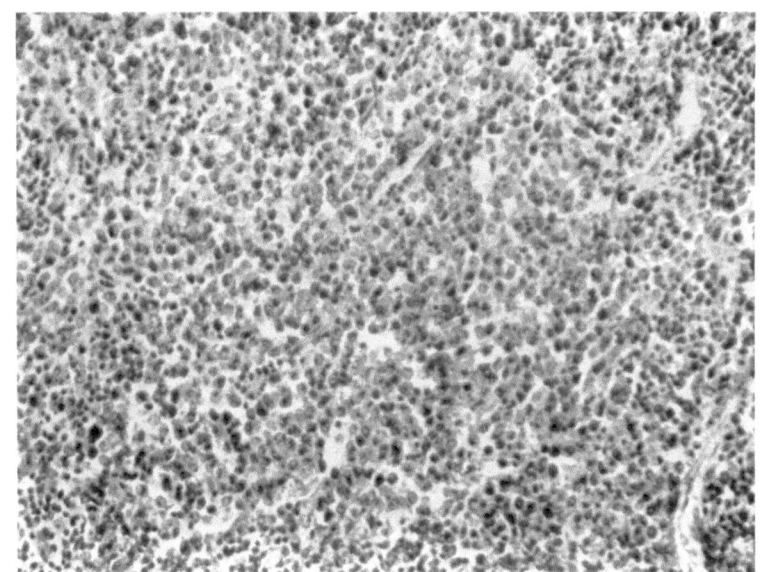

Fig. 153. × 200.   F 14 83—67

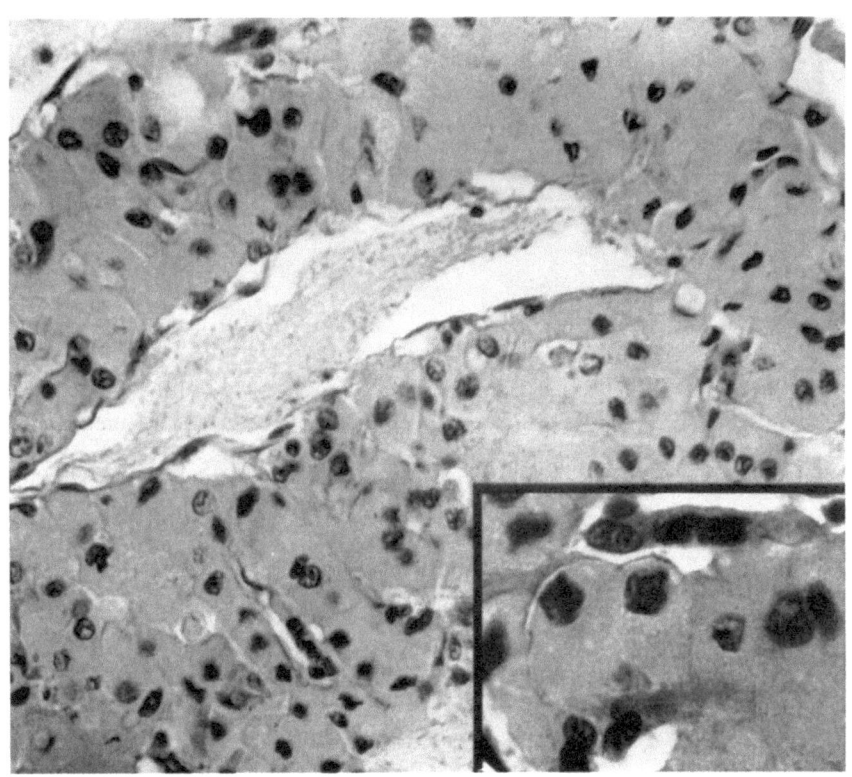

Fig. 154. × 395.   F 14 91—75

16. **Parathyroid**   **Parathyroïde**   **Паращитовидная железа**

Nebenschilddrüse   **Paratiroides**   Glandula parathyreoidea   (194.1)

155	Chief cell adenoma	Adénome à cellules principales	Аденома из главных клеток
	Hauptzelladenom	Adenoma de células principales	Adenoma principocellulare

156	Clear cell adenoma	Adénome à cellules claires	Светлоклеточная аденома
	Hellzelliges Adenom	Adenoma de células claras	Adenoma clarocellulare

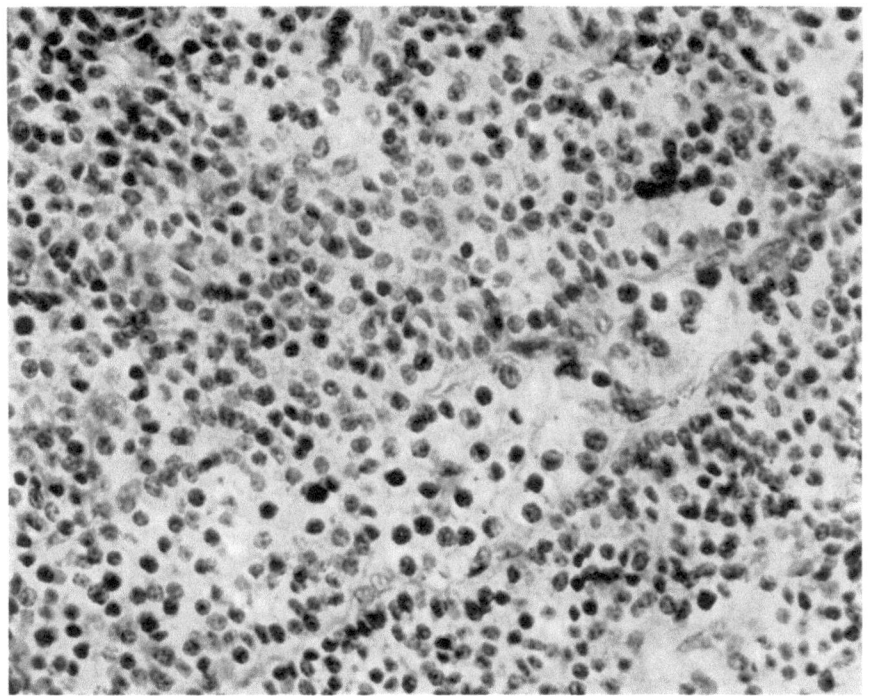

Fig. 155.   × 400.   F 15 35—20

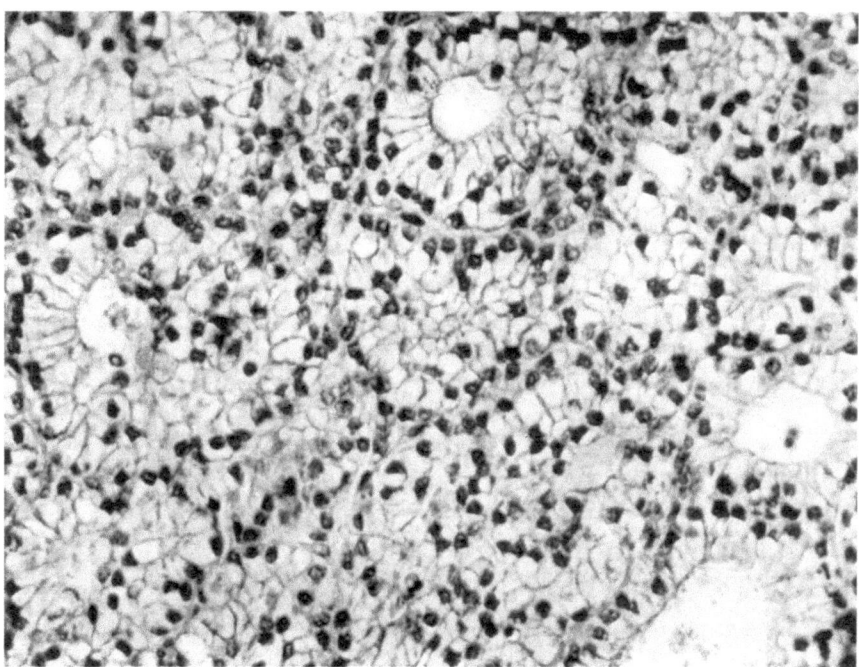

Fig. 156.   F 15 45—29

157 Acinous adenoma   Adénome acineux   Ацинозная аденома

Acinöses Adenom   Adenoma acinoso   Adenoma acinosum

158 Oxyphilic adenoma   Adénome à cellules   Оксифильная аденома
Oncocytic adenoma   acidophiles   Онкоцитарная аденома
Adénome oncocytaire

Oxyphiles Adenom   Adenoma oxífilo   Adenoma acidophile
Onkocytäres Adenom   Adenoma oncocítico   Adenoma oncocyticum

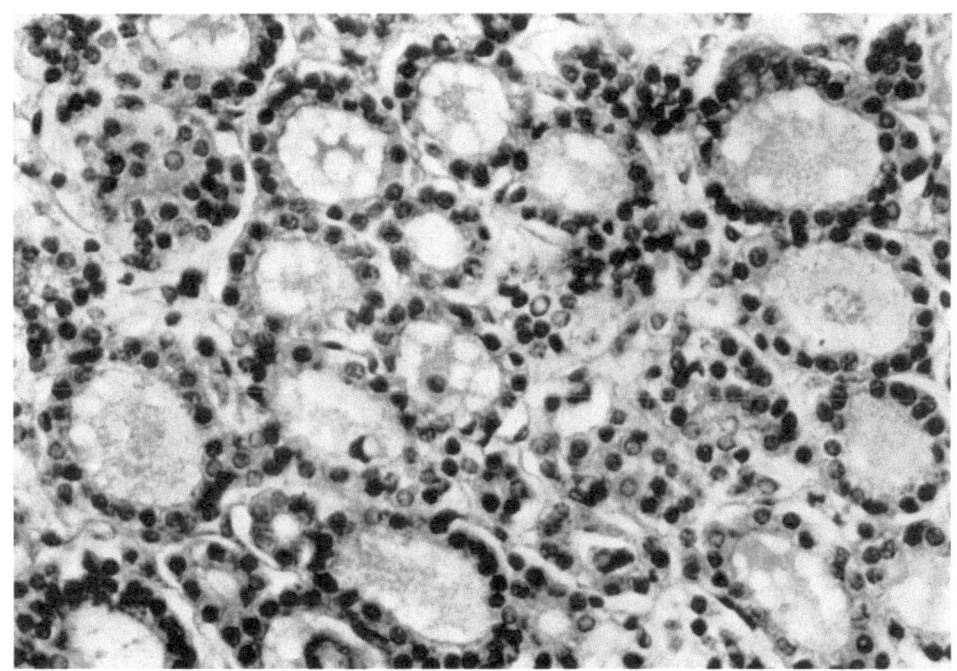

Fig. 157. × 400.   F 15 43—28

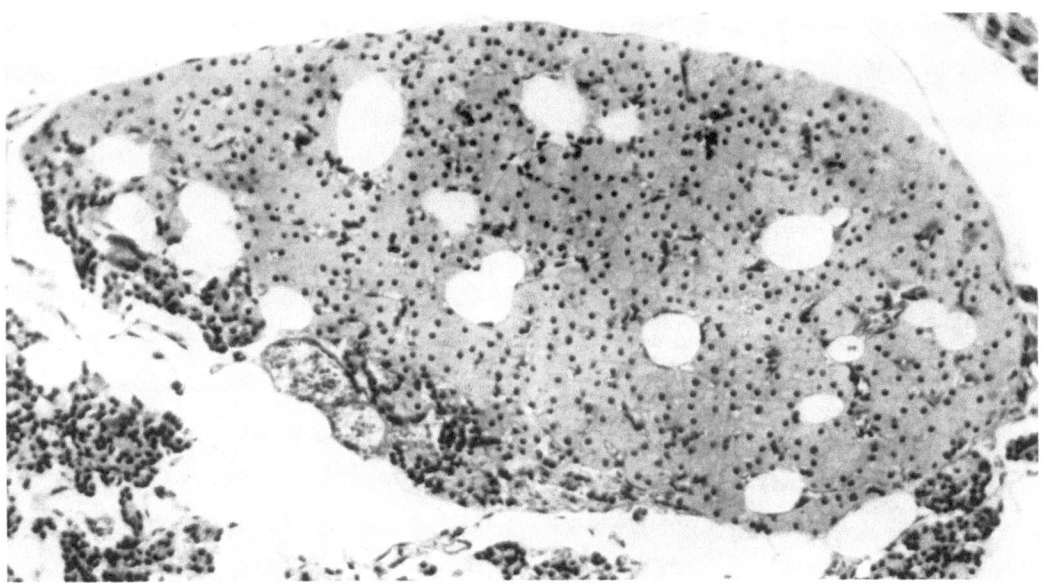

Fig. 158. × 165.   F 15 11—4

159 Trabecular carcinoma	Epithélioma trabéculaire	Трабекулярная карцинома
Trabeculäres Carcinom	Carcinoma trabecular	Carcinoma trabeculare

---

17. **Pineal gland**	**Glande pinéale (Epiphyse)**	**Шишковидная железа**	
Zirbeldrüse	**Glándula pineal**	Corpus pineale	(194.4)

---

160 Pinealoma	Pinéalome	Пинеалома
Pinealom	Pinealoma	Pinealoma

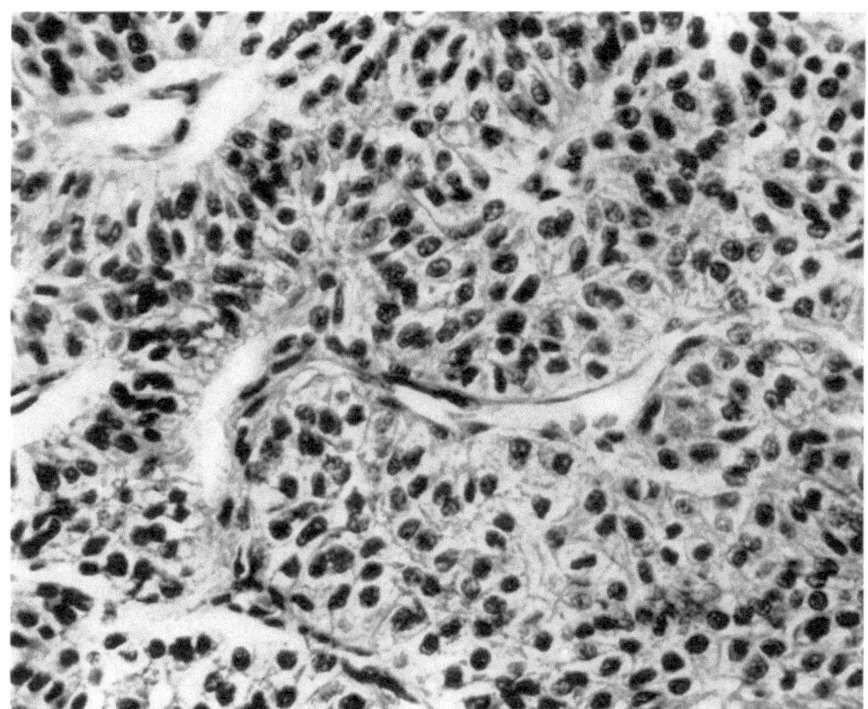

Fig. 159. × 400.   F 15 53—35

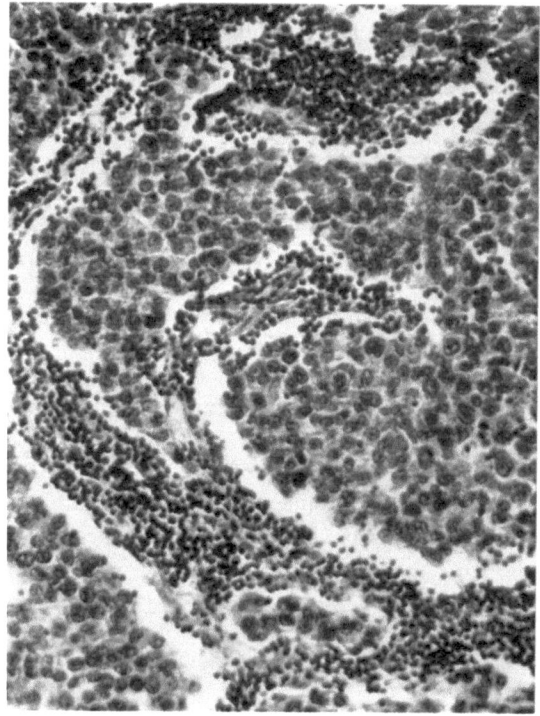

Fig. 160. × 175.   F 35 127—123

18. **Hypophysis** **Hypophyse** **Гипофиз**

Hypophyse **Hipófisis** **Hypophysis** (194.3)

| 161 | Diffuse chromophobe adenoma | Adénome à cellules chromophobes diffus | Диффузная хромофобная Аденома |
| | Diffuses chromophobes Adenom | Adenoma cromófobo difuso | Adenoma chromophobes diffusum |

| 162 | Sinusoidal chromophobe adenoma | Adénome à cellules chromophobes sinusoïdal | Синусоидальная хромофоб ная Аденома |
| | Sinusoidales chromophobes Adenom | Adenoma cromófobo sinusoidal | Adenoma chromophobes sinusoidale |

| 163 | Papillary chromophobe adenoma | Adénome à cellules chromophobes papillaire | Папиллярная хромофобная Аденома |
| | Papilläres chromophobes Adenom | Adenoma cromófobo papilífero | Adenoma chromophobes papilliferum |

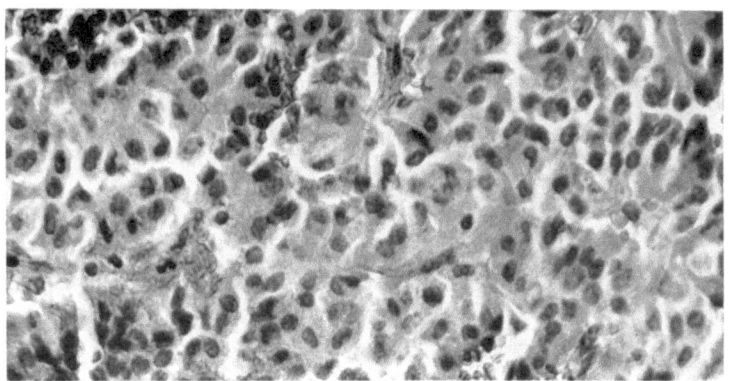

Fig. 161. × 350.

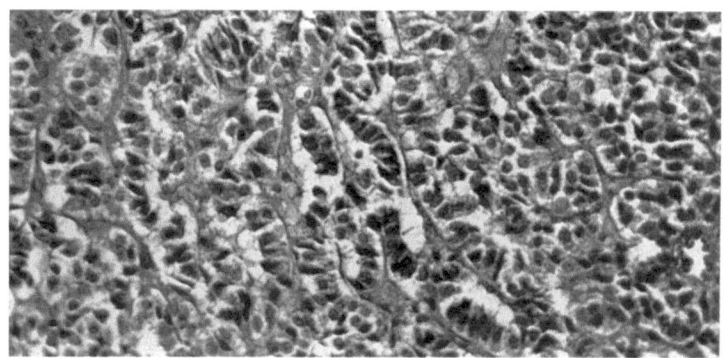

Fig. 162. × 235. F 36 33—29

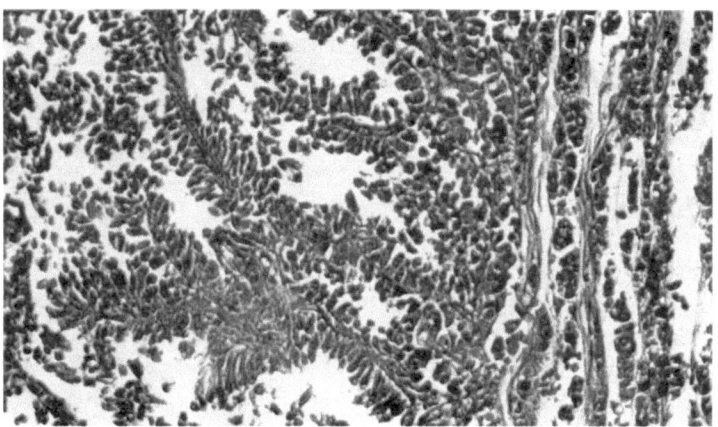

Fig. 163. × 165. F 36 35—33

164	Oxyphilic adenoma	Adénome à cellules acidophiles	Оксифильная аденома
	Oxyphiles Adenom	Adenoma oxífilo	Adenoma acidophile

165	Papillary oxyphilic adenoma	Adénome à cellules acidophiles papillaire	Папиллярная оксифильная Аденома
	Papilläres oxyphiles Adenom	Adenoma oxífilo papilífero	Adenoma acidophile papilliferum

166	Basophil adenoma	Adénome à cellules basophiles	Базофильная аденома
	Basophiles Adenom	Adenoma basófilo	Adenoma basophile

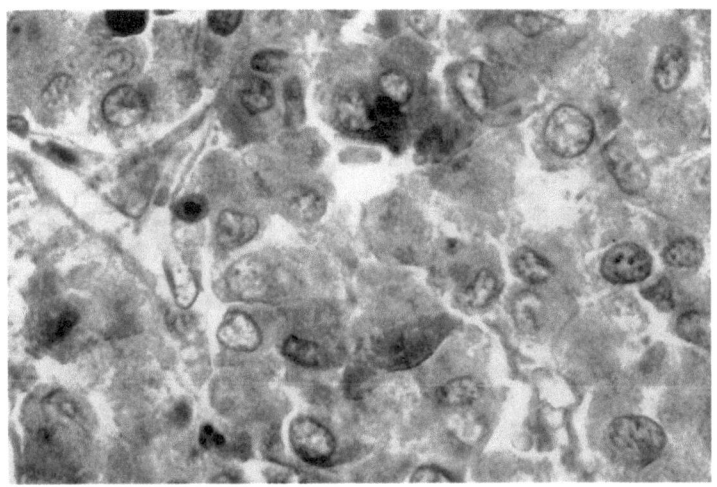

Fig. 164. ×920.   F 36 45—40

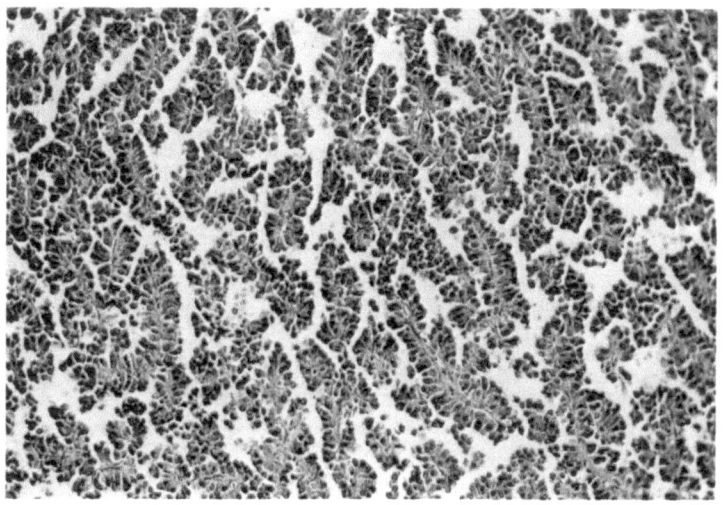

Fig. 165. ×120.   F 36 53—47

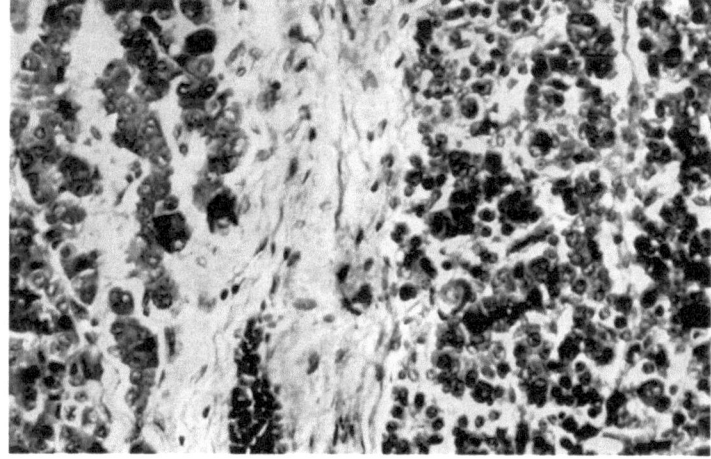

Fig. 166.   Zülch 530—385

167 Craniopharyngioma   Craniopharyngiome   Краниофарингиома
     Adamantinoma of cranio-   Adamantinome du canal
        pharyngeal duct   pharyngo-hypophysaire

     Craniopharyngiom   Craniofaringioma   Craniopharyngioma

168 Chromophobe carcinoma   Epithélioma chromophobe Хромофобная карцинома

     Chromophobes Carcinom   Carcinoma cromófobo   Carcinoma chromophobes

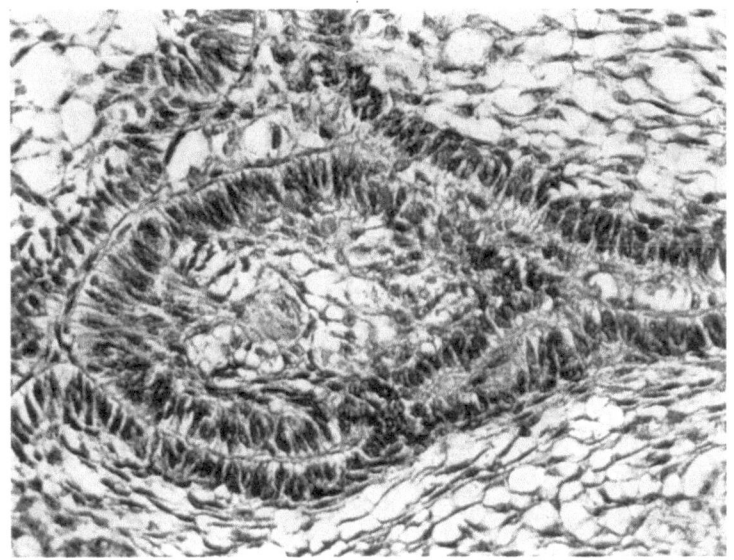

Fig. 167. ×325.   F 36 71—58

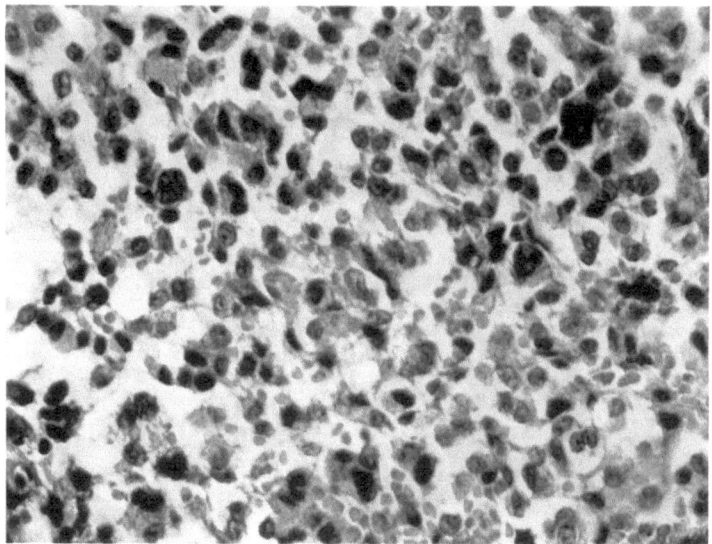

Fig. 168. ×430.   F 36 41—35

19. Suprarenal gland   Surrénale   **Надпочечник**

Nebenniere   Suprarrenal   Glandula suprarenalis   (194.0)

169   Cortical adenoma   Adénome cortical   Аденома коры

Rindenadenom   Adenoma cortical   Adenoma corticale

170   Phaeochromocytoma   Phéochromocytome   Феохромоцитома

Phaeochromocytom   Feocromocitoma   Phaeochromocytoma

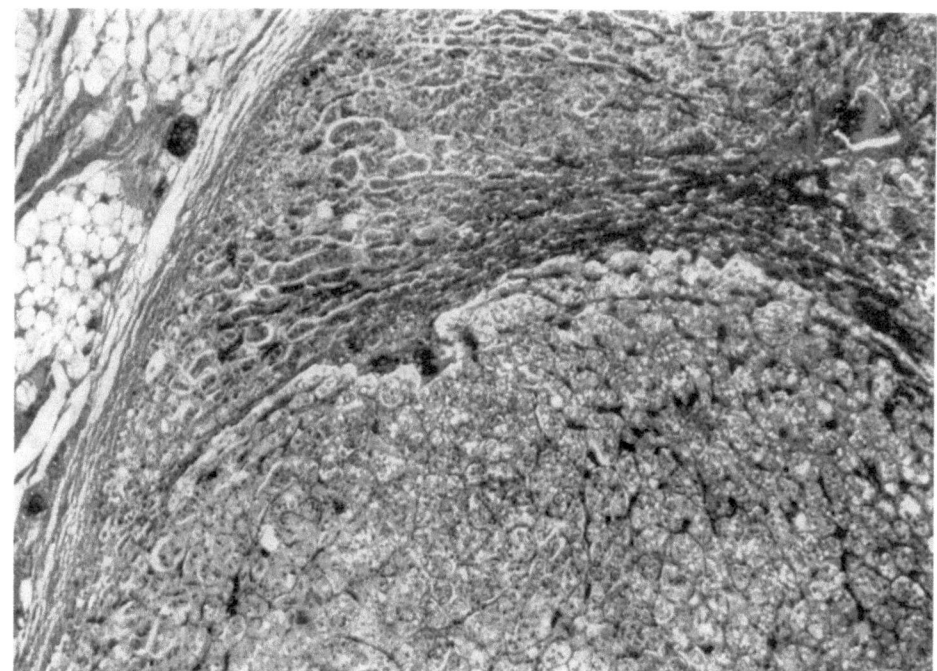

Fig. 169. × 100.   F 29 10—4

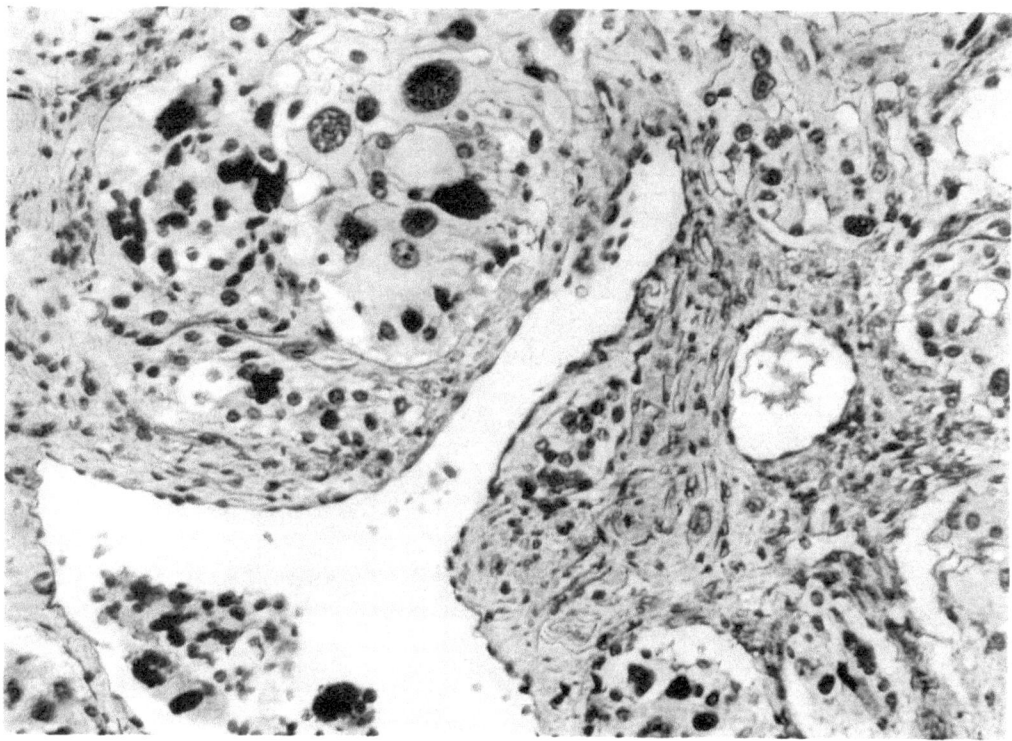

Fig. 170.   F 6 44—51

171 Cortical carcinoma   Epithélioma cortical   Рак коры (гипернефрома)

     Rindencarcinom   Carcinoma cortical   Carcinoma corticale

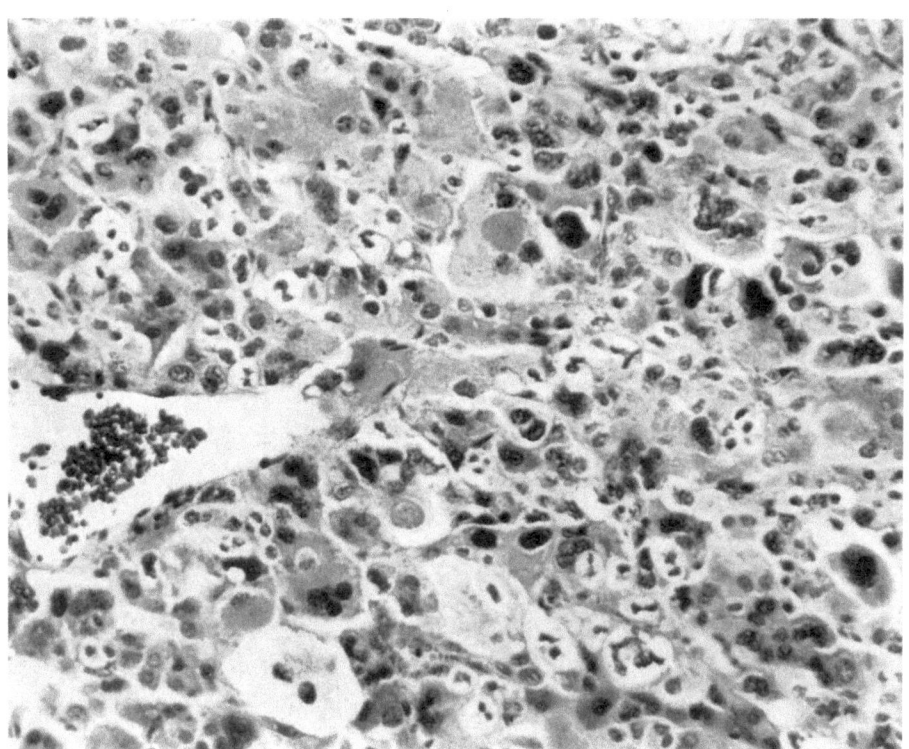

Fig. 171.　× 225.

F 29 25—19

III.

Tumors of melanin-forming tissue (172)

Tumeurs du système mélanogène

Опухоли меланинобразующей ткани

Tumoren des melaninbildenden Gewebes

Tumores de tejidos formadores de melanina

Tumores thelae melaninifacientes

172 Blue nevus   Naevus bleu   Синий невус

     Blauer Naevus   Nevus azul   Naevus coeruleus

173 Intradermal pigmented   Naevus pigmentaire intra- Интрадермальный
     nevus   dermique   пигментный невус

     Intradermaler Pigment-   Nevus pigmentado   Naevus pigmentosus
     Naevus   intradérmico   intradermalis

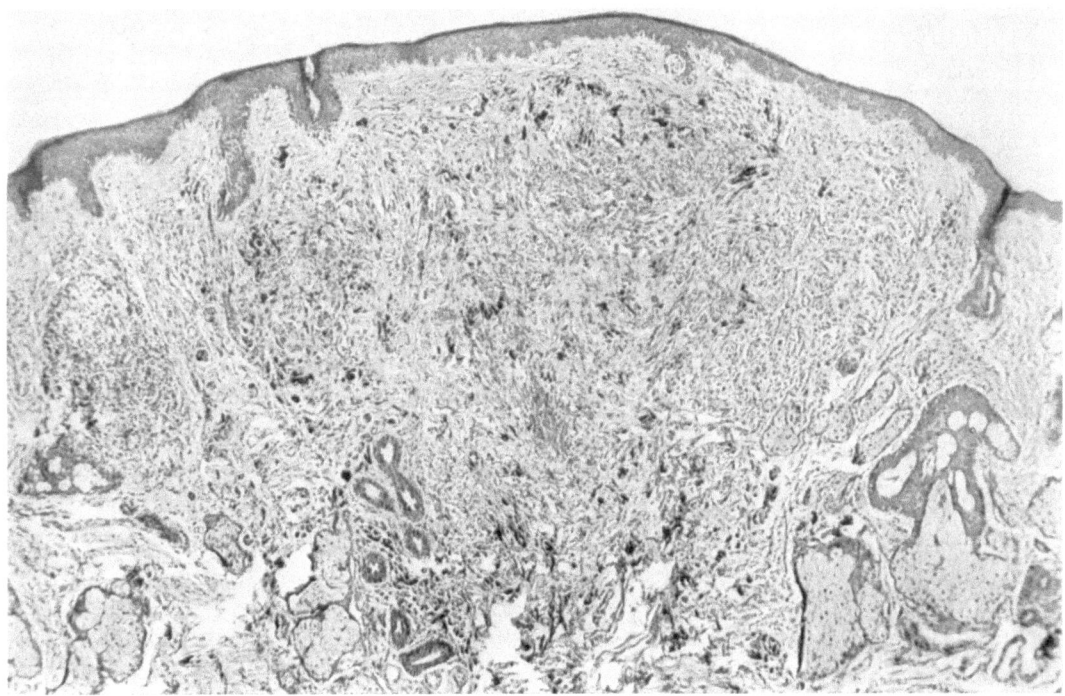

Fig. 172. ×48.   F 3 109—74

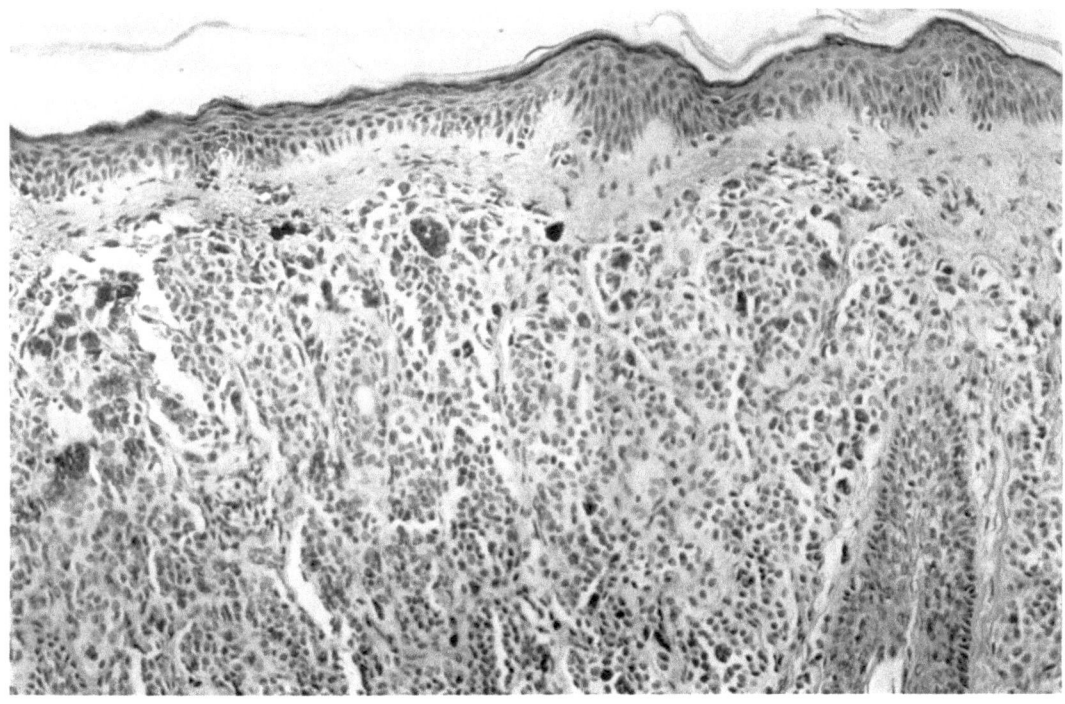

Fig. 173. ×186.   F 3 65—22

174 Compound pigmented
nevus

Komplexer Pigment-
Naevus

Naevus pigmentaire
complexe

Nevus pigmentado
compuesto

Комплексный пигментный
невус

Naevus pigmentosus
complexus

175 Junctional pigmented
nevus

Intraepidermaler Pigment-
Naevus

Naevus pigmentaire
jonctionnel

Nevus pigmentado
intraepidérmico

Пограничный пигментный
невус

Naevus pigmentosus
junctivus

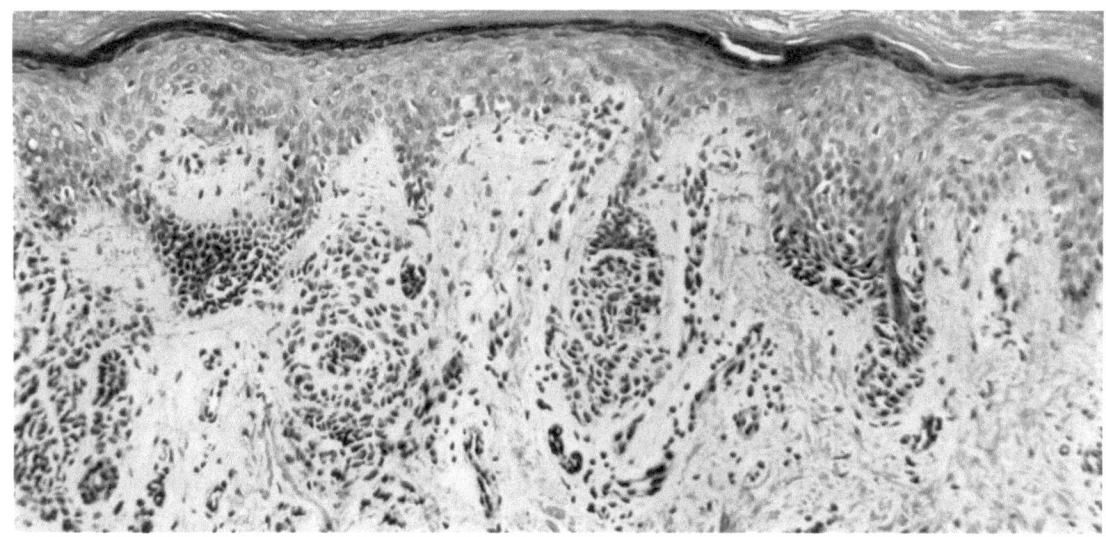

Fig. 174. × 150.   F 3 73—33

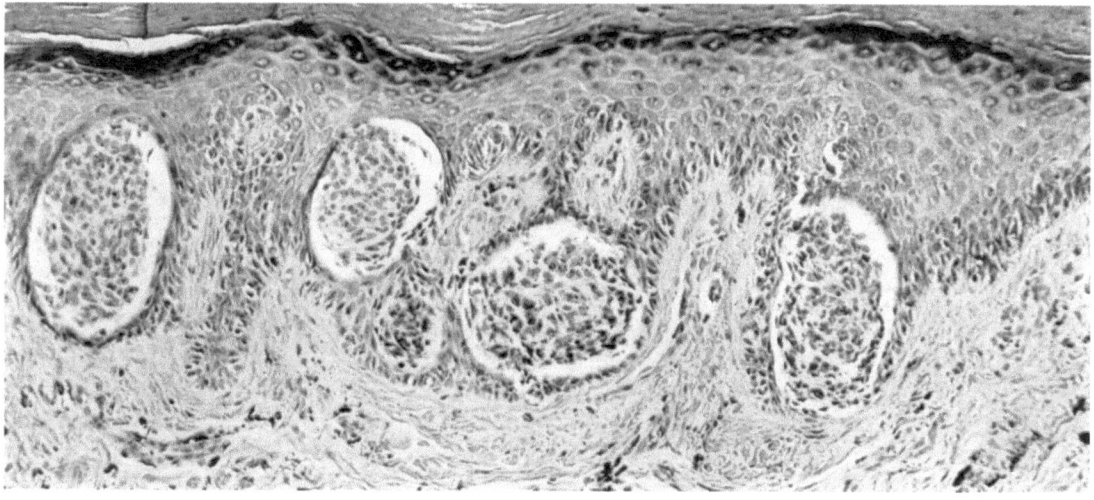

Fig. 175. × 150.   F 3 73—32

12*

176 Papillary pigmented nevus   Naevus pigmentaire   Папиллярный пигментный
                                    verruqueux   невус

     Papillärer Pigment-Naevus   Nevus pigmentado papilí-   Naevus pigmentosus
                                    fero   papilliferus

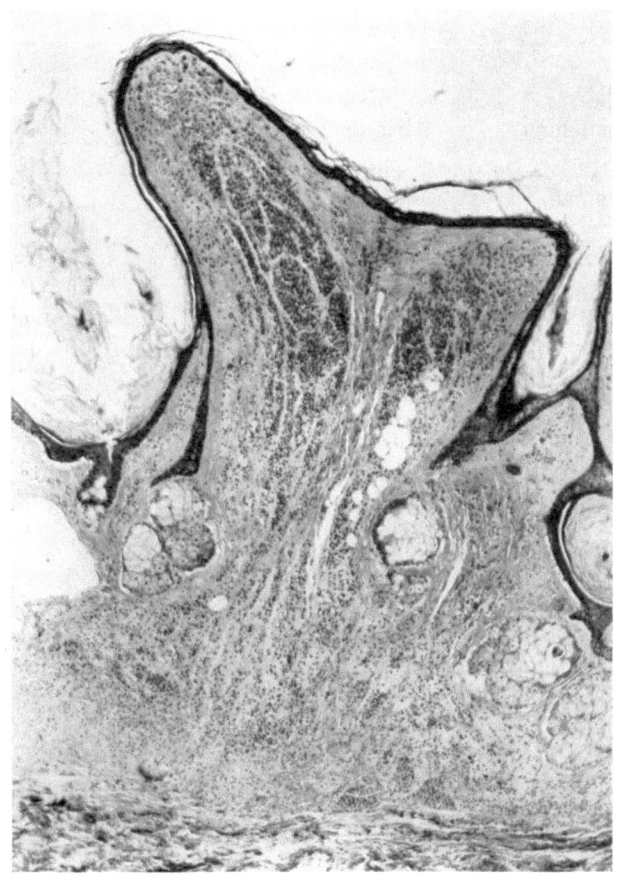

Fig. 176. × 39.   v. A. 495—597

177 Cuboidal cell malignant
     melanoma
     (Melanocarcinoma)

     Epitheloidzelliges bös-
     artiges Melanom
     (Melanocarcinom)

Mélanome malin à cellules
cubiques
(Mélanocarcinome)

Melanoma maligno
de células cúbicas
(Melanocarcinoma)

Злокачественная эпители-
оидноклеточная меланома
(Меланокарцинома)

Melanoma malignum
cuboidocellulare
(Melanocarcinoma)

178 Fusiform cell malignant
     melanoma
     (Melanosarcoma)

     Spindelzelliges bösartiges
     Melanom
     (Melanosarkom)

Mélanome malin à cellules
fusiformes
(Mélanosarcome)

Melanoma maligno de
células fusiformes
(Melanosarcoma)

Злокачественная веретено-
клеточная меланома
(Меланосаркома)

Melanoma malignum
fusicellulare
(Melanosarcoma)

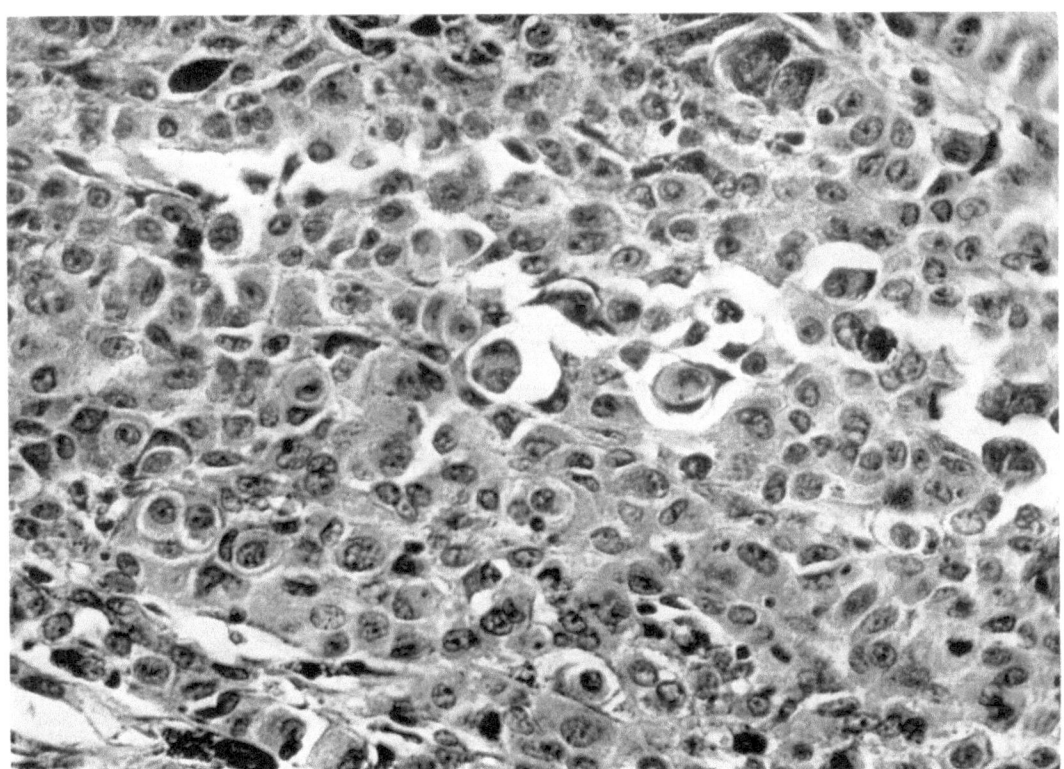

Fig. 177. × 600.   F 3 91—57

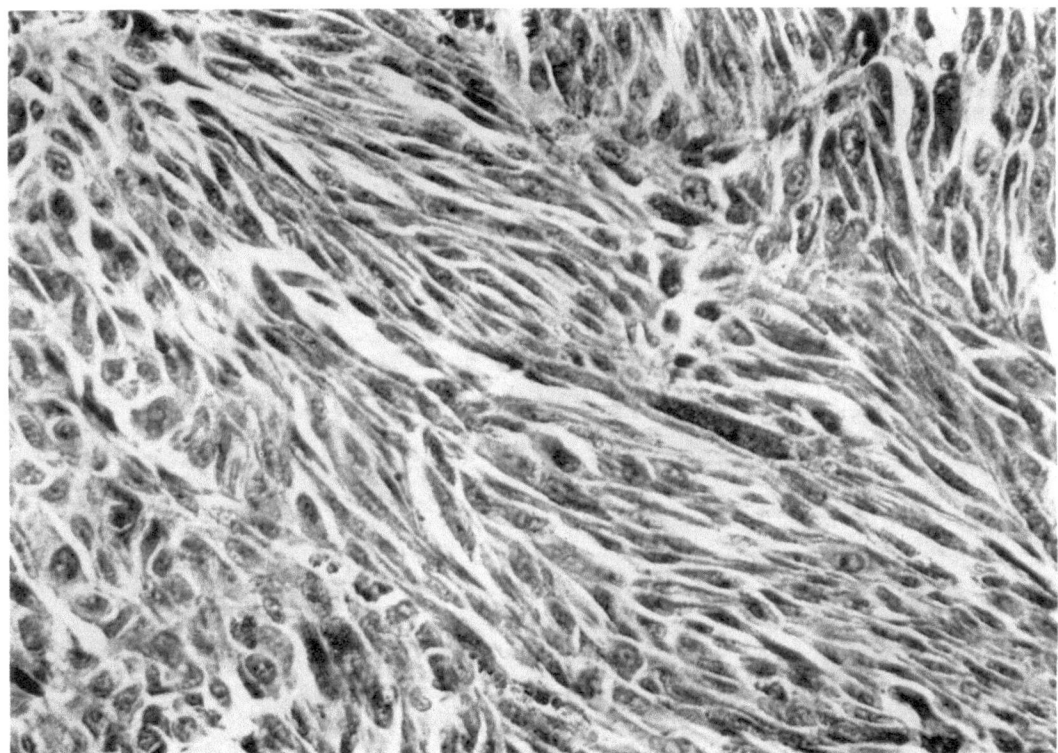

Fig. 178. × 600.   F 3 93—60

IV.

Tumors of nerve tissues and associated structures

Tumeurs des tissus nerveux et des structures tissulaires associés

Опухоли нервной ткани и ее оболочек

Tumoren des Nervengewebes und seiner Hüllen

Tumores del tejido nervioso y estructuras asociadas

Tumores thelae nervosae, etc.

1.   Nerve cells   Cellules nerveuses   Нервные клетки

   Nervenzellen   Células nerviosas   Cellulae nervosae   (191)

179   Ganglioneuroma   Ganglioneurome   Ганглионеврома
      Gangliocytoma   Gangliocytome   Ганглиоцитома
      Ganglioglioma   Gangliogliome   Ганглиоглиома

      Ganglioneurom   Ganglioneuroma   Ganglioneuroma
      Gangliocytom   Gangliocitoma   Gangliocytoma
      Gangliogliom   Ganglioglioma   Ganglioglioma

180   Ganglioneuroblastoma   Glanglioneuroblastome   Ганглионевробластома
      Malignant ganglioneuroma   Ganglioneurome malin   Злокачественная
      Malignant gangliocytoma   Gangliocytome malin   ганглионеврома
      Malignant ganglioglioma   Gangliogliome malin   Злокачественная
                                                               ганглиоцитома
                                                           Злокачественная
                                                               ганглиоглиома

      Ganglioneuroblastom   Ganglioneuroblastoma   Ganglioneuroblastoma
      Bösartiges Ganglioneurom   Ganglioneuroma maligno   Ganglioneuroma malignum
      Malignes Gangliocytom   Gangliocitoma maligno   Gangliocytoma malignum
                                  Ganglioma maligno   Ganglioglioma malignum

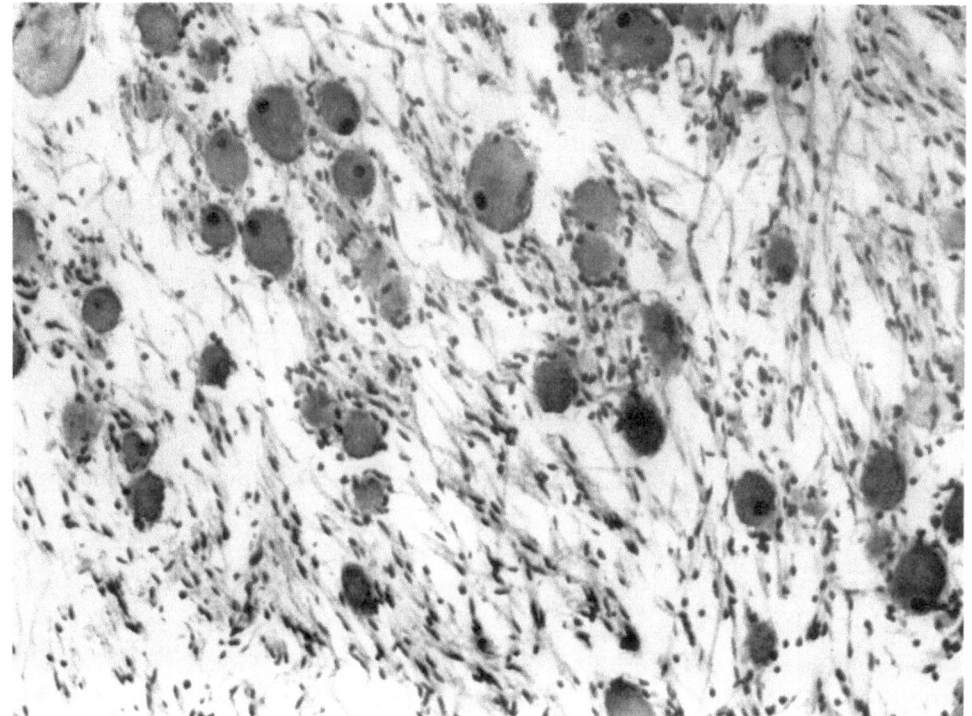

Fig. 179. × 200.   F 29 39—31

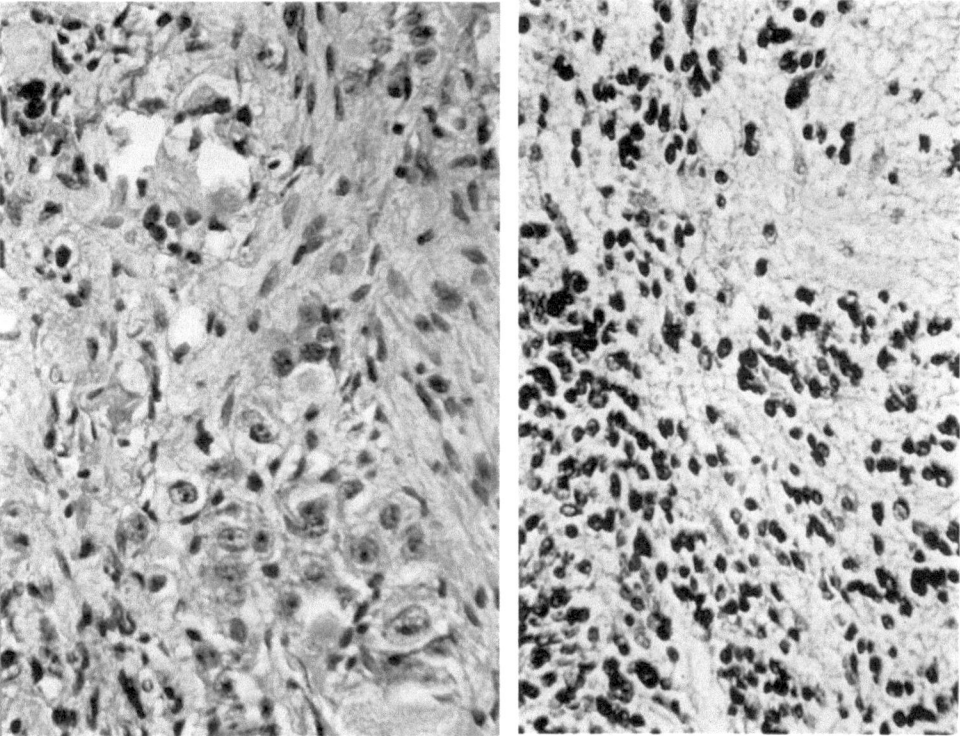

Fig. 180. × 300.

181 Sympathicogonioma   Sympathogoniome   Симпатогониома

   Sympathicogoniom   Simpáticogonioma   Sympathogonioma

182 Sympathicoblastoma   Sympathoblastome   Симпатобластома
   Neuroblastoma

   Sympathicoblastom   Simpáticoblastoma   Sympathoblastoma
             Neuroblastoma

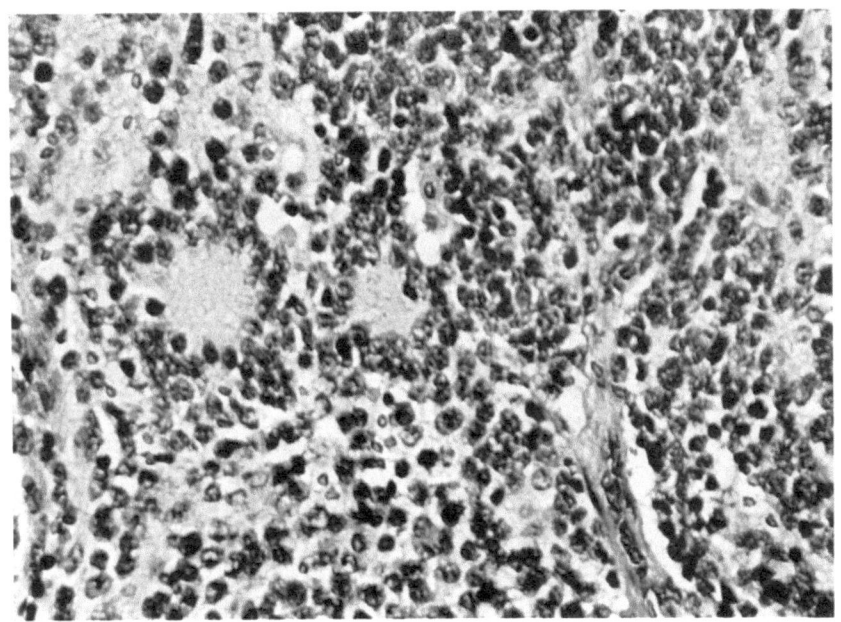

Fig. 181. × 350.

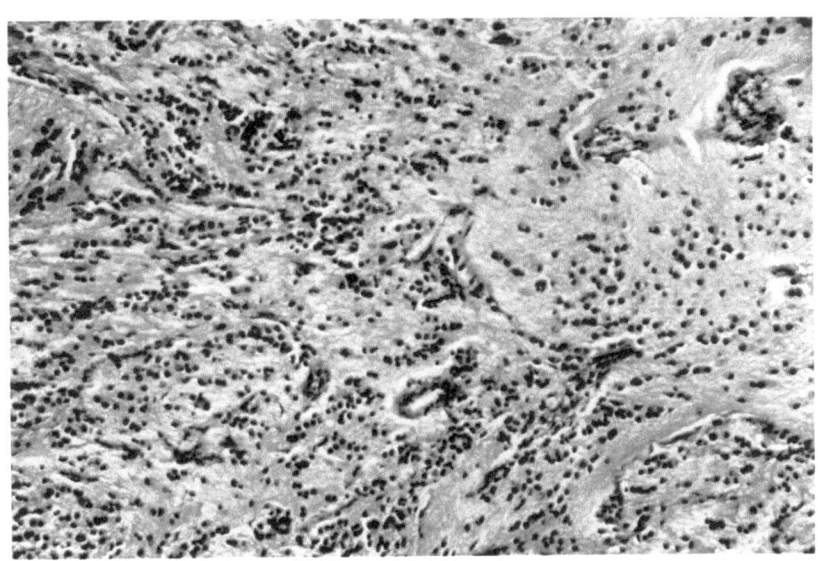

Fig. 182. × 120.

2. Neuroepithelium   Neuroépithélium   **Невроэпителий**

    Neuroepithel   Neuroepitelio   Neuroepithelium   (191)

---

183   Epithelial ependymoma   Ependymome épithélial   Эпителиальная Эпендимома

      Epitheliales Ependymom   Ependimoma epitelial   Ependymoma epitheliale

184   Papillary ependymoma   Ependymome papillaire   Папиллярная Эпендимома

      Papilläres Ependymom   Ependimoma papilífero   Ependymoma papilliferum

185   Cellular ependymoma   Ependymome cellulaire   Клеточная Эпендимома

      Celluläres Ependymom   Ependimoma celular   Ependymoma cellulare

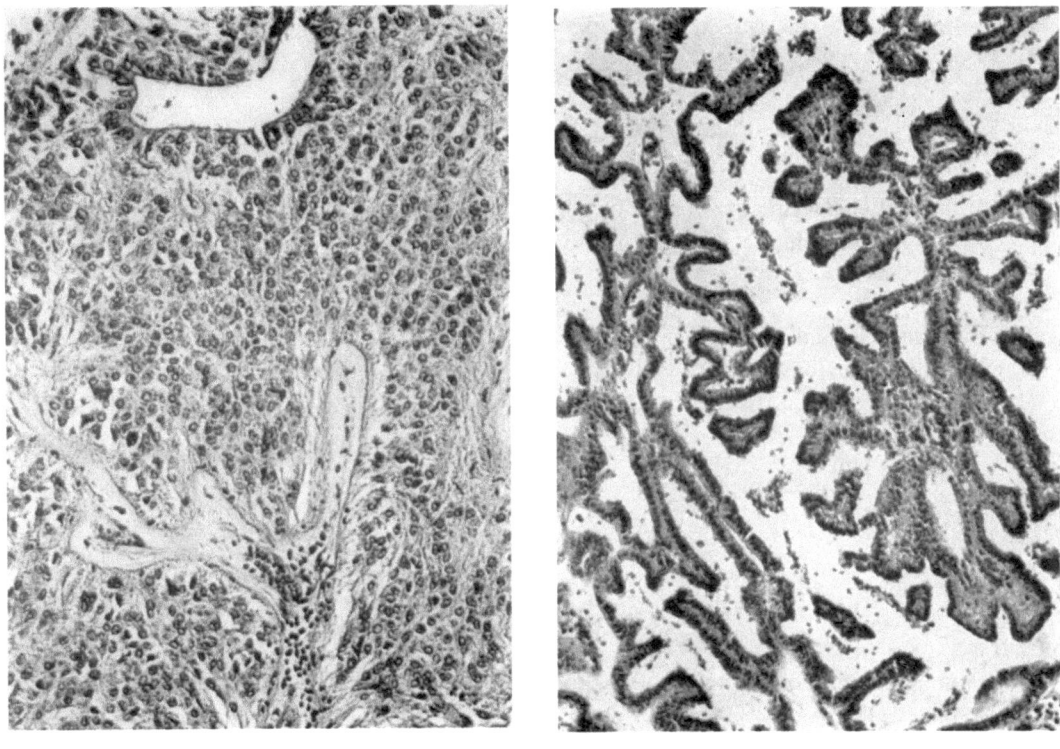

Fig. 183. × 140.   F 35 53—41   Fig. 184. × 100.   F 35 55—45

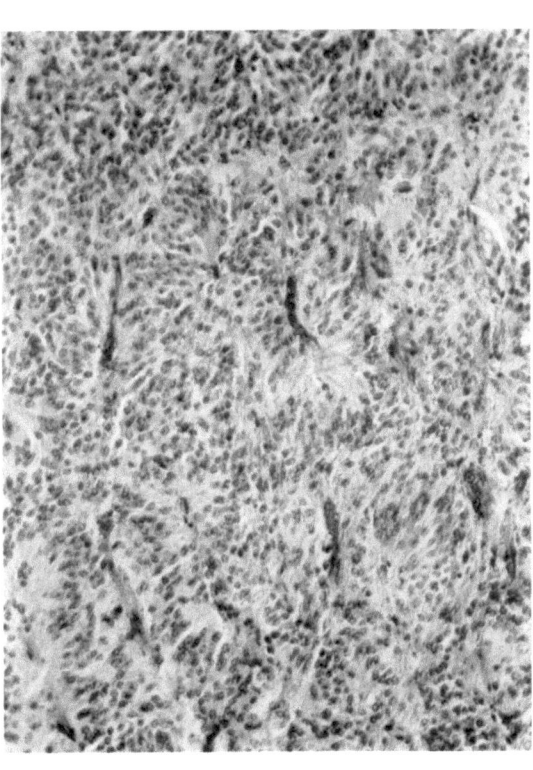

Fig. 185. × 150.   F 35 55—47

186   Malignant ependymoma
Ependymoblastoma

Ependymome malin
Ependymoblastome

Злокачественная
эпендимома
Эпендимобластома

Bösartiges Ependymom
Ependymoblastom

Ependimoma maligno
Ependimoblastoma

Ependymoma malignum
Ependymoblastoma

187   Papilloma of choroid plexus
Plexuspapilloma

Papillome du plexus
choroïde

Папиллома хороидального
сплетения
Плексуспапиллома

Papillom des Plexus
chorioideus
Plexuspapillom

Papiloma de los plexos
coroideos
Plexuspapiloma

Papilloma plexus chorioidei

188   Olfactory neuroepithelioma

Neuroépithéliome olfactif
Esthésio-neuro-épithéliome

Невроэпителиома
обонятельная

Olfactorius-Neuroepi-
theliom

Neuroepitelioma olfatorio

Neuroepithelioma olfac-
torium

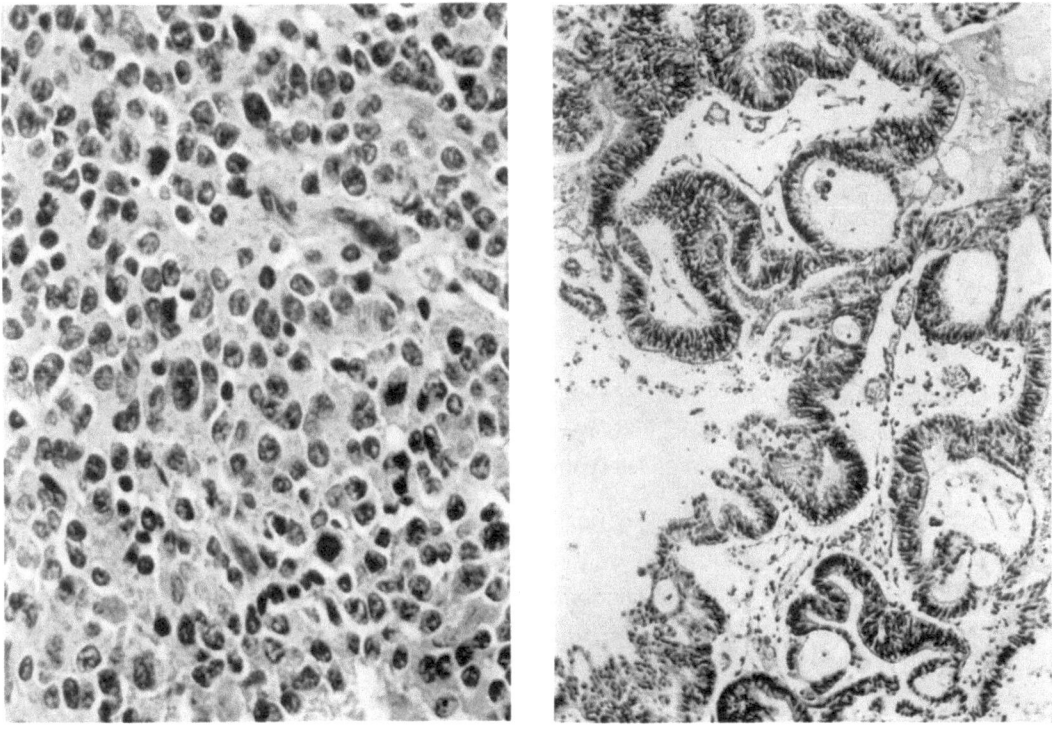

Fig. 186. × 400.   F 35 57—52   Fig. 187. × 100.   F 35 55—48

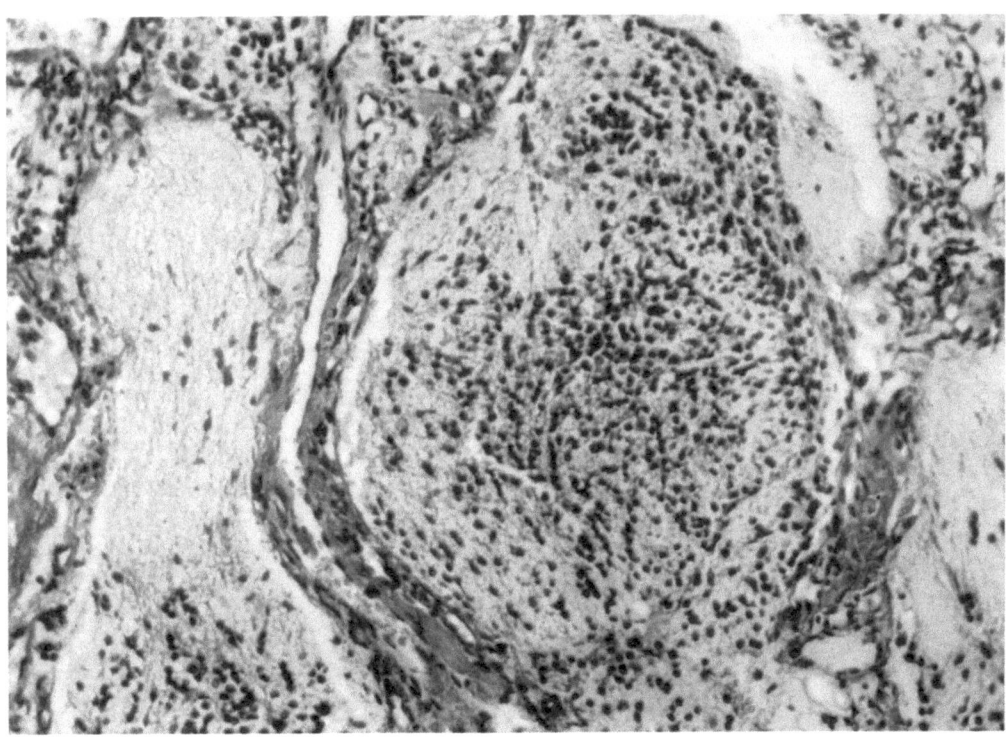

Fig. 188.   F 6 52—55

3. **Eye** **Œil** **Глаз**

Auge **Ojo** **Oculus** (190)

189	Medulloepithelioma of ciliary epithelium Diktyoma	Médulloépithéliome du corps ciliaire Dictyome	Медуллоэпителиома цилиарного эпителия Диктиома
	Medulloepitheliom des Ciliar-Epithels Diktyom	Meduloepitelioma de epitelio ciliar Dictioma	Medulloepithelioma cilio-epitheliale Diktyoma

190	Neuroepithelioma with true rosettes Retinoblastoma with true rosettes	Neuro-epithéliome avec rosettes véritables Rétinoblastome avec rosettes véritables	Невроэпителиома Ретинобластома с истинными розетками
	Retinoblastom mit Rosettenbildung	Neuroepitelioma con rosetas verdaderas Retinoblastoma con rosetas verdaderas	Neuroepithelioma cum corollis veris Retinoblastoma cum corollis veris

191	Neuroepithelioma without true rosettes Retinoblastoma without true rosettes	Neuro-epithéliome sans rosettes véritables Rétinoblastome sans rosettes véritables	Невроэпителиома Ретино бластома без истинных розеток
	Retinoblastom ohne Rosettenbildung	Neuroepitelioma sin rosetas verdaderas Retinoblastoma sin rosetas verdaderas	Neuroepithelioma sine corollis veris Retinoblastoma sine corollis veris

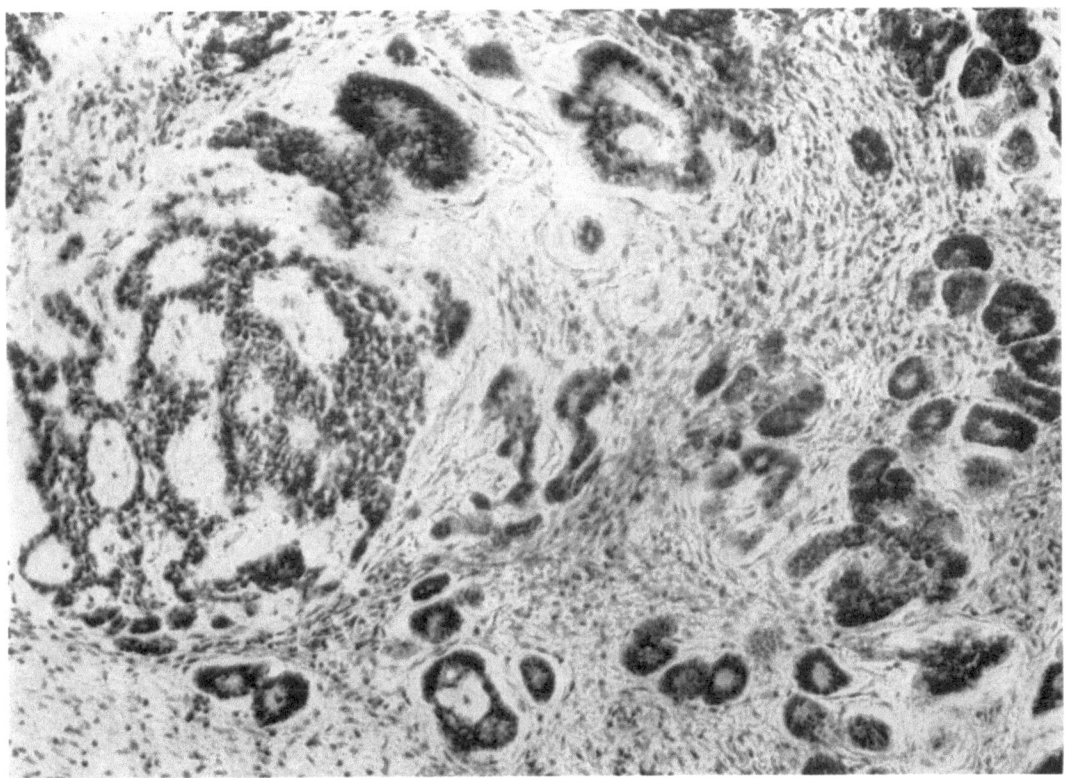

Fig. 189. F 38 29—16

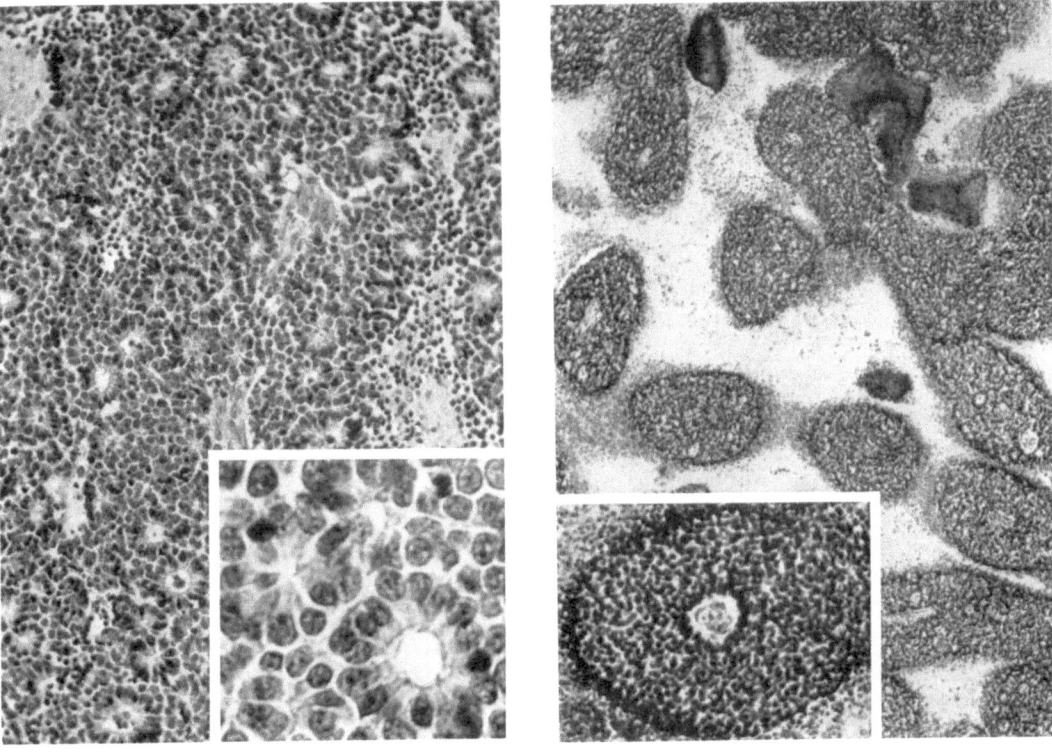

Fig. 190. × 55. F 38 49—28 Fig. 191. × 160. F 38 49—29

13*

196

---

4. **Glia** **Glie** **Глия**
   Glia **Glia** **Glia** (191)

---

192 Fibrillary astrocytoma Astrocytome fibrillaire Фибриллярная Астроцитома

   Fibrilläres Astrocytom Astrocitoma fibrilar Astrocytoma fibrillare

193 Protoplasmatic astrocytoma Astrocytes «engraissés» Протоплазматическая
   Gemistocytic astrocytoma Astrocytome protoplasmique Астроцитома
                             Astroblastome Гигантоклеточная
                                            Астроцитома

   Protoplasmatisches Astrocitoma protoplasmático Astrocytoma protoplas-
      Astrocytom Astrocitoma gemistocítico maticum
   Astroblastom Astroblastoma

194 Astrocytoma of the nose Astrocytome du nez Астроцитома
   Nasal glioma Gliome nasal Глиома носа

   Astrocytom der Nase Astrocitoma de la nariz Astrocytoma nasi
   Nasales Gliom Glioma nasal Glioma nasale

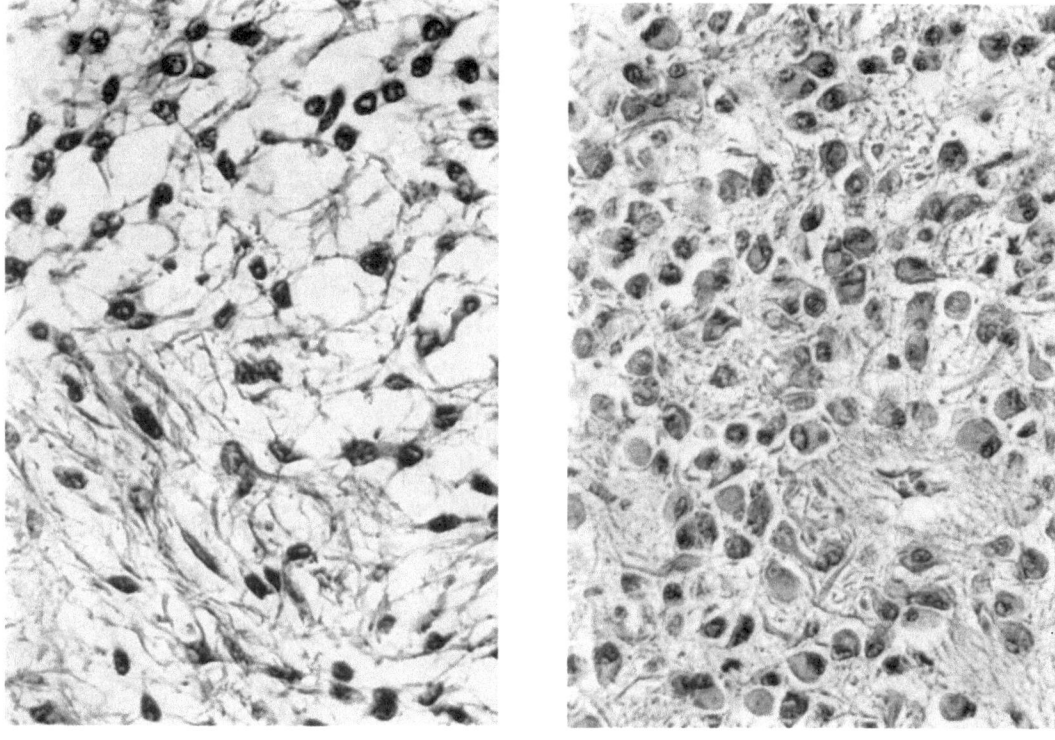

Fig. 192. ×400.   F 35 29—14   Fig. 193.   F 35 31—18

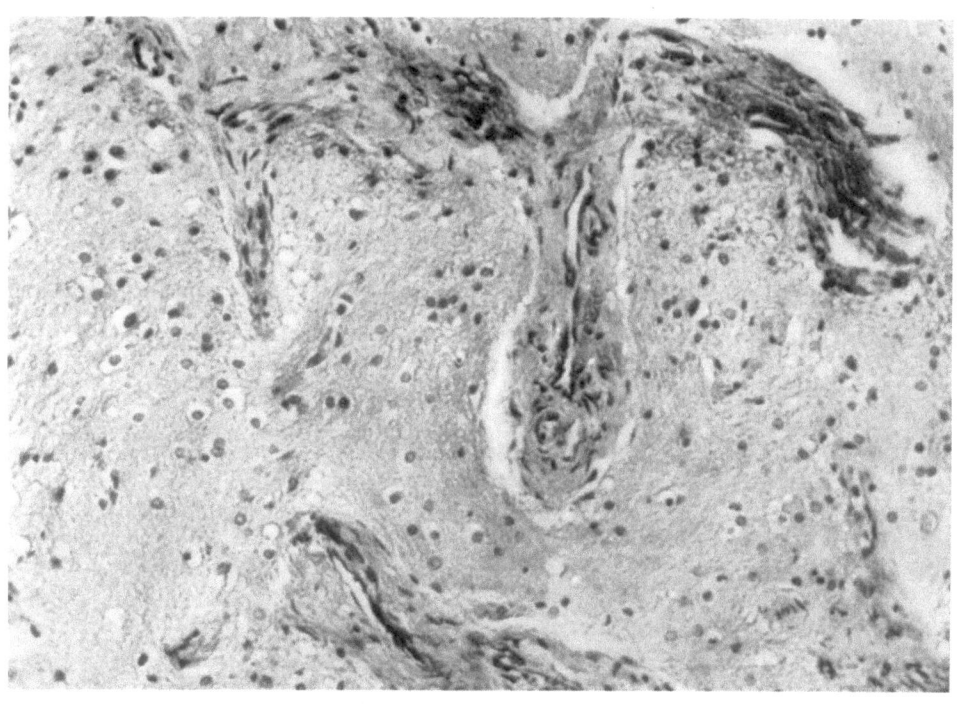

Fig. 194.   F 6 51—54

195	Oligodendroglioma	Oligodendrogliome	Олигодендроглиома
	Oligodendrogliom	Oligodendroglioma	Oligodendroglioma
196	Multiform glioblastoma	Glioblastome multiforme	Мультиформная глиобластома
	Multiformes Glioblastom	Glioblastoma multiforme	Glioblastoma multiforme
197	Polar spongioblastoma	Spongioblastome	Полярная спонгиобластома
	Spongioblastom	Espongioblastoma polar	Spongioblastoma
198	Medulloblastoma	Médulloblastome	Медуллобластома
	Medulloblastom	Meduloblastoma	Medulloblastoma

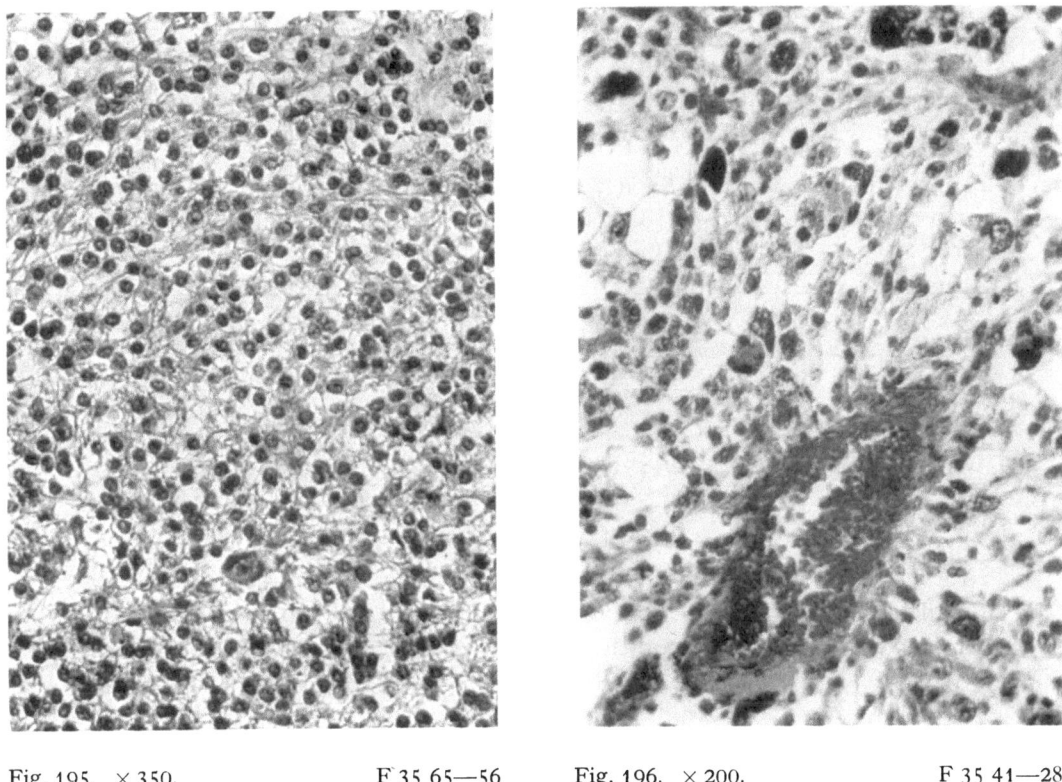

Fig. 195. × 350.   F 35 65—56

Fig. 196. × 200.   F 35 41—28

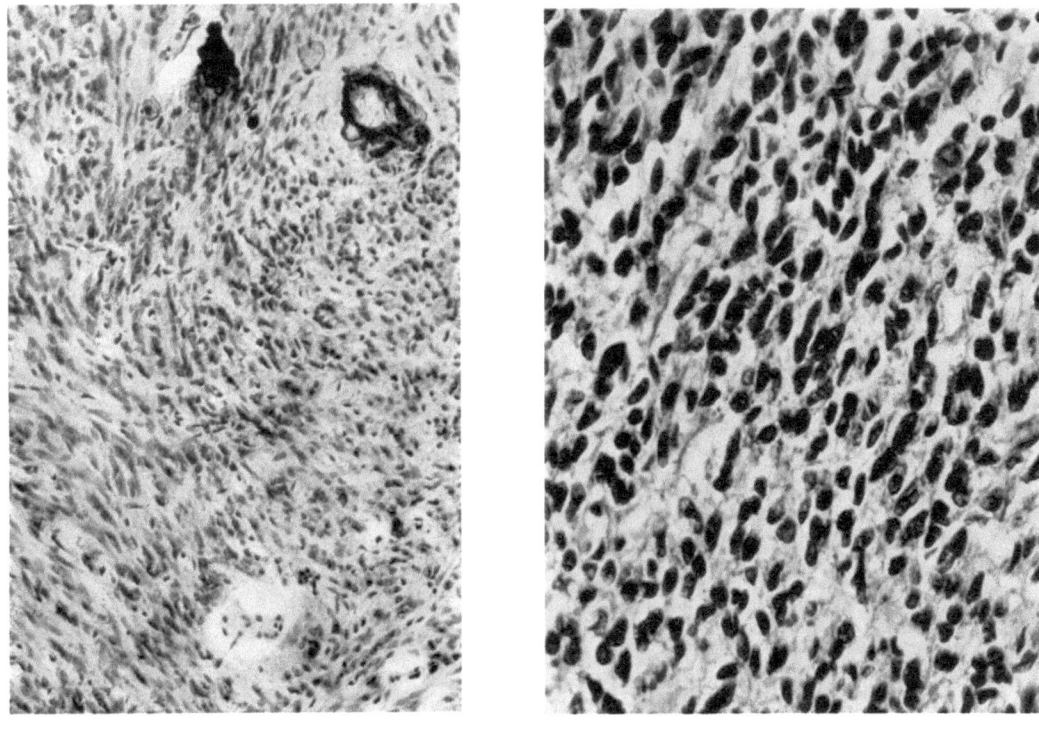

Fig. 197. × 90.   Zülch 158—74a

Fig. 198. × 400.   F 35 75—65

5. **Peripheral and cranial nerves**

Nerfs périphériques et gaines nerveuses

Периферические и черепномозговые нервы

Periphere Nerven und Nervenscheiden

Nervios craneales y periféricos

Nervi peripherici et tunicarum nervorum (192)

199 Neurinoma	Neurinome	Невринома
Neurilemoma	Neurilémome	Неврилемома
Schwannoma	Schwannome	Шваннома
Neurinom	Neurinoma	Neurinoma
Neurilemom	Neurilemoma	Neurilemoma
Schwannom	Schwannoma	Schwannoma

200 Neurofibroma*	Neurofibrome*	Неврофиброма*
Neurofibrom*	Neurofibroma*	Neurofibroma

---

* For sarcomas arising from neurofibromas see V/1.
* Pour les sarcomes issus de neurofibromes, voir V/1.
* о саркомах на почве неврофиброматоза см. V/1.
* Sarcome ausgehend von Neurofibromen s. V/1.
* Ver V/1 para los sarcomas que tienen origen en neurofibromas.

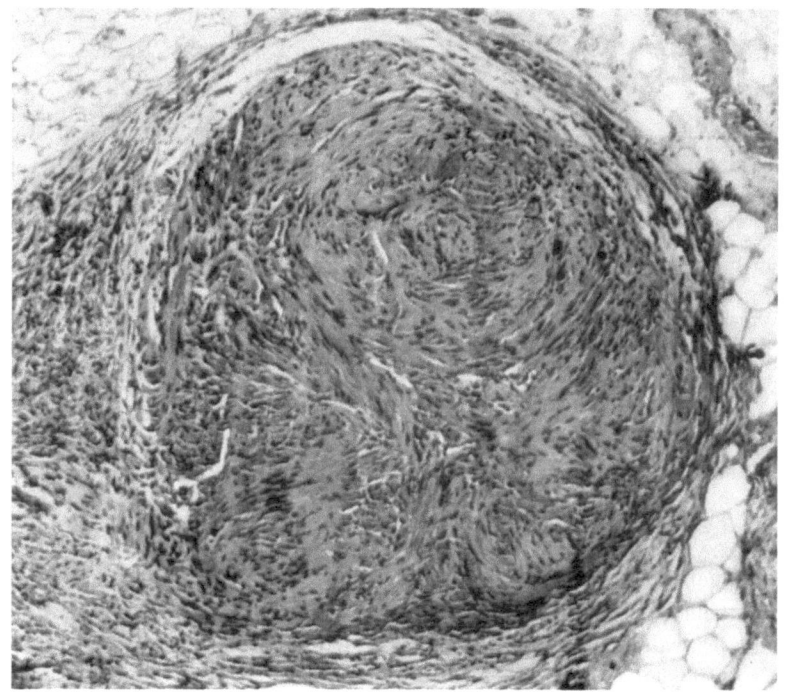

Fig. 199. F 6 20—12

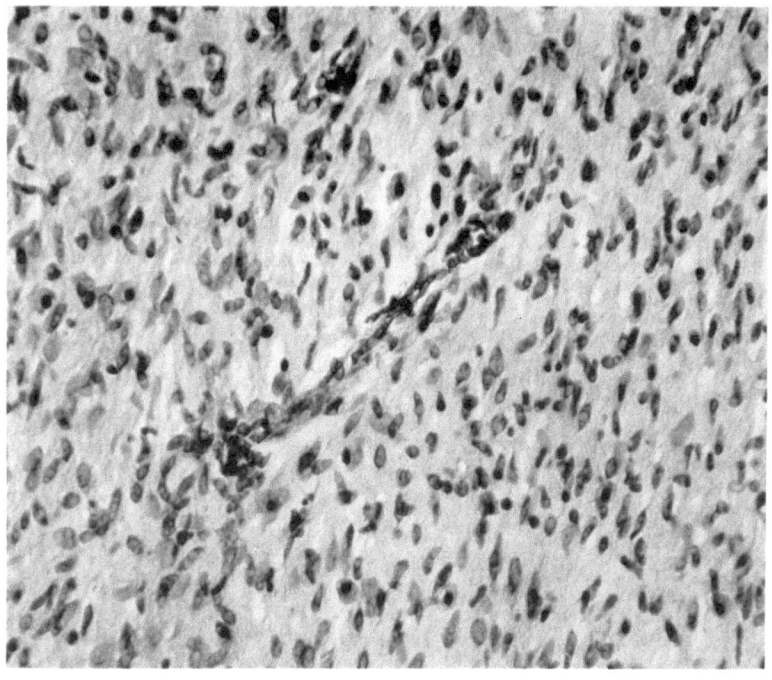

Fig. 200. × 300.

201	Malignant neurinoma	Neurinome malin	Злокачественная невринома
	Malignant neurilemoma	Neurilémome malin	Злокачественная
	Malignant Schwannoma	Schwannome malin	неврилемома
			Злокачественная шваннома
	Bösartiges Neurinom	Neurinoma maligno	Neurinoma malignum
	Bösartiges Neurilemmom	Neurilemoma maligno	Neurilemoma malignum
	Bösartiges Schwannom	Schwannoma maligno	Schwannoma malignum

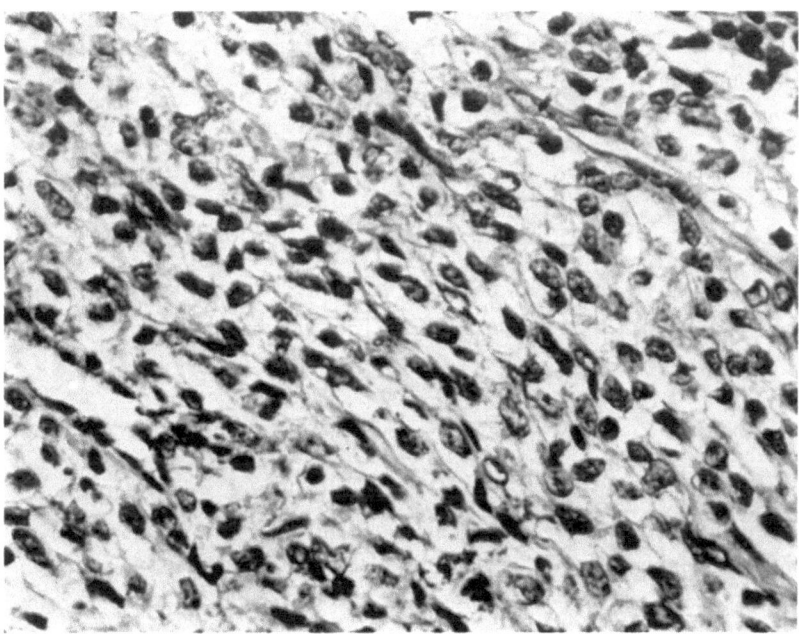

Fig. 201.　× 600.　　　　　　　　　　　　　　　　　F 24 49—35

6. Meninges   Méninges   Мозговые оболочки

   Meningen   Meninges   Meninges   (192)

---

202 Epithelioid meningioma   Méningiome épithéloïde   Эпителиоидная Менингиома
     Meningotheliomatous   Méningiome   Менингоэпителиоматозная
       menigioma   méningothéliomateux   Менингиома
     Endotheliomatous   Méningiome   Эндотелиоматозная
       meningioma   endothéliomateux   Менингиома

     Epitheloides Meningiom   Meningioma epitelíoide   Meningioma epitheloides
                                   Meningioma   Meningioma
                                     meningoteliomatoso   meningotheliomatosum
                                   Meningioma endotelioma-
                                     toso

203 Fibroblastic meningioma   Méningioma à cellules   Фибробластическая
     Fibromatous meningioma   fusiformes   Менингиома
                                   Méningiome fibromateux   Фиброматозная
                                                                    Менингиома

     Fibroblastisches Meningiom   Meningioma fibroblástico   Meningioma fibroblasticum
                                   Meningioma fibromatoso

204 Psammomatous   Méningiome psammomateux   Псаммоматозная
       meningioma   Менингиома

     Psammöses Meningiom   Meningioma psamomatoso   Meningeoma
                                                                    psammomatosum

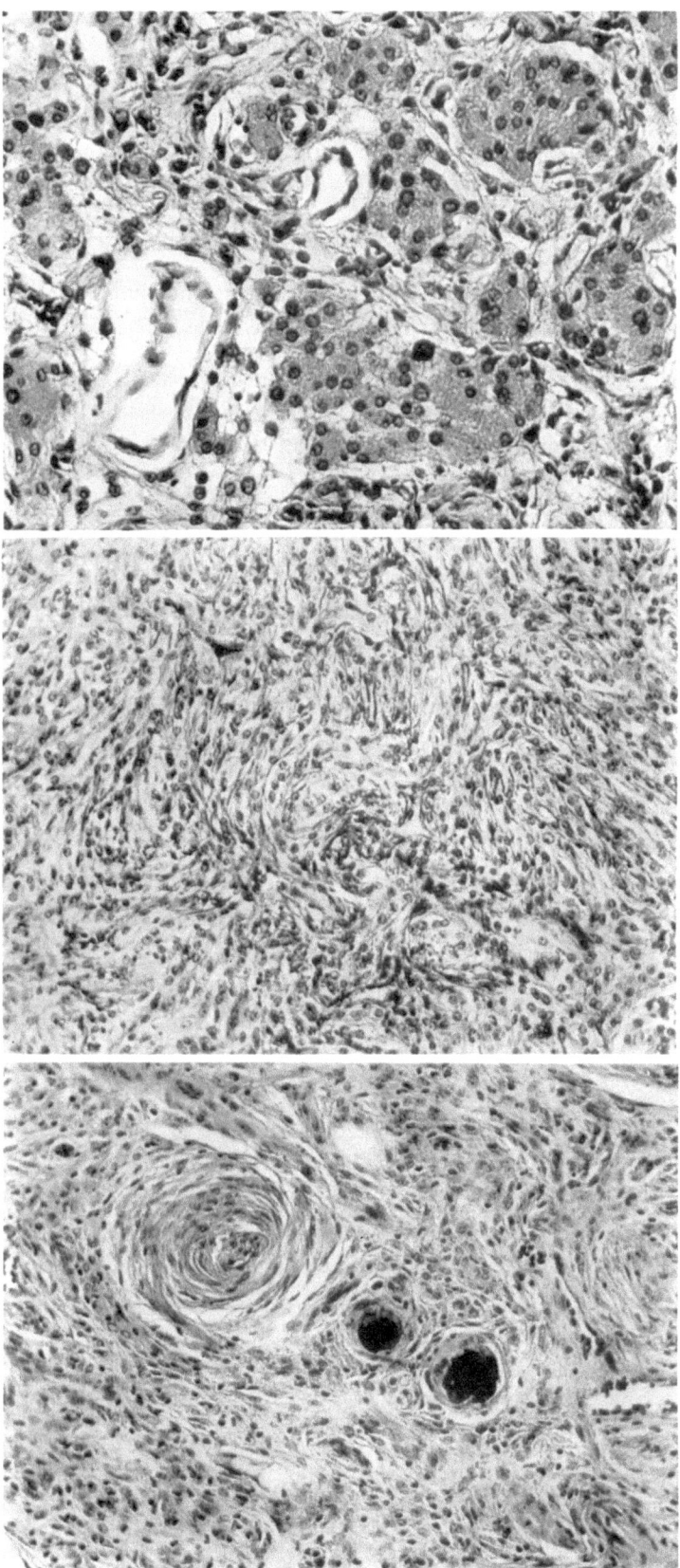

Fig. 202. ×200.
F 35 107—98

Fig. 203. ×135.
F 35 111—106

Fig. 204. ×165.
F 35 111—104

206

7.	Vascular structures of central nervous system	Structures vasculaires du système nerveux central	Сосудистые новообразования в ЦНС	
	Gefäßtumoren des Zentralnervensystems	Estructuras vasculares del sistema nervioso central	Structurae vasculares systematis nervosi centralis	(191)

205	Hemangioma of cerebellum v. Hippel-Lindau's disease	Hémangiome du cervelet Maladie de Hippel-Lindau	Гемангиома мозжечка болезнь Гиппель-Линдау
	Hämangiom des Kleinhirns v. Hippel-Lindausche Krankheit	Hemangioma del cerebelo Enfermedad de von Hippel-Lindau	Haemangioma cerebelli Morbus v. Hippel-Lindau

8.	Paraganglia	Paraganglions	Параганглии	
	Paraganglien	Paraganglios	Paraganglia	(192)

206	Non-chromaffin paraganglioma Carotid body tumor Glomus caroticum tumor Chemodectoma	Paragangliome non chromaffine Paragangliome carotidien et similaires	Нехромаффиновая параганглиома Опухоль каротидного тела Опухоль каротидного гломуса Хемодектома
	Nichtchromaffines Paragangliom Glomus caroticum-Tumor	Paraganglioma no cromafínico Tumor del corpúsculo carotídeo Tumor del glomus caroticum Quemodectoma	Paraganglioma non-chromaffine Tumor glomeris carotici

Some very rare and therefore controversial tumors and terms have not been included such as "astroblastoma", "malignant meningioma", "malignant plexus papilloma", "monstrocellular sarcoma" etc.

Quelques trés rares tumeurs et termes controversés n'ont pas été cités tels que «astroblastomcs», «méningiome malin», «papillome malin du plexus choroïde», «sarcome à cellules monstrueuses» etc.

Некоторые очень редкие и вызывающие споры опухоли и термины, как «астробластома», «злокачественная менингиома», «злокачетвенная папиллома сплетения», «гигантоклеточная саркома» и т. п. в список не включены.

Einige sehr seltene und daher strittige Tumoren und Bezeichnungen, wie z. B. „Astroblastom", „malignes Meningeom", „malignes Plexuspapillom", „monstrozelluläres Sarkom" etc. wurden nicht aufgeführt.

Algunos tumores y términos muy raros y por lo tanto motivos de polémica, no han sido incluídos, tales como "astroblastoma", "meningioma maligno", "papiloma maligno de los plexos coroideos", „sarcoma de células monstruosas", etc.

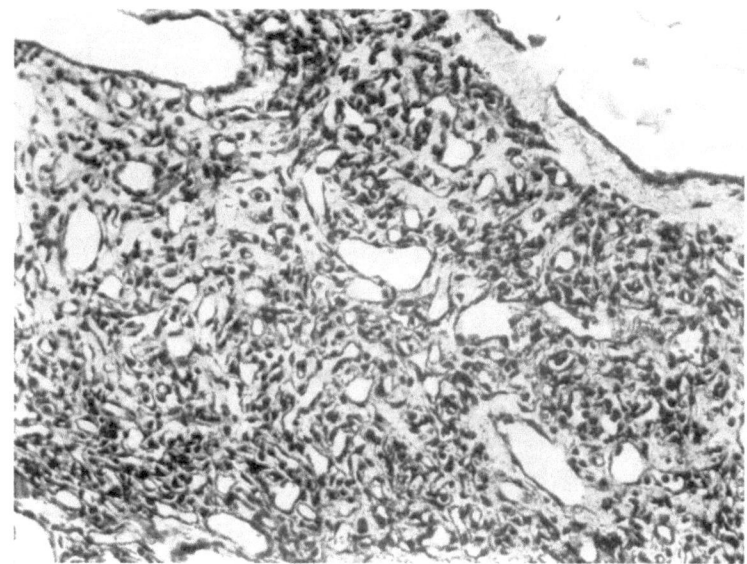

Fig. 205.   × 165.   F 35 95—85

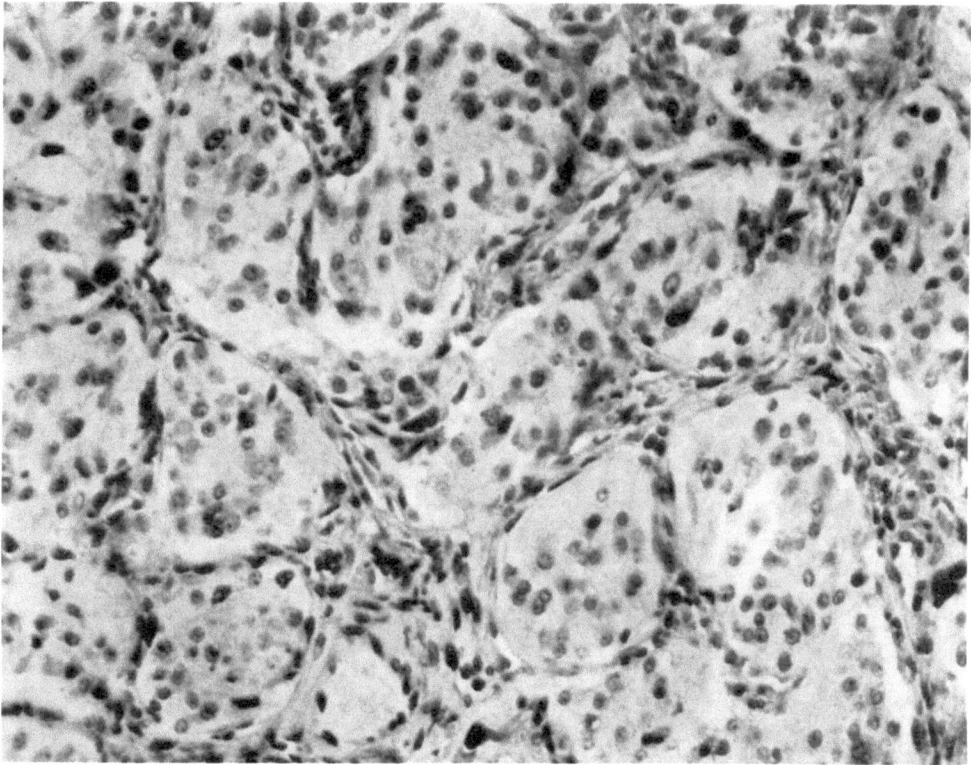

Fig. 206.   × 300.   F 16 19—7

V.

Mesenchymal tumors

Tumeurs mésenchymateuses

Мезенхимальные опухоли

Mesenchymale Tumoren

Tumores mesenquimales

Tumores mesenchymales

1.	Fibrous tissue	Tissu fibreux	Мезенхима	
	Bindegewebe	Tejido fibroso	Thela fibrosa	(171)

207	Fibroma	Fibrome	Фиброма
	Fibrom	Fibroma	Fibroma

208	Desmoid	Tumeur desmoïde	Десмоид
	Invading fibroma	Fibrome envahissant	Инвазивная фиброма
	Desmoid	Desmoide	Tumor desmoides
	Invasives Fibrom	Fibroma invasor	Fibroma invadens

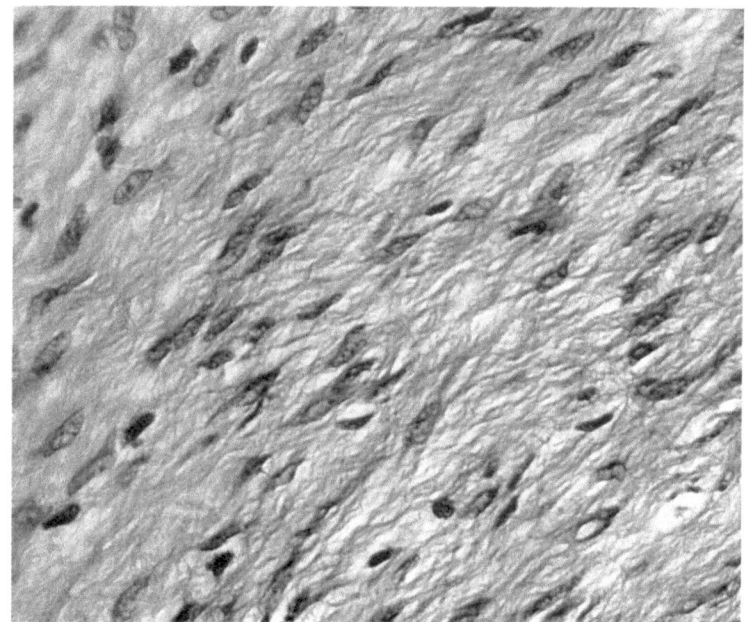

Fig. 207. × 400.   F 4 207—205

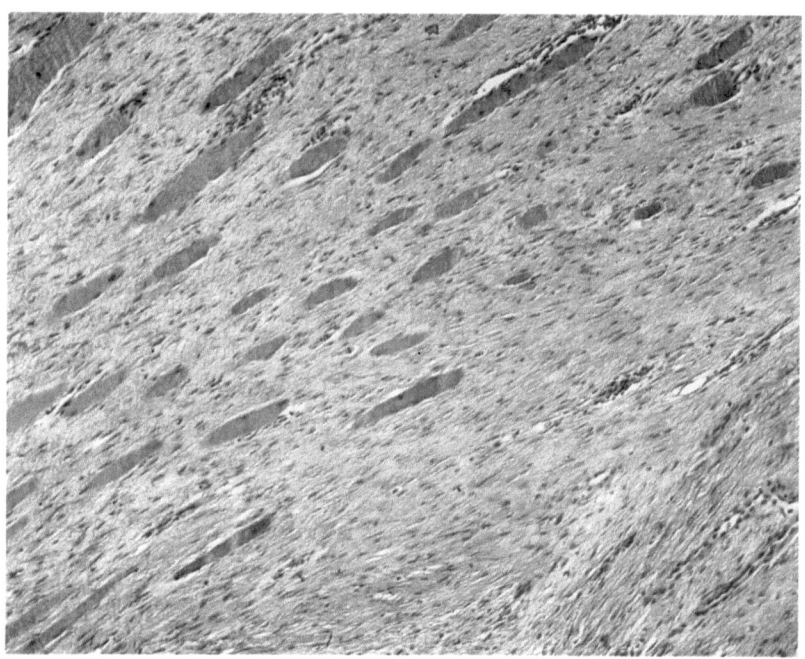

Fig. 208.   A—R 1195—743

212

209   Xanthoma   Xanthome   Ксантома
      Xanthom   Xantoma   Xanthoma

210   Xanthofibroma   Xanthofibrome   Ксантофиброма
      Fibroxanthoma   Fibroxanthome   Фиброксантома
      Histiocytoma   Histiocytome   Гистиоцитома

      Xanthofibrom   Xantofibroma   Xanthofibroma
      Fibroxanthom   Fibroxantoma   Fibroxanthoma
      Histiocytom   Histiocitoma   Histiocytoma
                            Hemangioma esclerosante

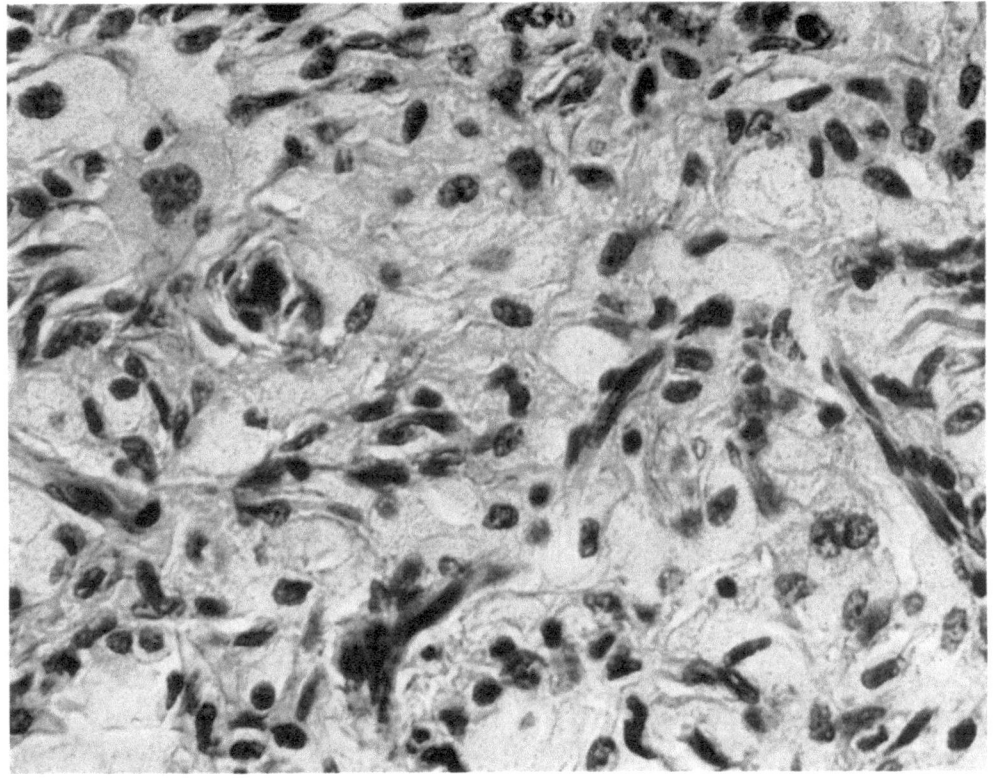

Fig. 209. × 602.   F 5 27—8

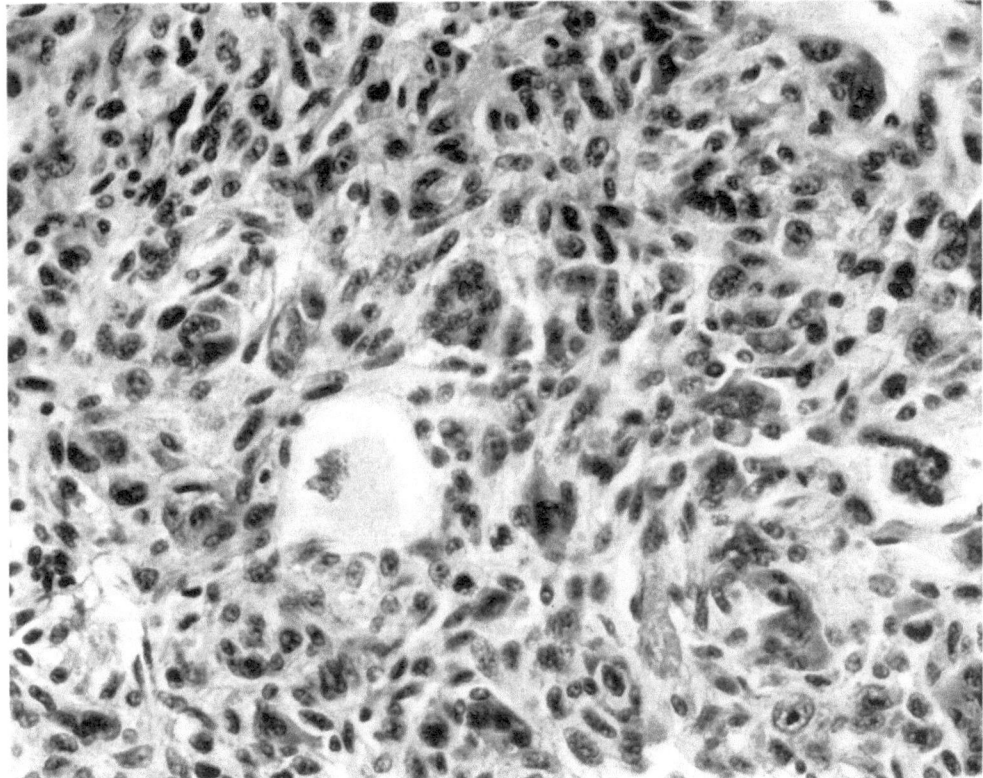

Fig. 210. × 335.   F 2 285—218

211 Subepidermal nodular
    fibrosis

Subepidermale noduläre
    Fibrose

Fibrose nodulaire sous-
    épidermique

Fibrosis Nodular Subepi-
    dérmica

Субэпидермальный
    узловатый фиброз

Fibrosis subepidermoidalis
    nodularis

212 Dermatofibrosarcoma
    protuberans

Dermatofibrosarcoma
    protuberans

Dermatofibrosarcome
    expansif (Fibrosarcome
    de Darier-Ferrand)

Dermatofibrosarcoma
    protuberante

Дерматофибросаркома
    (протуберанс)

Dermatofibrosarcoma
    protuberans

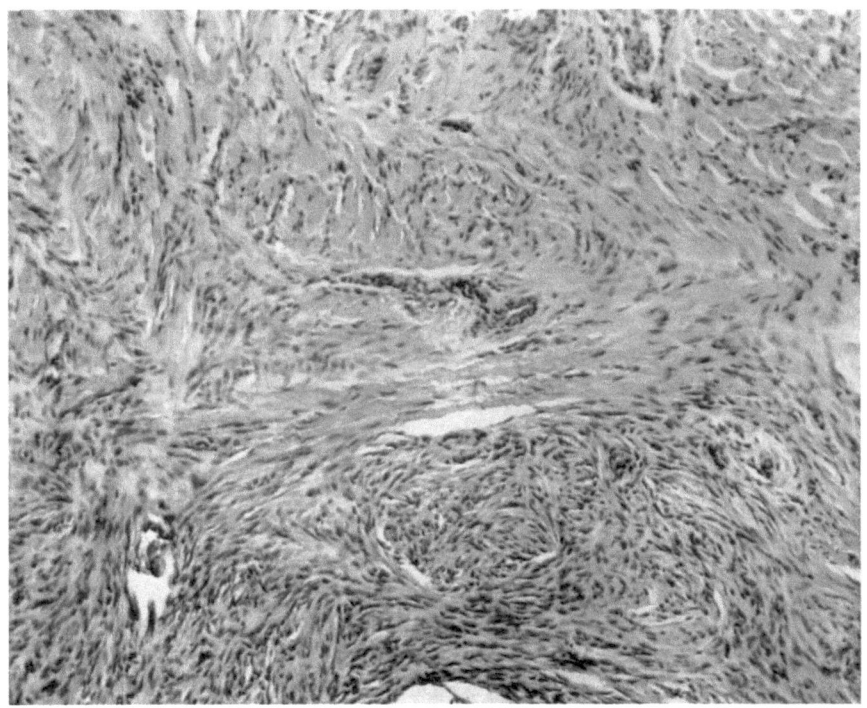

Fig. 211. × 100.

F 2 291—227

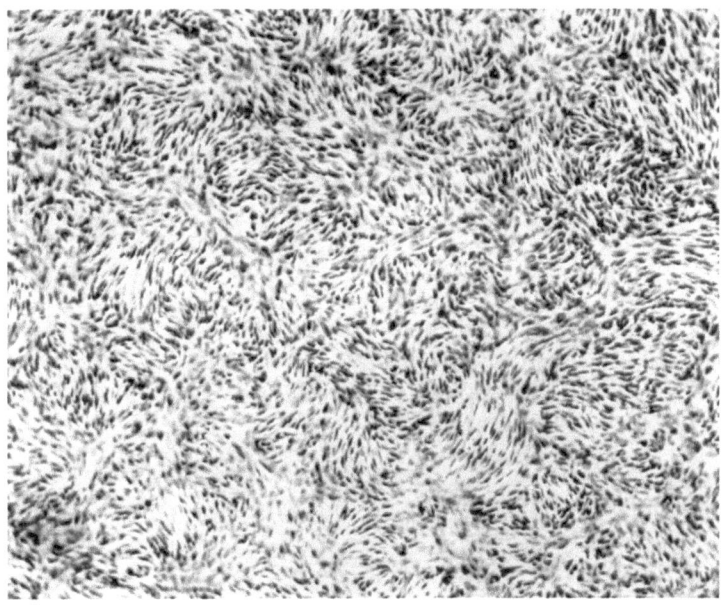

Fig. 212. × 290.

F 2 297—233

213 Fibrosarcoma   Fibrosarcome   Фибросаркома

Fibrosarkom   Fibrosarcoma   Fibrosarcoma

214 Alveolar soft part sarcoma   Sarcome alvéolaire des parties molles   Альвеолярная саркома мягких тканей

Alveoläres Weichteilsarkom   Sarcoma alveolar de tejidos blandos   Sarcoma alveolare molle

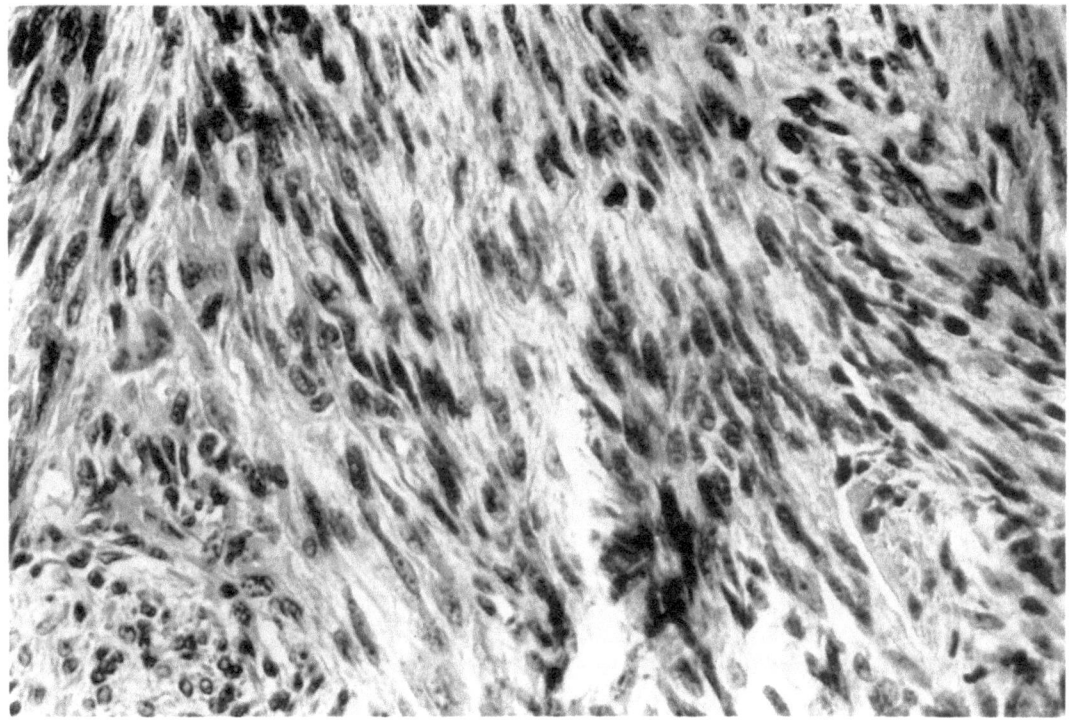

Fig. 213. × 511.   F 5 75—45

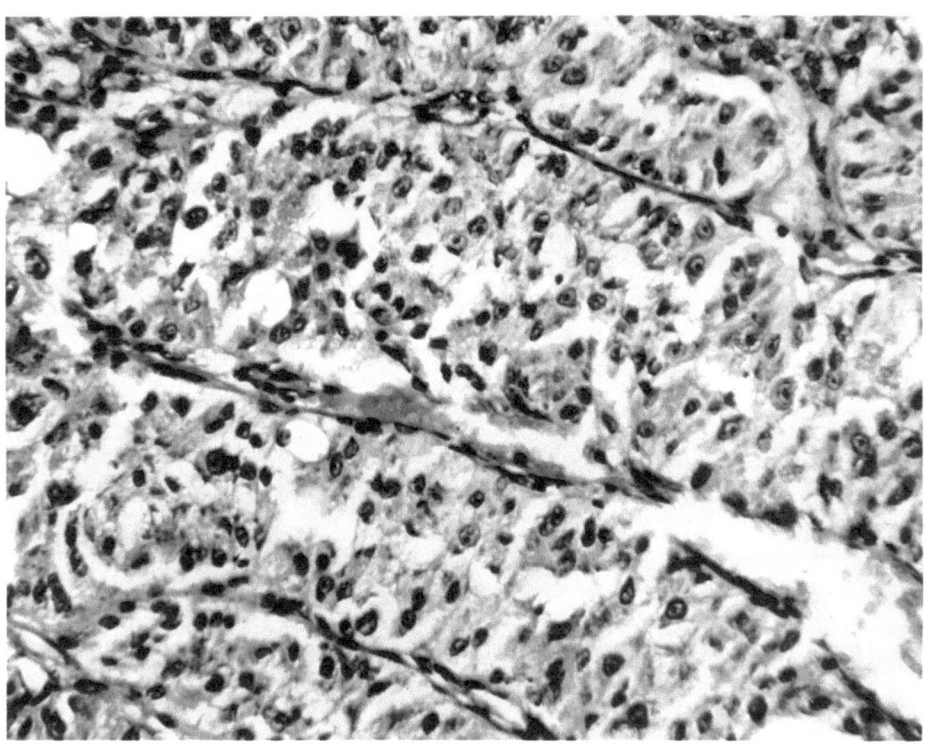

Fig. 214. × 300.

2. Mucoid tissue   Tissu mucoïde   **Слизеобразующая ткань**

   Schleimbildendes Gewebe   Tejido mucoide   Thela mucoides   (171)

3. Fat tissue   Tissu adipeux   **Жировая ткань**

   Fettgewebe   Tejido adiposo   Thela adiposa   (171)

215   Myxoma   Myxome   Миксома

      Myxom   Mixoma   Myxoma

216   Lipoma   Lipome   Липома

      Lipom   Lipoma   Lipoma

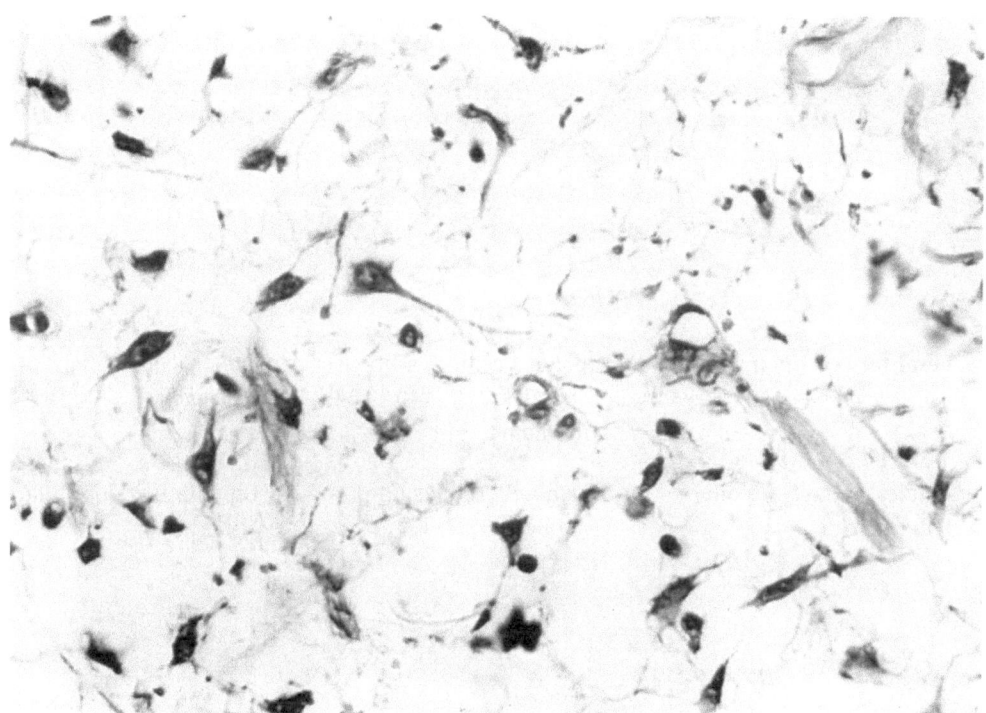

Fig. 215.   F 5 77—48

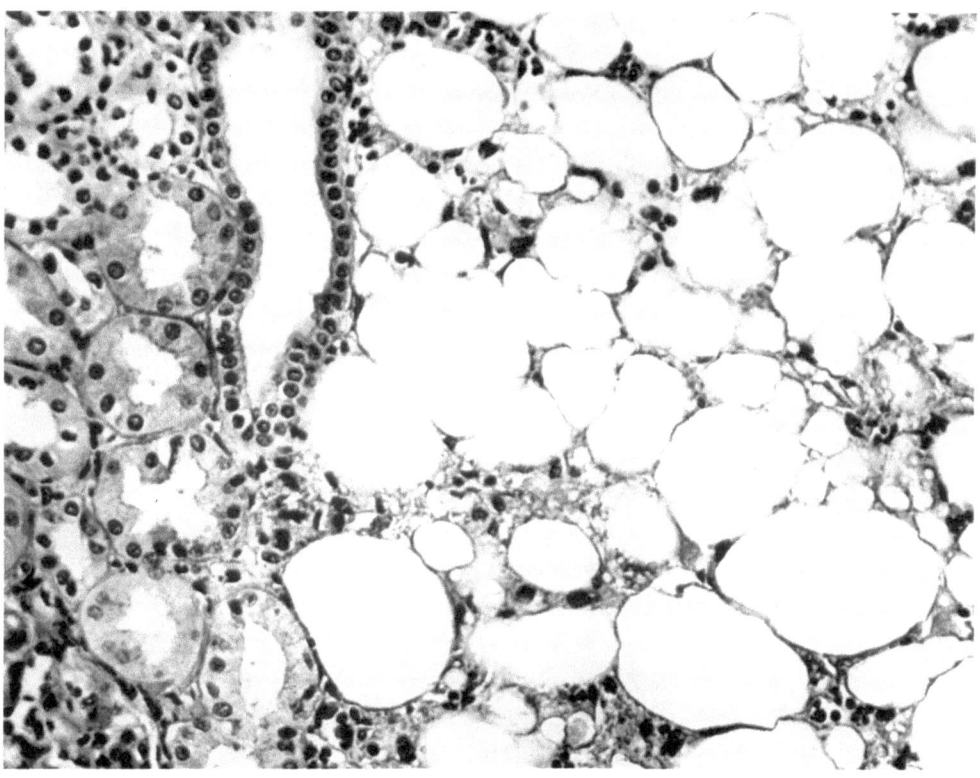

Fig. 216. × 275.   F 30 127—110

217 Fetal fat cell lipoma

Lipome à cellules adipeuses
foetales
Hibernome

Фетальная липома
Гибернома

Fetales Fettzell-Lipom
Hibernom

Lipoma de células adiposas
fetales
Hibernoma

Lipoma foetalocellulare
Hibernoma

218 Liposarcoma

Liposarcome

Липосаркома

Liposarkom

Liposarcoma

Liposarcoma

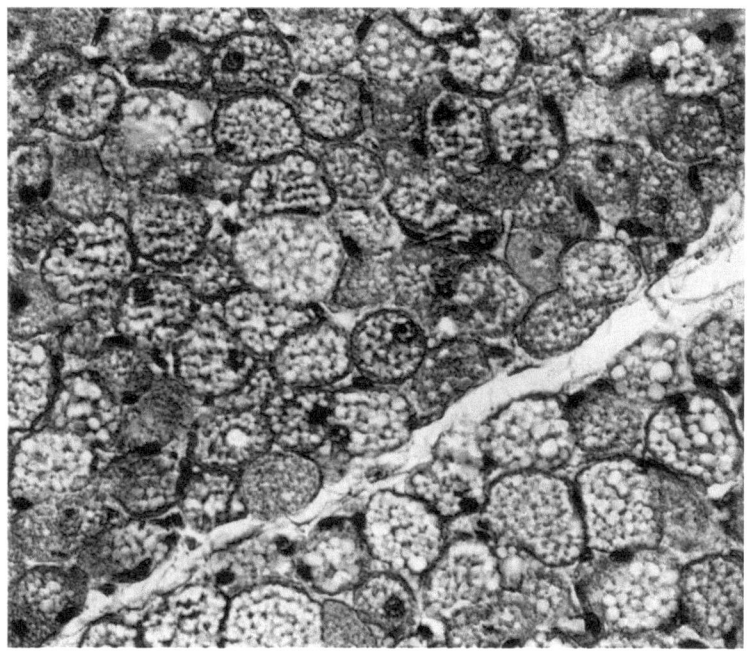

Fig. 217. × 480.   A 852—915

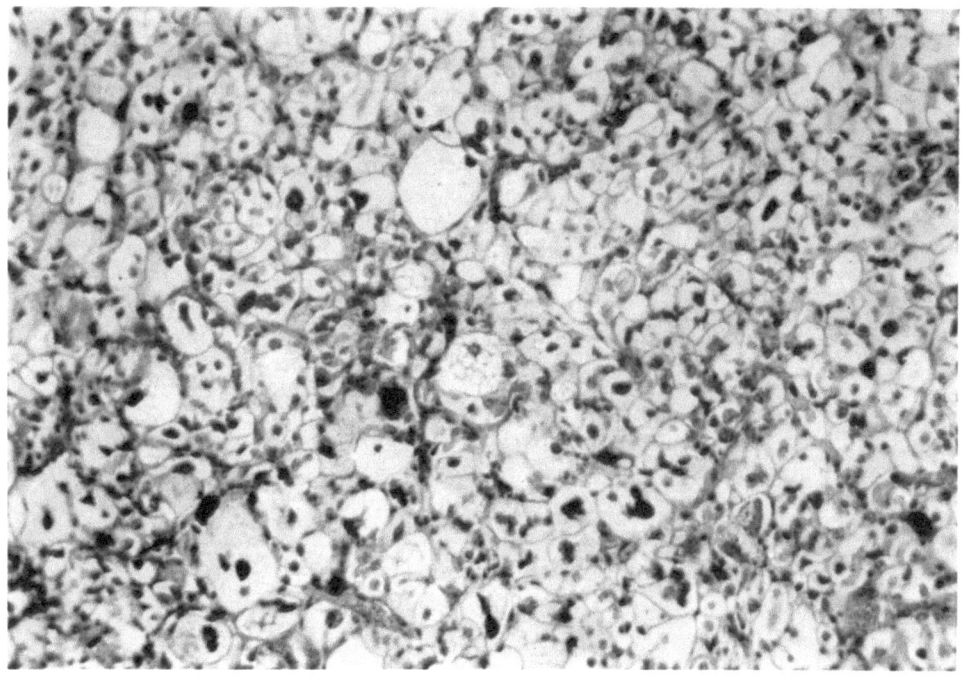

Fig. 218.   F 34 77—44

4.	Muscle tissue	Tissu musculaire	Мышечная ткань	
	Muskelgewebe	Tejido muscular	Thela muscularis	(171)

219	Leiomyoma	Léiomyome	Лейомиома
	Leiomyom	Leiomioma	Leiomyoma

220	Rhabdomyoma	Rhabdomyome	Рабдомиома
	Rhabdomyom	Rabdomioma	Rhabdomyoma

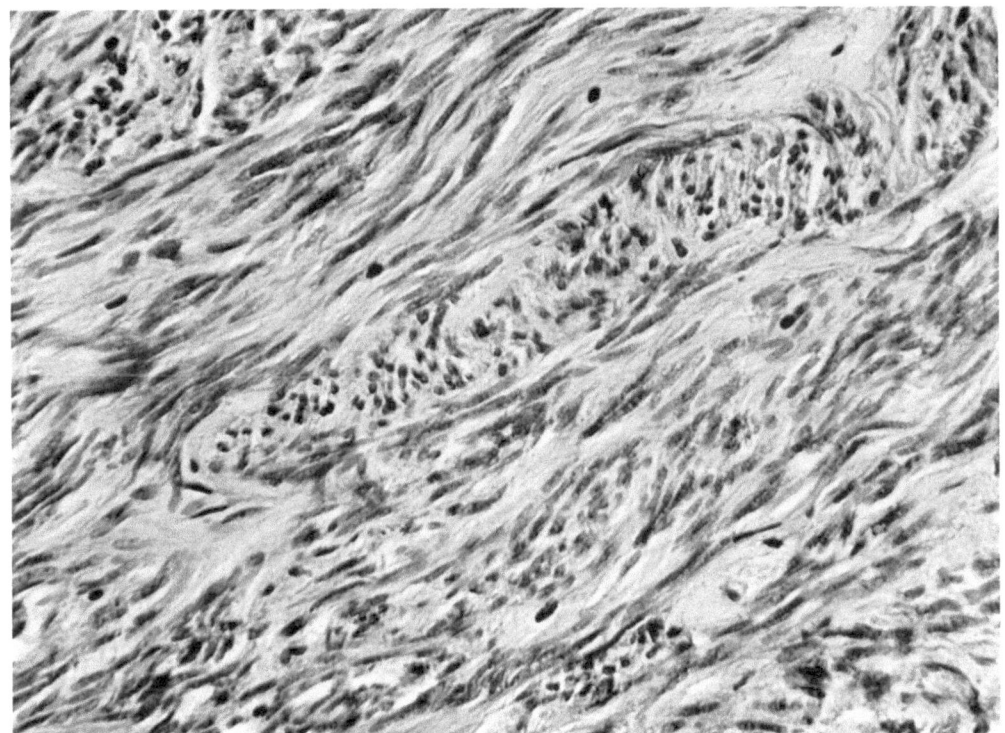

Fig. 219. × 350.

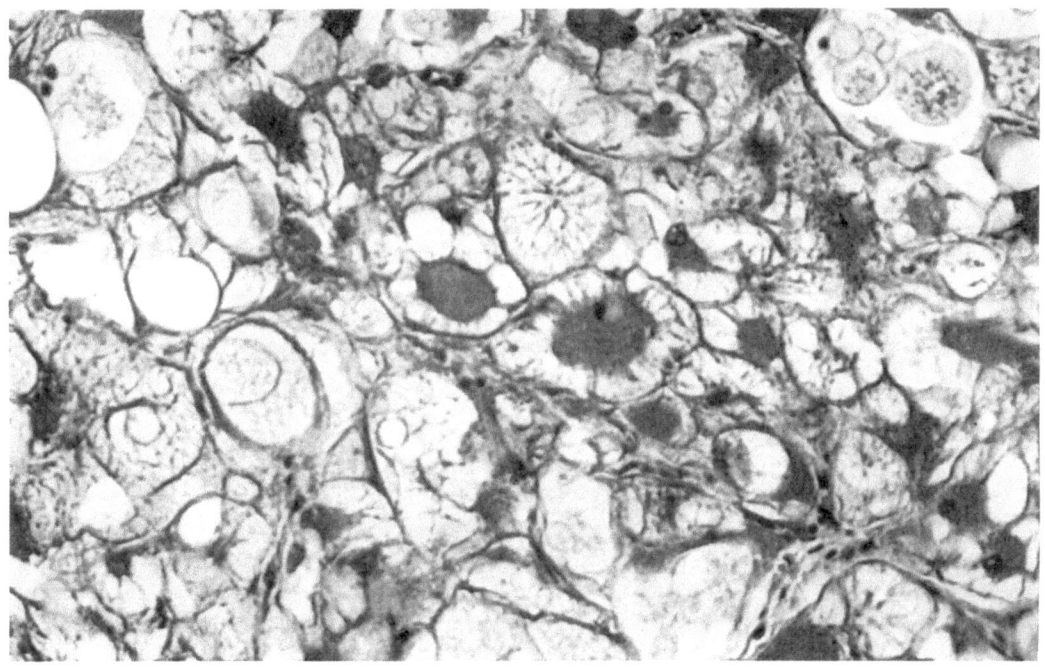

Fig. 220.

221   Granular cell myoblastoma   Myoblastome à cellules   Зернистоклеточная
                                               granuleuses   миобластома (мио-
                                                                                                   бластомиома)

       Gekörnt-zelliges Myobla-   Mioblastoma de células   Myoblastoma granulo-
         stom (Myoblastenmẏom)   granulosas   cellulare

222   Leiomyosarcoma   Léiomyosarcome   Лейомиосаркома

       Leiomyosarkom   Leiomiosarcoma   Leiomyosarcoma

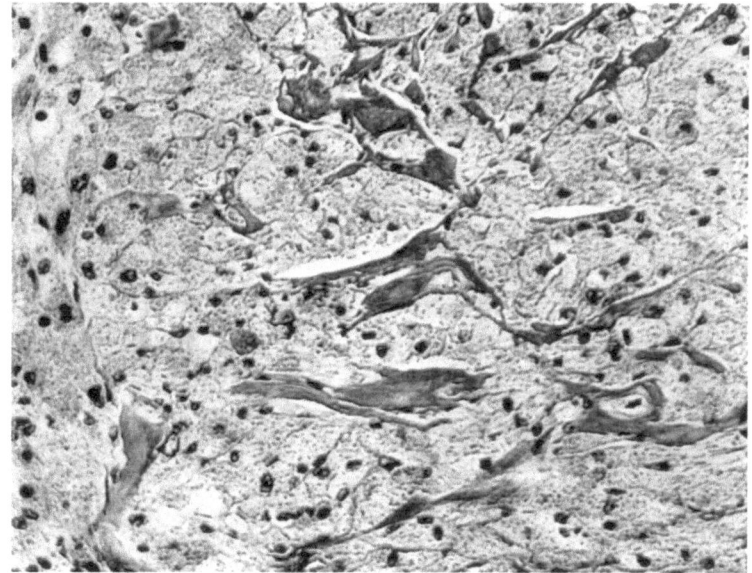

Fig. 221. × 226.   F 5 43—20

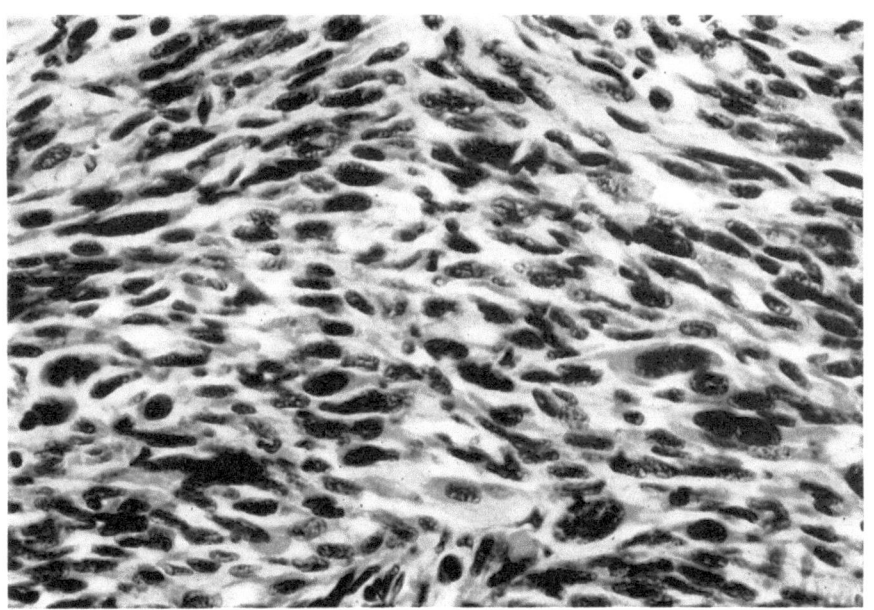

Fig. 222. × 300.

223 Rhabdomyosarcoma   Rhabdomyosarcome   Рабдомиосаркома
       alveolar   alveolaire
       botryoid   botryoïde

     Rhabdomyosarkom   Rabdomiosarcoma   Rhabdomyosarcoma
                                 alveolar   alveolare
                                 botrioide   bothryoides

224 Malignant granular cell   Myoblastome malin à   Злокачественная зернисто-
       myoblastoma   cellules granuleuses   клеточная миобластома
                                                           (Злокачественная мио-
                                                           бластомиома)

     Bösartiges gekörnt-zelliges   Mioblastoma maligno de   Myoblastoma granulo-
       Myoblastom (Malignes   células granulosas   cellulare malignum
       Myoblastenmyom)

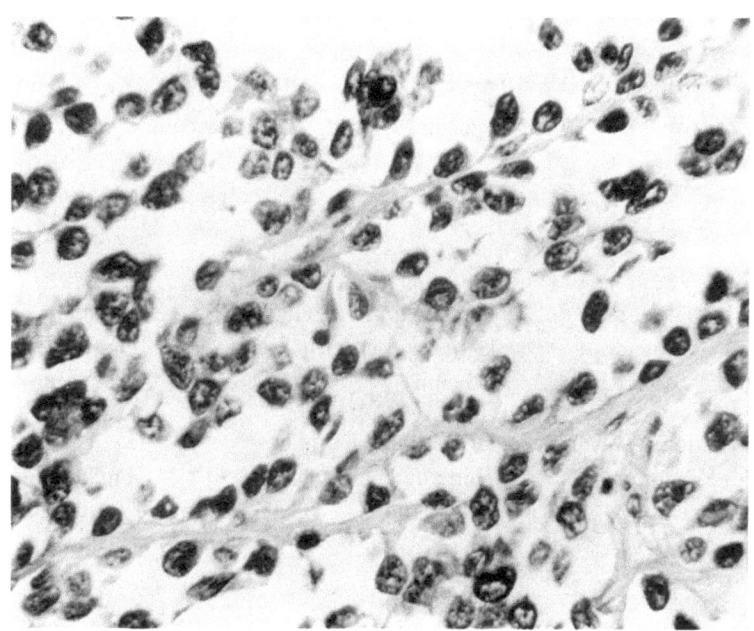

Fig. 223.   × 770.   A 859—926

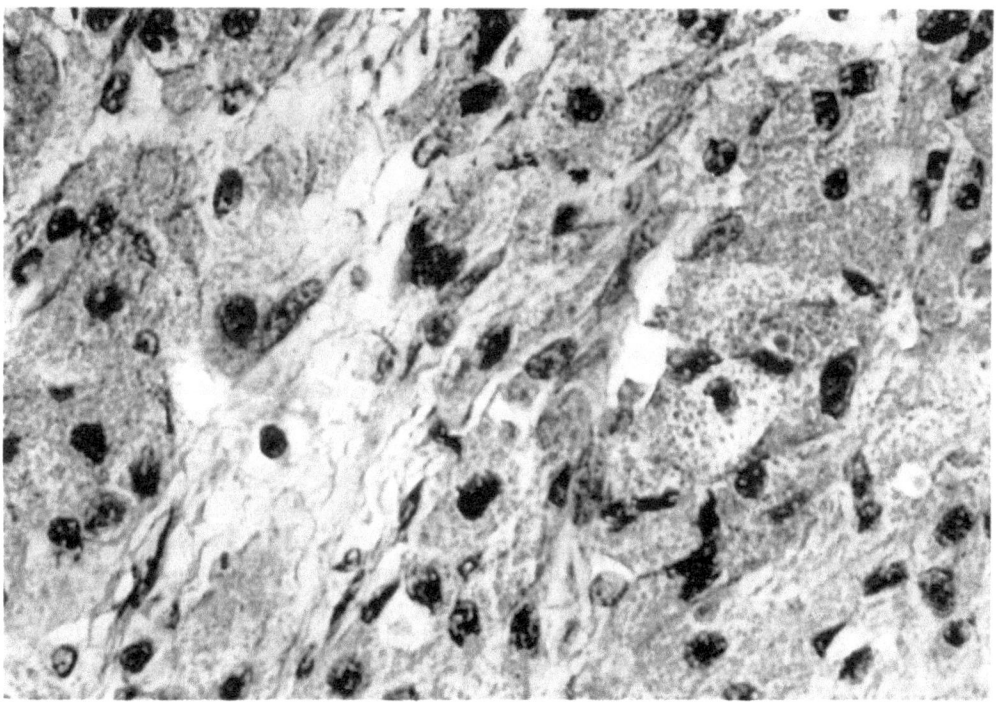

Fig. 224.   × 600.   F 5 97—60

15*

5. Vascular tissue   Tissu vasculaire   Сосуды

     Gefäße   Tejido vascular   Thela vascularis   (171)

225	Capillary hemangioma Benign hemangioendo- thelioma	Hémangiome capillaire Hémangio-endothéliome bénin	Капиллярная гемангиома Доброкачественная гемангиоэндотелиома
	Capilläres Hämangiom Gutartiges Hämangio- endotheliom	Hemangioma capilar Hemangioendotelioma benigno	Haemangioma capillare Haemangioendothelioma benignum
226	Cavernous (venous) hemangioma Cavernoma	Hémangiome caverneux (veineux) Cavernome	Кавернозная гемангиома Кавернома
	Kavernöses Hämangiom Kavernom	Hemangioma cavernoso Cavernoma	Haemangioma cavernosum (venosum) Cavernoma
227	Arterial hemangioma Arteriovenous angioma Hemangioma racemosum	Hémangiome artériel Angiome artério-veineux Hémangiome racémeux	Артериальная гемангиома Артериовенозная ангиома Рацемозная гемангиома
	Arterielles Hämangiom Arterio-venöses Angiom Haemangioma racemosum	Hemangioma arterial Angioma arteriovenoso Hemangioma racemoso	Haemangioma arteriale Angioma arteriovenosum Haemangioma racemosum

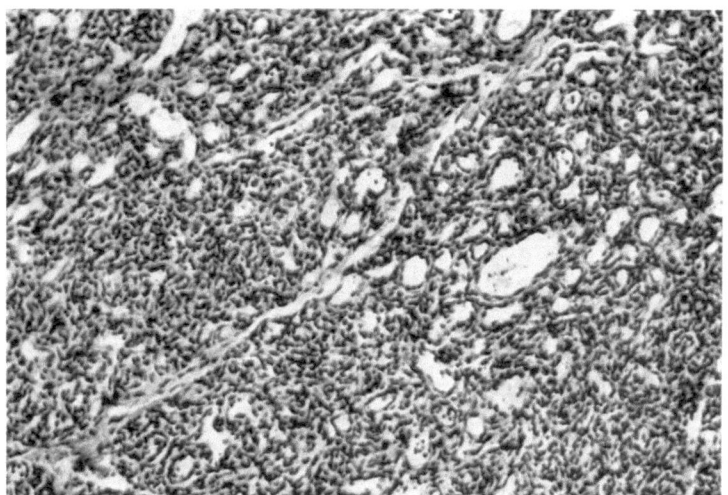

Fig. 225. × 120.
F 7 55—41

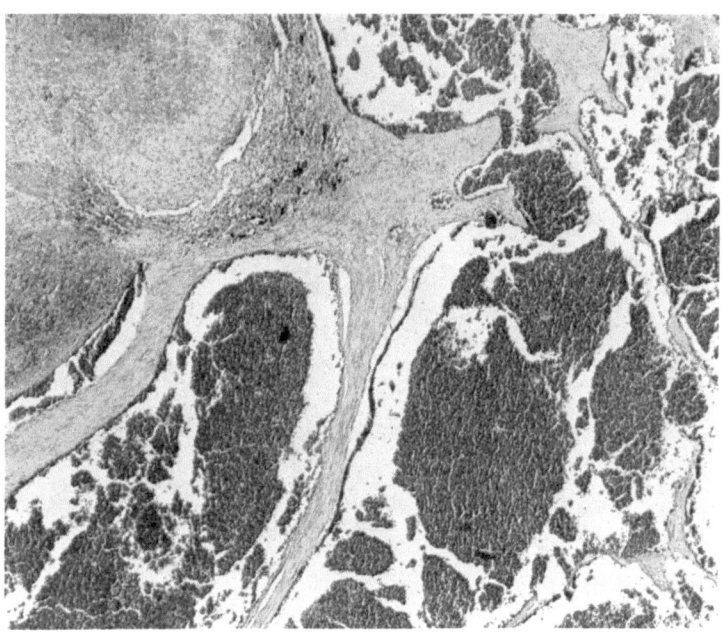

Fig. 226. × 300.

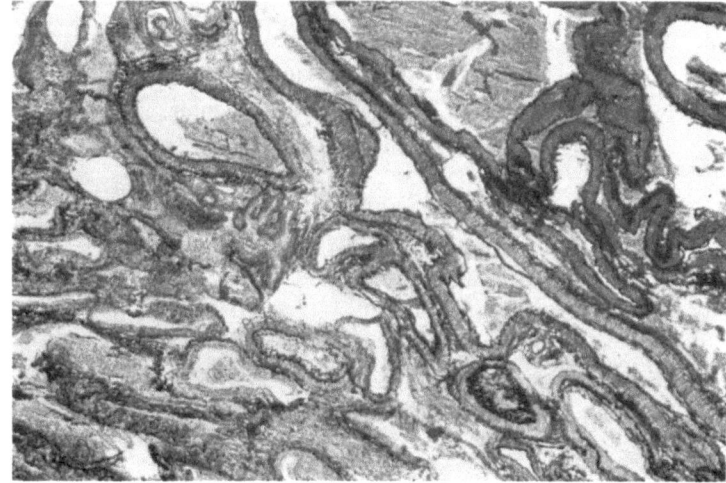

Fig. 227.
F 7 59—45

228 Lymphangioma
Cystic hygroma

Lymphangiom
Cystisches Hygrom

Lymphangiome
Hygroma cystique

Linfangioma
Higroma quístico

Лимфангиома
Кистозная гигрома

Lymphangioma
Hygroma cysticum

229 Glomus tumor
Glomangioma

Glomus-Tumor
Glomangiom

Tumeur glomique
Glomangiome

Tumor glómico
Glomangioma

Гломическая опухоль
Гломангиома

Glomus tumor
Glomangioma

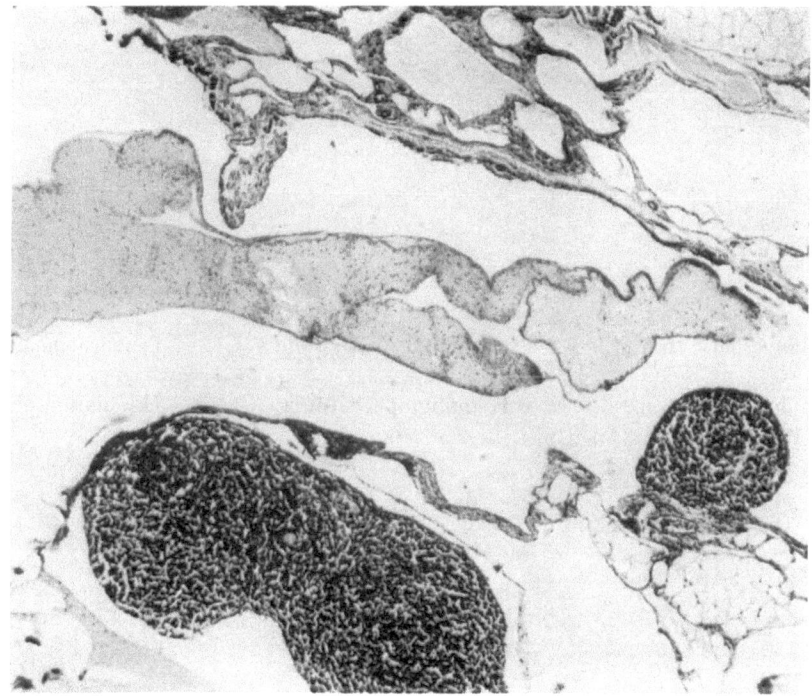

Fig. 228. × 48. F 24 27—15

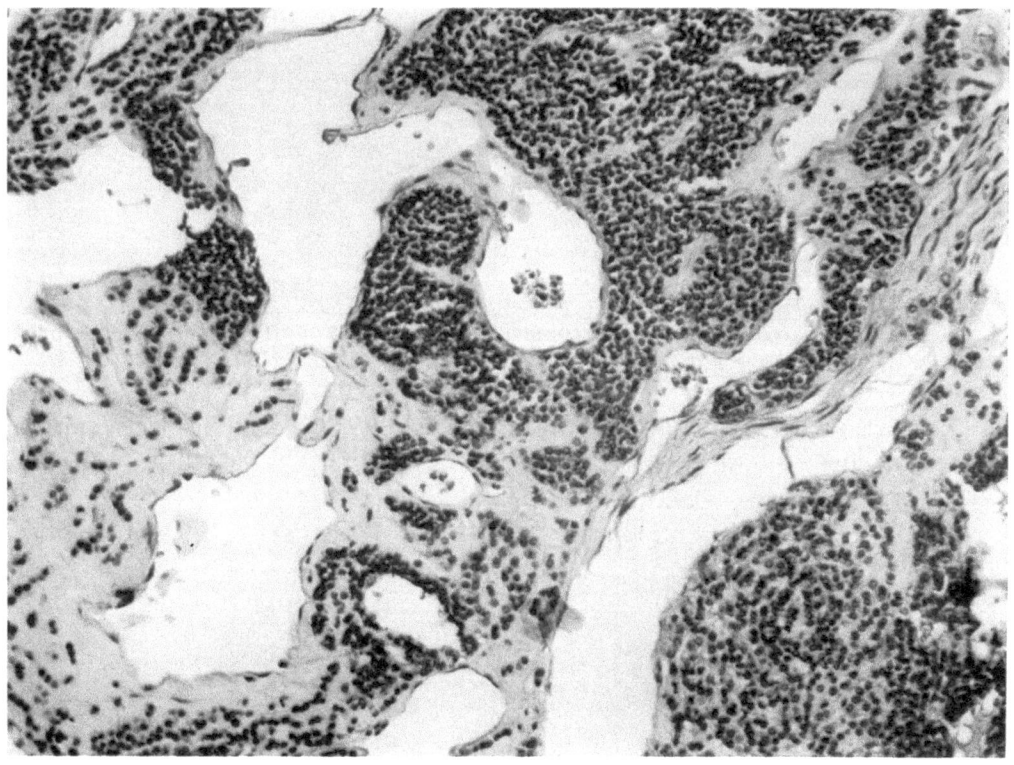

Fig. 229. × 180. F 21 41—25

230 Hemangiopericytoma Hémangio-péricytome Гемангиоперицитома

   Hämangiopericytom Hemangiopericitoma Haemangiopericytoma

231 Hemorrhagic sarcoma Sarcome hémorragique Геморрагическая саркома
   (Kaposi)   (Kaposi)   (Капози)

   Hämorrhagisches Sarkom Sarcoma hemorrágico Sarcoma haemorrhagicum
   (Kaposi)   (Kaposi)   (Kaposi)

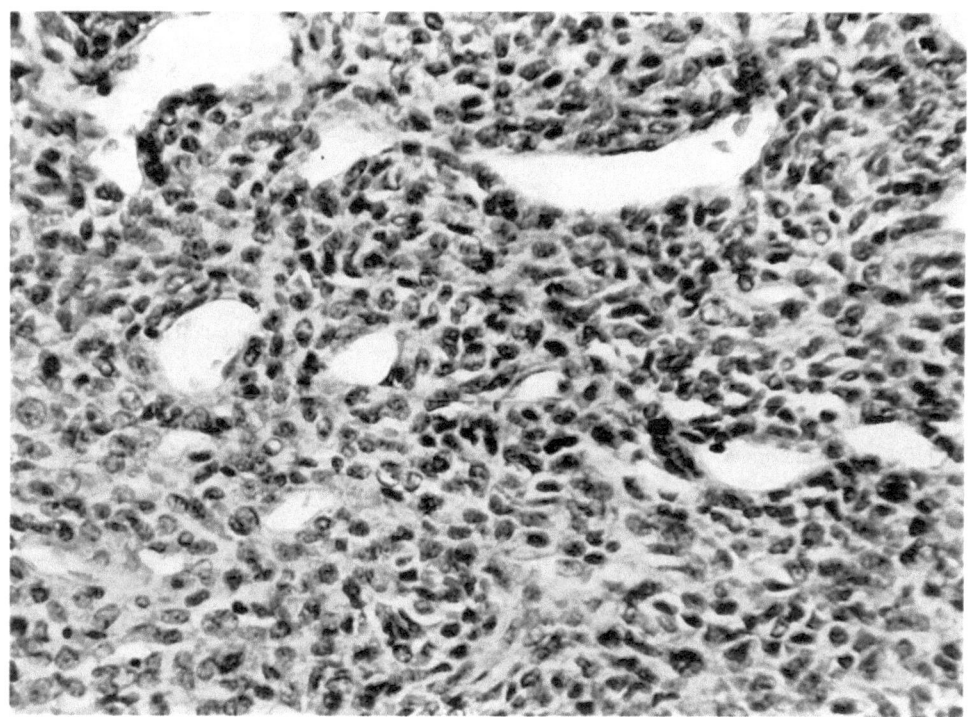

Fig. 230. ×. 350.

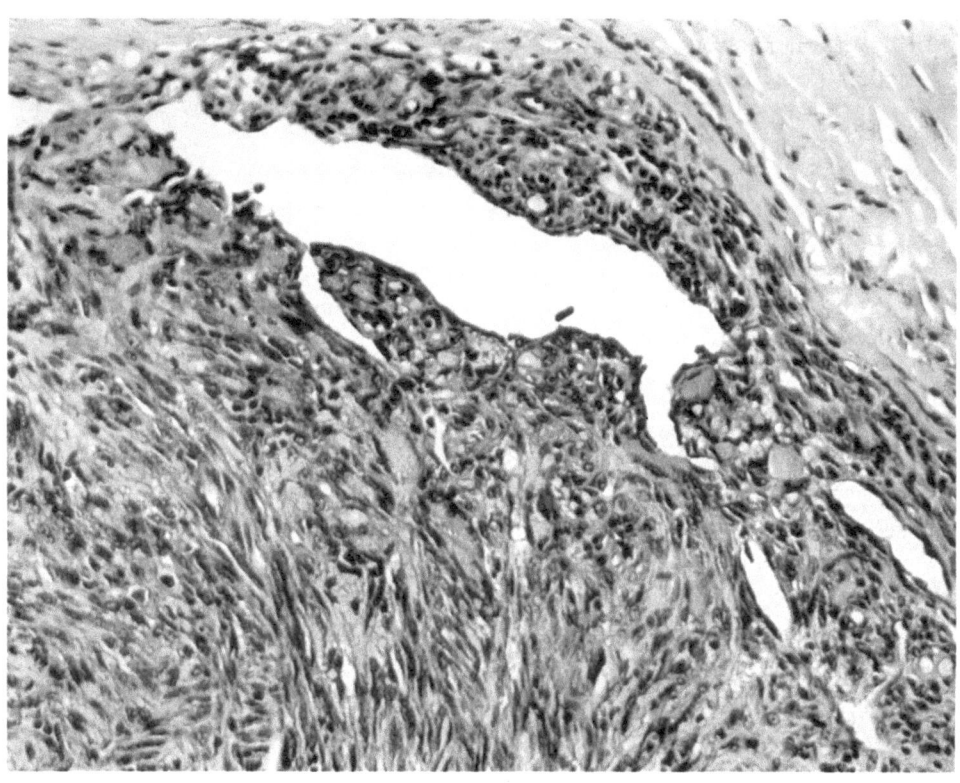

Fig. 231. × 310.

232	Malignant hemangioendothelioma Hemangiosarcoma	Hémangio-endothéliome malin Hémangiosarcome	Злокачественная гемангиоэндотелиома Гемангиосаркома
	Bösartiges Hämangioendotheliom Hämangiosarkom	Hemangioendotelioma maligno Hemangiosarcoma	Haemangioendothelioma malignum Haemangiosarcoma
233	Malignant hemangiopericytoma	Hémangio-péricytome malin	Злокачественная гемангиоперицитома
	Bösartiges Hämangiopericytom	Hemangiopericitoma maligno	Haemangiopericytoma malignum

Some benign and malignant mesenchymal tumors may contain different components such as muscular, fibrous, mucoid, vascular, and fat tissue. Such tumors should be called according their components e.g. myofibroma, myxoliposarcoma etc.

Certaines tumeurs mésenchymateuses bénignes et malignes peuvent contenir différents composants tissulaires tels que tissus musculaire, fibreux, mucoïde, vasculaire ou adipeux. Ces tumeurs devront être intitulées selon leurs constituants p. ex. myofibrome, myxoliposarcome etc.

Некоторые доброкачественные и злокачественные мезенхимные опухоли могут содержать разные компоненты, как напр. мышечную, соединительную, слизеобразующую, сосудистую, жировую ткани. Такие опухоли должны называться соответственно их тканевому составу, как напр. миофиброма, миксолипосаркома и т. п.

Manche mesenchymalen Tumoren können verschiedene Anteile enthalten, wie z. B. Muskel-, Schleim-, Gefäß- und Fett-Gewebe. Solche Tumoren sollten entsprechend ihren Anteilen etwa als „Myofibrom", „Myxoliposarkom" etc. bezeichnet werden.

Algunos tumores mesenquimales benignos y malignos pueden contener diferentes componentes, tales como tejido muscular, fibroso, mucoide, vascular y adiposo. Tales tumores deben ser denominados de acuerdo con sus componentes: ej. miofibroma, mixoliposarcoma, etc.

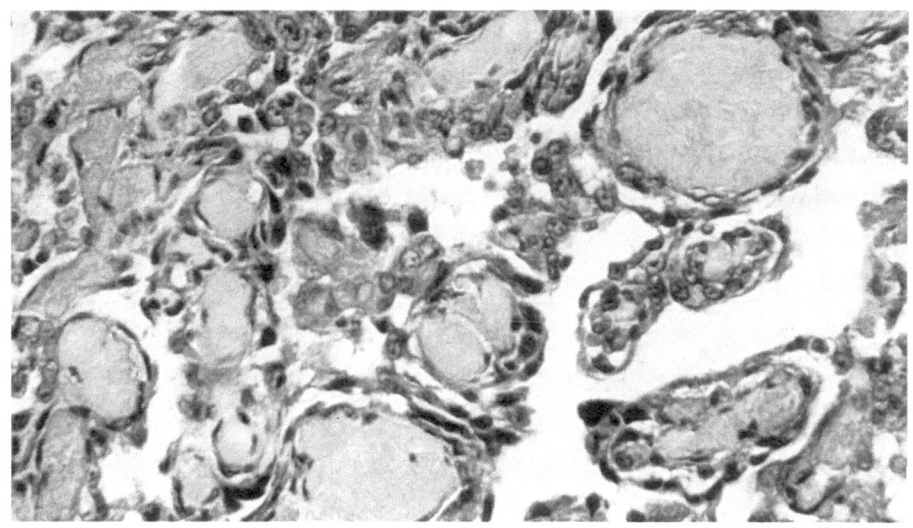

Fig. 232. × 350.   F 4 245—253

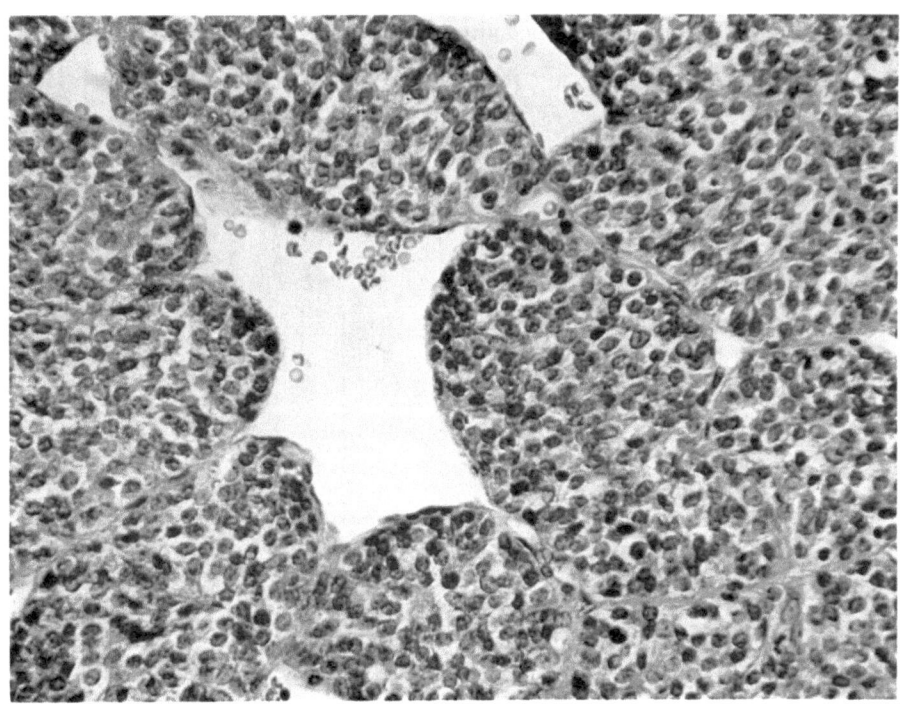

Fig. 233. × 350.

6. **Skeletal tissues**
(Bone, cartilage, notochord)

Tissus squelettogènes
(Os, cartilage, chorde dorsale)

Скелет
(Кости, хрящ, хорда)

Skelet
(Knochen, Knorpel, Chorda)

Tejidos del esqueleto
(Huesos, cartílagos, notocorda)

Thelae ossium
(Os, cartilago, chorda)

(170)

234   Chondroma
Enchondroma

Chondrom
Enchondrom

Chondrome
Enchondrome

Condroma
Encondroma

Хондрома
Энхондрома

Chondroma
Enchondroma

235   Osteochondroma

Osteochondrom

Ostéo-chondrome

Osteocondroma

Остеохондрома

Osteochondroma

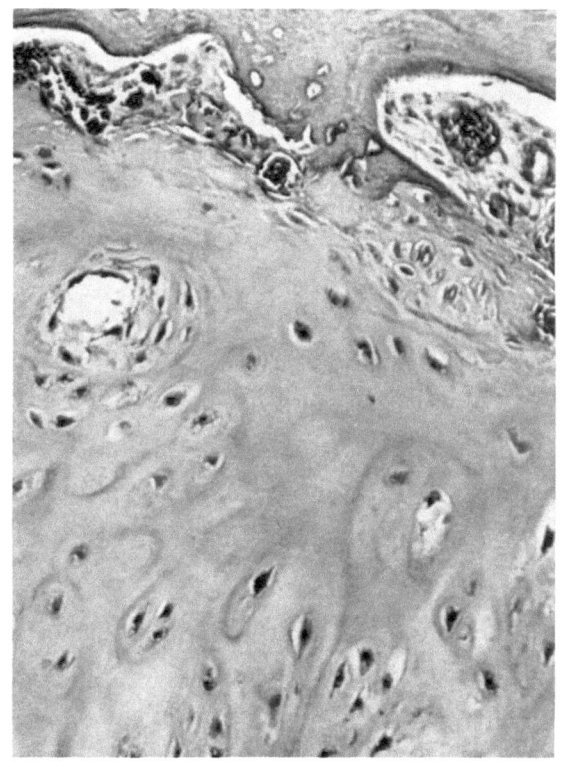

Fig. 234.　× 175.　　　　　　　　　F 4 55—47

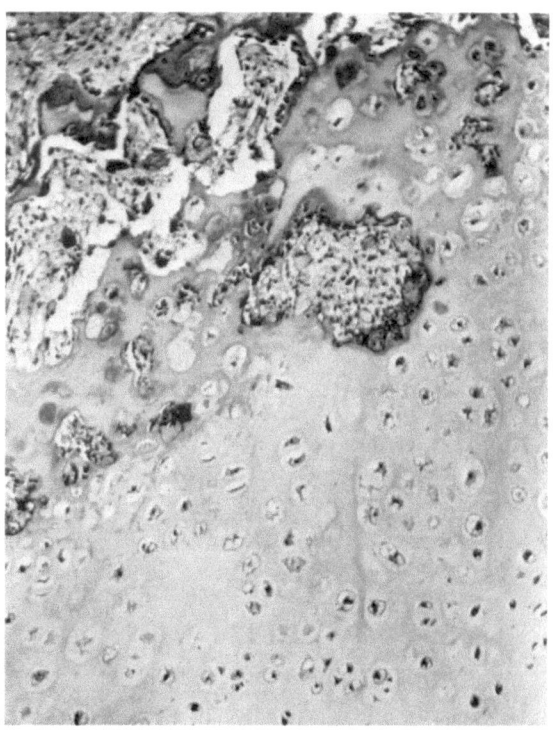

Fig. 235.　× 125.　　　　　　　　　F 4 49—36

236 Chondroblastoma (benign) (Codman)

Chondroblastome (bénin) (Codman)

Хондробластома (доброкачественная) (Кодмэн)

Chondroblastom (gutartig)

Condroblastoma (benigno)

Chondroblastoma (benignum)

237 Chondromyxoid fibroma

Fibrome chondro-myxoïde

Хондромиксоидная фиброма

Chondromyxoides Fibrom

Fibroma condromixoide

Fibroma chondromyxoides

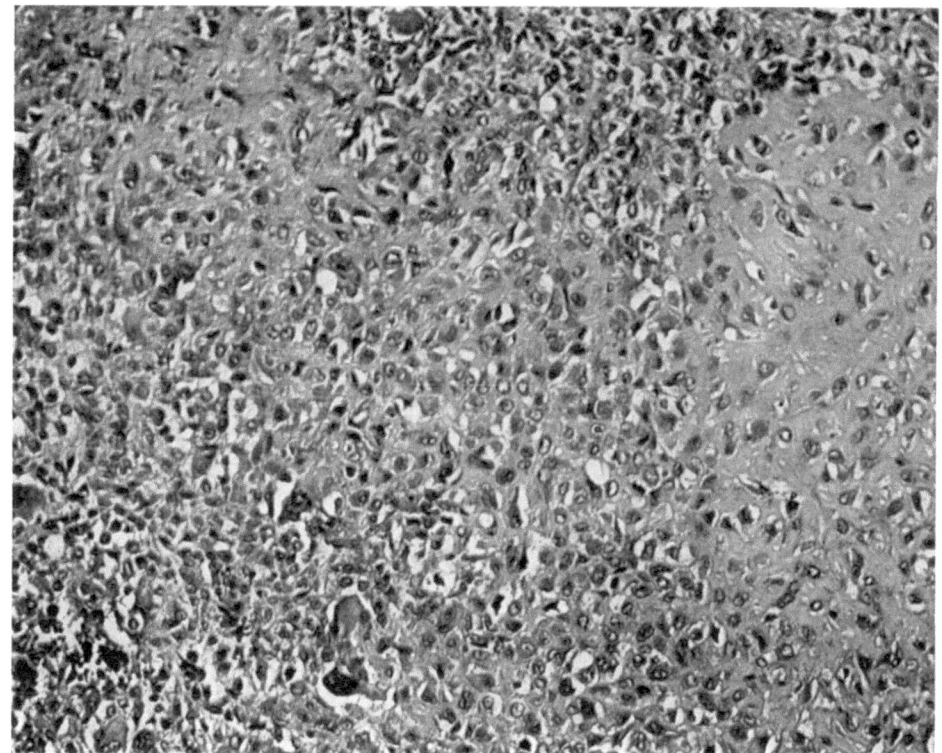

Fig. 236.   × 165.   F 4 29—8

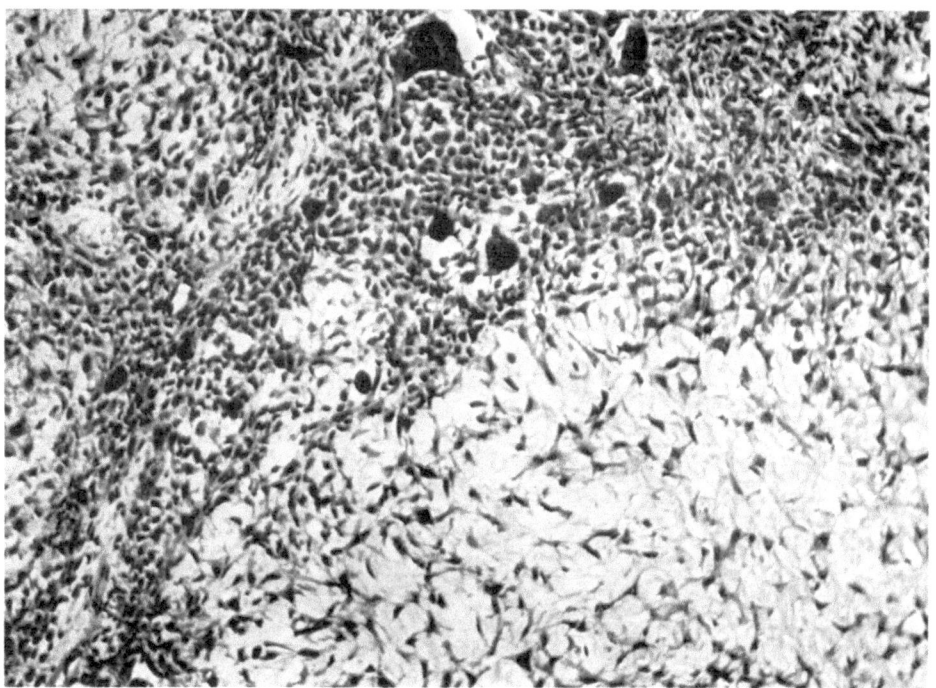

Fig. 237.   × 150.   F 4 43—27

238 Osteoma	Ostéome	Остеома
Osteom	Osteoma	Osteoma

239 Osteoid-Osteoma	Ostéome ostéoïde	Остеоидная остеома
Osteoidosteom	Osteoma osteoide	Osteoma osteoides

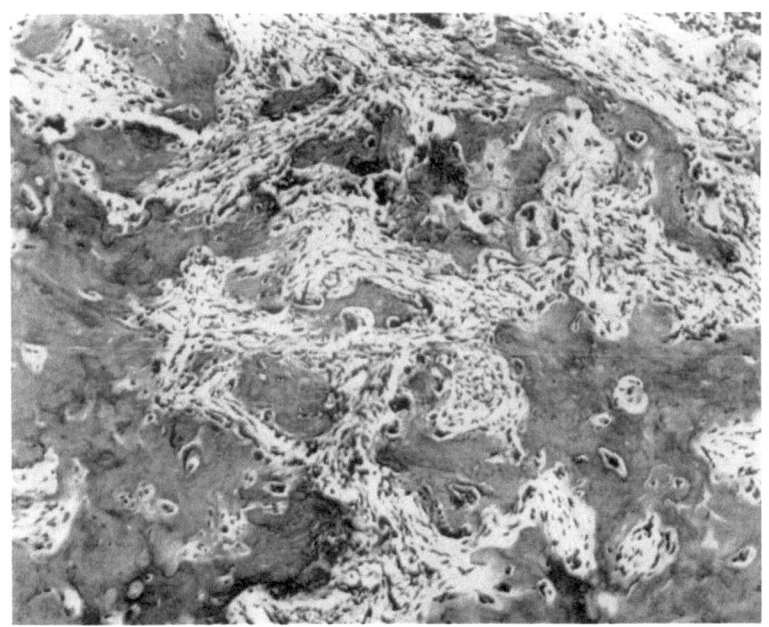

Fig. 238. × 400.   Li 84—40B

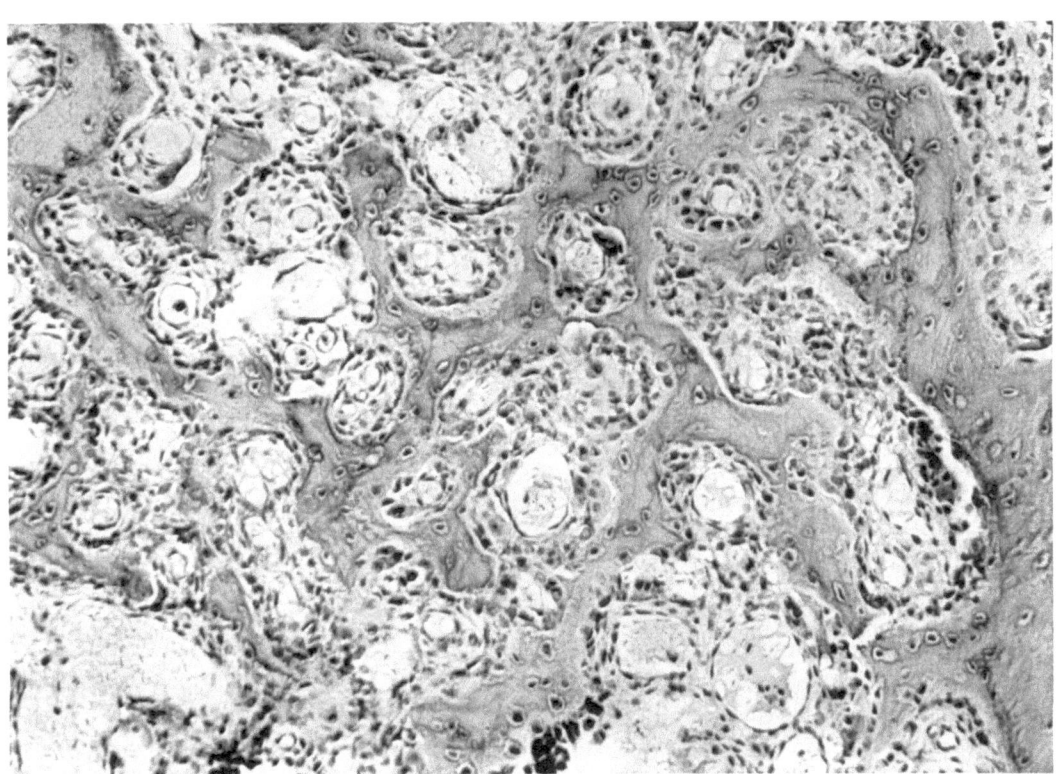

Fig. 239. × 175.   F 4 105—92

240 Non-osteogenic fibroma Fibrome non ostéogénique Неостеогенная фиброма
Metaphyseal fibrous defect «Metaphyseal fibrous Фиброзный дефект
defect» метафиза

Nichtosteogenes Fibrom Fibroma no osteogénico Fibroma non osteogenes
Fibröser Metaphysendefekt Defecto fibroso metafisario Defectum metaphysis
fibrosum

241 Giant cell tumor* Tumeur à cellules géantes* Гигантоклеточная опухоль*
Osteoclastoma Ostéoclastome Остеокластома
Myelogenic giant cell tumor Tumeur à myéloplaxes Миэлогенная гигантокле-
точная опухоль

Riesenzelltumor (Epulis)* Tumor de células gigantes* Tumor gigantocellularis
Osteoklastom Osteoclastoma (Epulis)
Myelogener Riesenzell- Tumor mielogénico de Osteoclastoma
tumor células gigantes

---

* Giant cell tumors may behave as malignant neoplasms. Only when fibrosarcomatous changes occur can the diagnosis of malignancy be made with confidence.

* La tumeur à cellules géantes peut avoir un comportement malin. Le diagnostic de malignité ne peut être posé qu'en présence d'un stroma fibro-sarcomateux.

* Малигнизация гигантоклеточных опухолей — возможно. Только при наличии изменений типа фибросаркомы можно с уверенностью утверждать злокачественность процесса.

* Riesenzelltumoren können sich wie maligne Geschwülste verhalten. Die Diagnose der Malignität kann aber nur mit einiger Sicherheit gestellt werden, wenn fibrosarkomatöse Veränderungen vorhanden sind.

* Los tumores de células gigantes pueden comportarse como neoplasias malignas. Sólo cuando occuren cambios fibrosarcomatosos el diagnóstico de malignidad se puede hacer con certeza.

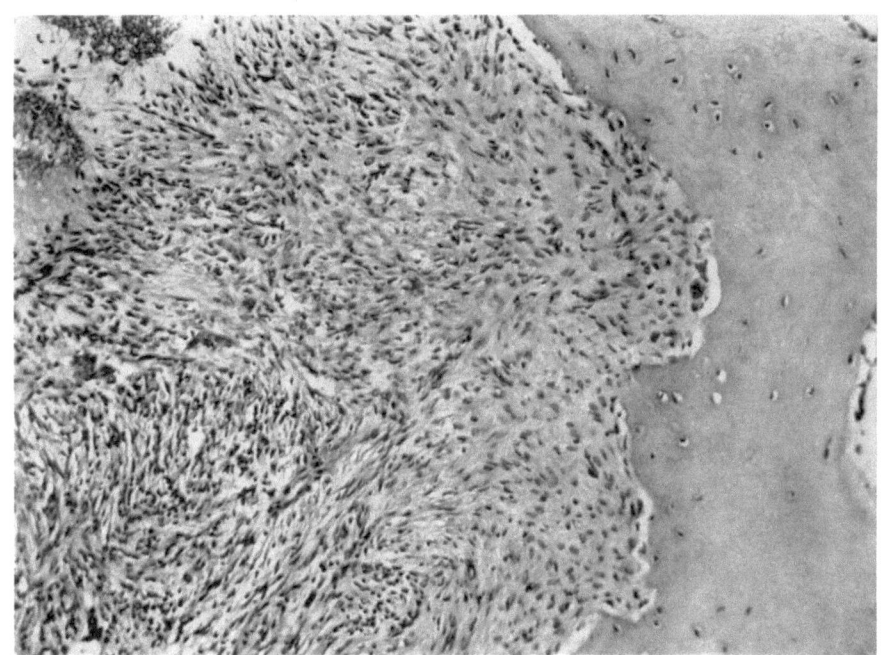

Fig. 240. × 120.   F 4 317—318

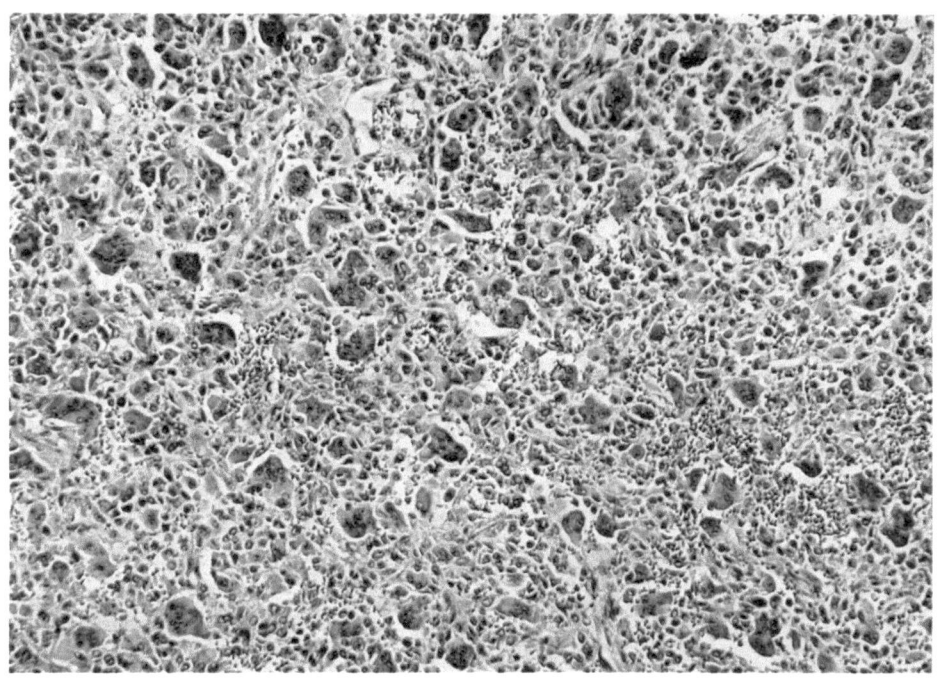

Fig. 241. × 150.

244

Osteogenic sarcoma (244—247):
Sarcome ostéogénique (244—247):
Остеогенная саркома (244—247):
Osteogenes Sarkom (244—247):
Sarcoma osteogénico (244—247):
Sarcoma osteogenes (244—247):

242	Osteosarcoma	Sarcome ostéoïde	Остеоидная Саркома
	Osteoides Sarkom	Sarcoma osteoide	Sarcoma osteoides

243	Chondroid sarcoma	Sarcome chondroïde	Хондроидная Саркома
	Chondroides Sarkom	Sarcoma condroide	Sarcoma chondroides

244	Fibrous, mucoid sarcoma or combinations thereof	Sarcome fibreux ou mucoïde ou mixte	Фиброзная, мукозная, Саркома или их комбинации
	Fibröses, muköses Sarkom oder Kombination davon	Sarcoma fibroso, mucoide o combinado	Sarcoma fibrosum mucoides et combinationes

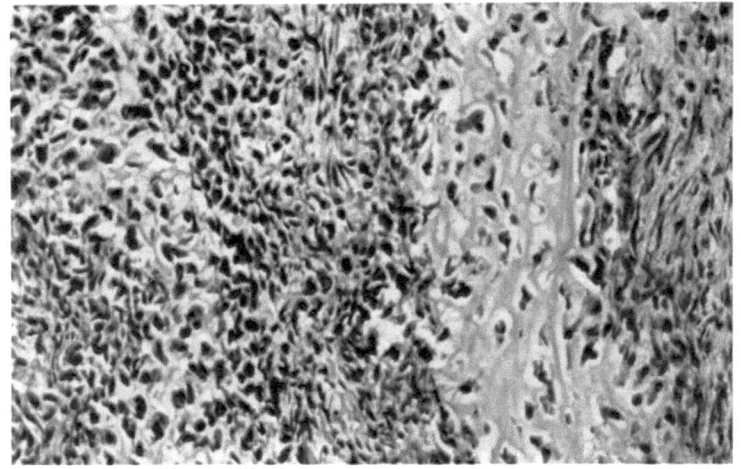

Fig. 242. × 180.   F 4 121—112

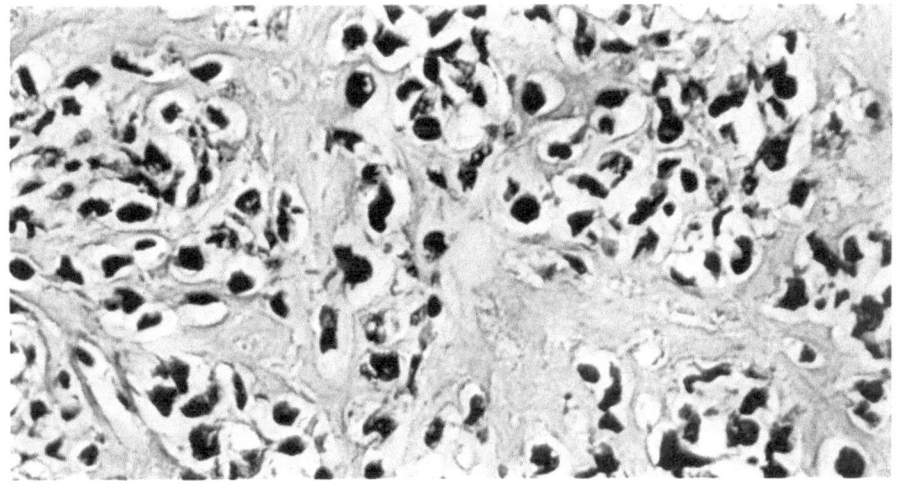

Fig. 243. × 300.   F 4 127—123

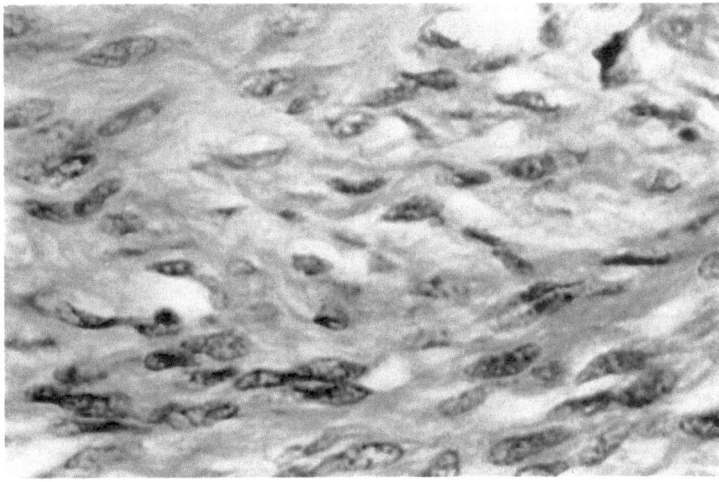

Fig. 244. × 615.   F 4 125—119

245 **Chondrosarcoma**   Chondrosarcome   Хондросаркома

Chondrosarkom   Condrosarcoma   Chondrosarcoma

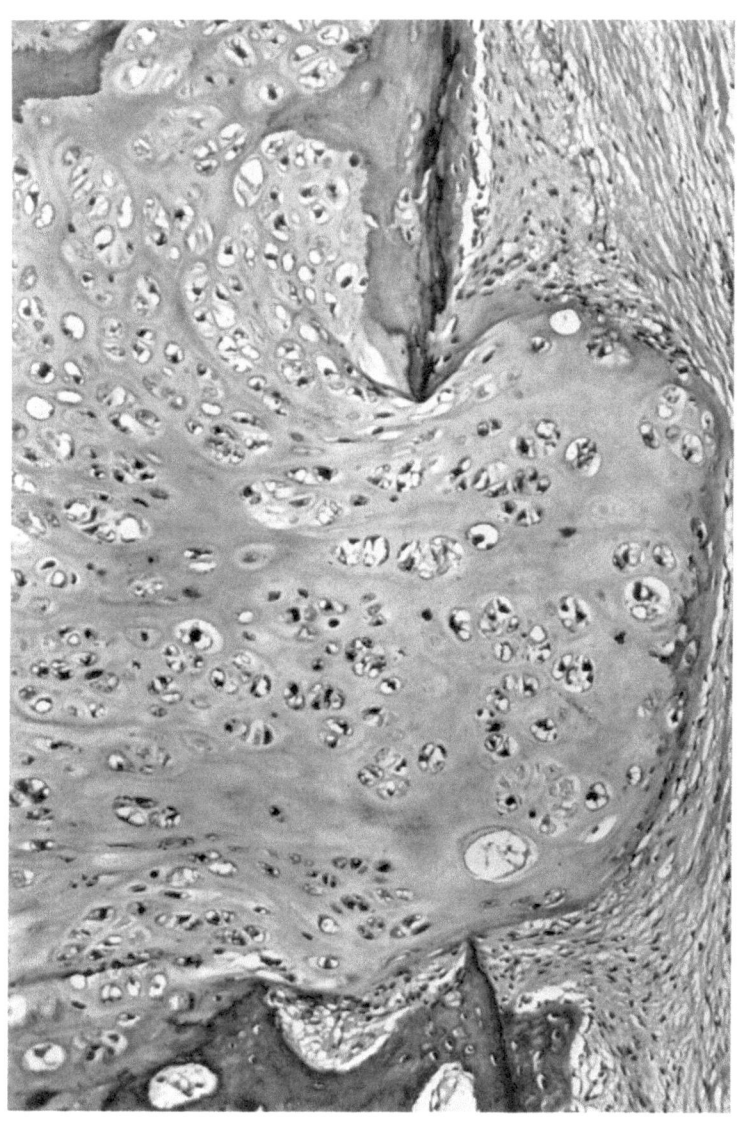

Fig. 245. × 125.   F 4 77—77

246 Ewing's sarcoma   Sarcome d'Ewing   Саркома Юинга

Ewing-Sarkom   Sarcoma de Ewing   Sarcoma Ewing

247 Chordoma   Chordome   Хордома

Chordom   Cordoma   Chordoma

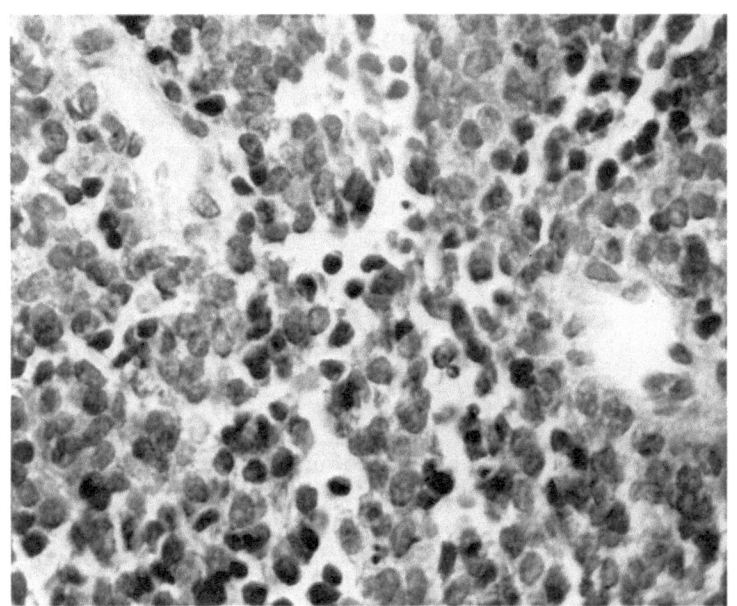

Fig. 246. × 550.   F 4 175—171

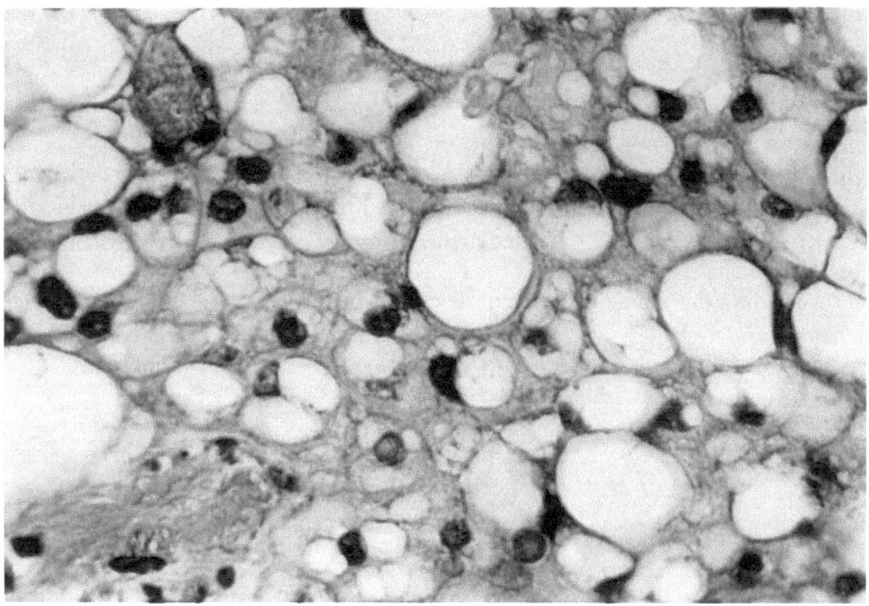

Fig. 247. × 600.   F 24 81—60

250

7.	Joints, tendon sheaths and bursae	Articulations, gaines tendineuses et bourses	Суставы, сухожильные влагалища и суставные сумки
	Gelenke, Sehnenscheiden und Schleimbeutel	Articulaciones, vainas tendinosas y bolsas serosas	Articulationes, vaginae synoviales et bursae (171)

248	Benign synovioma	Synoviome bénin	Доброкачественная синовиома
	Gutartiges Synoviom	Sinovioma benigno	Synovioma benignum

249	Giant cell tumor of tendon sheaths and joints	Tumeur à cellules géantes des gaines tendineuses et des articulations	Гигантоклеточная опухоль сухожильных влагалищ и суставов
	Riesenzelltumor der Sehnenscheiden und Gelenke	Tumor de células gigantes de vainas tendinosas y articulaciones	Tumor gigantocellularis tunicae synovialis

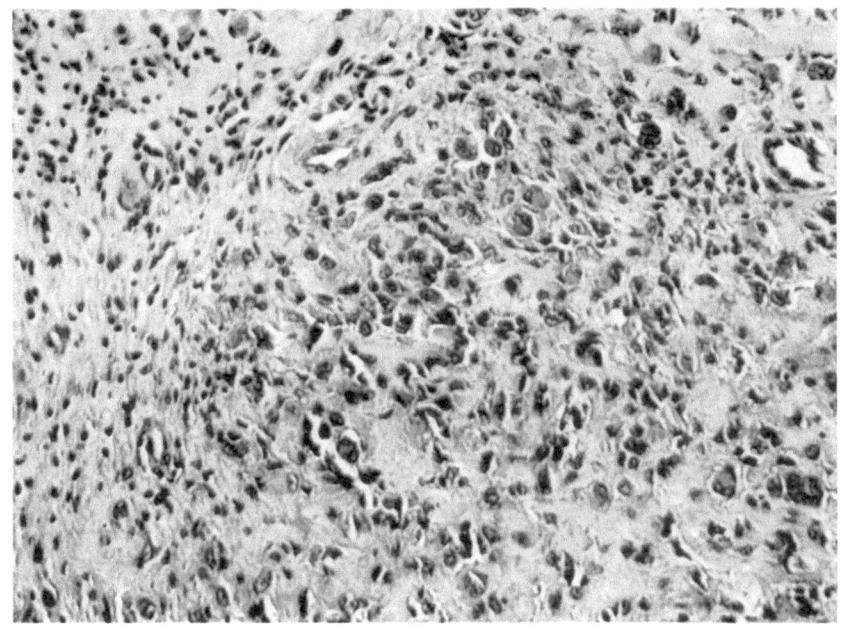

Fig. 248. × 226.   F 5 33—13

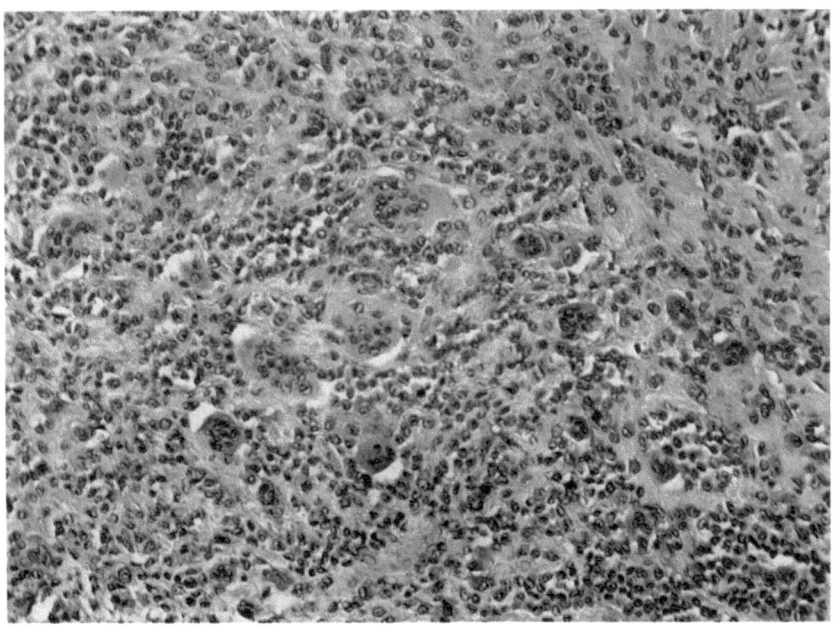

Fig. 249. × 200.   A 817—876

250 Synovial sarcoma   Sarcome synovial   Синовиальная саркома
    Malignant synovioma   Synoviome malin   Злокачественная синовиома

    Synovialsarkom   Sarcoma sinovial   Sarcoma synoviale
    Bösartiges Synoviom   Sinovioma maligno   Synovioma malignum

---

8. Serous cavities   Cavités séreuses   Серозные оболочки

    Seröse Häute   Cavidades serosas   Tunicæ serosae

---

251 Adenomatoid benign   Mésothéliome bénin   Аденоматоидная добро-
    mesothelioma   adénomatoïde   качественная мезотелиома

    Adenomatöses gutartiges   Mesotelioma benigno   Mesothelioma benignum
    Mesotheliom   adenomatoide   adenomatosum

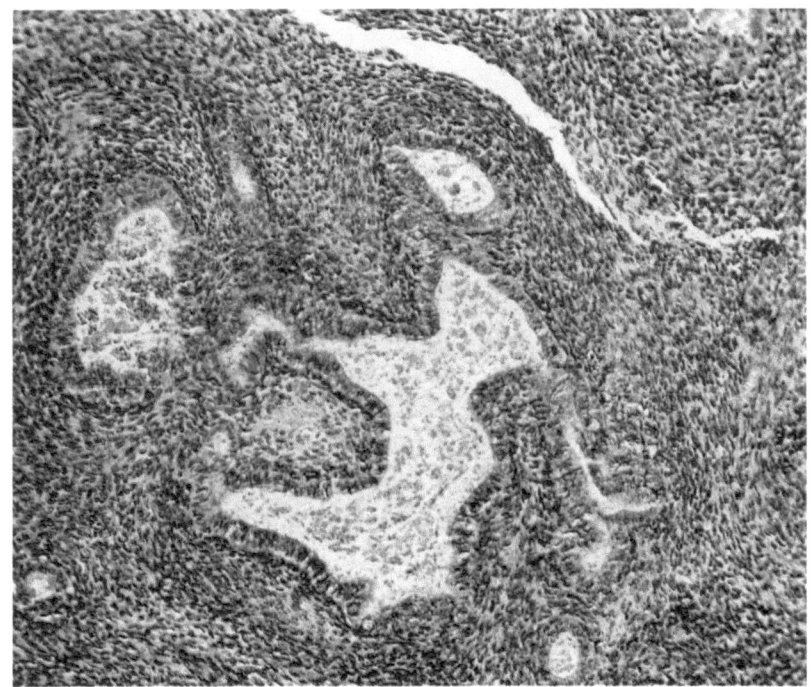

Fig. 250.   A—R 1190—739

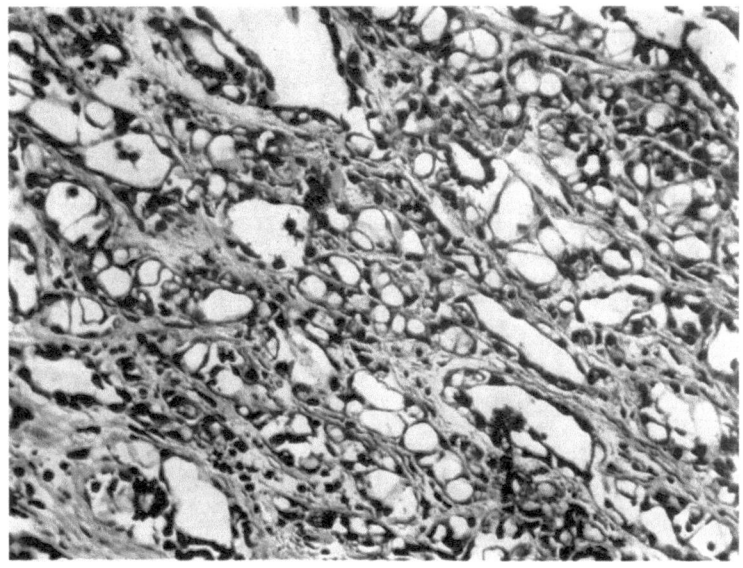

Fig. 251. × 105.   F 32 133—95

252 Papillary benign
    mesothelioma

    Papilläres gutartiges
    Mesotheliom

Mésotheliome benin
    papillaire

Mesotelioma benigno
    papilffero

Папиллярная добро-
    качественная мезотелиома

Mesothelioma benignum
    papilliferum

253 Fibrous benign
    mesothelioma

    Fibröses gutartiges
    Mesotheliom

Mésotheliome benin
    fibreux

Mesotelioma benigno
    fibroso

Фиброзная добро-
    качественная мезотелиома

Mesothelioma benignum
    fibrosum

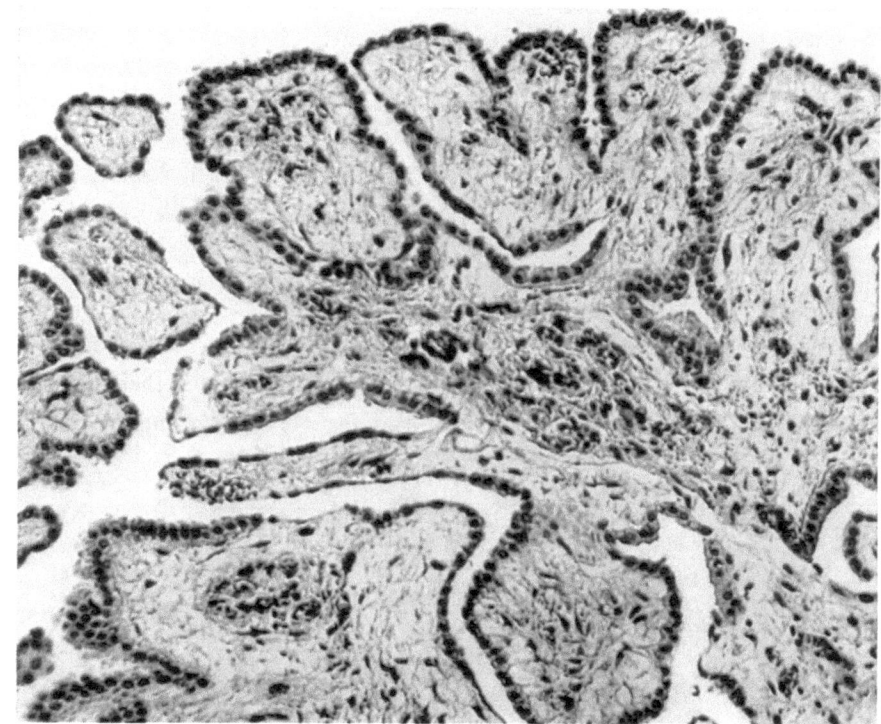

Fig. 252. × 120.   F 24 107—76

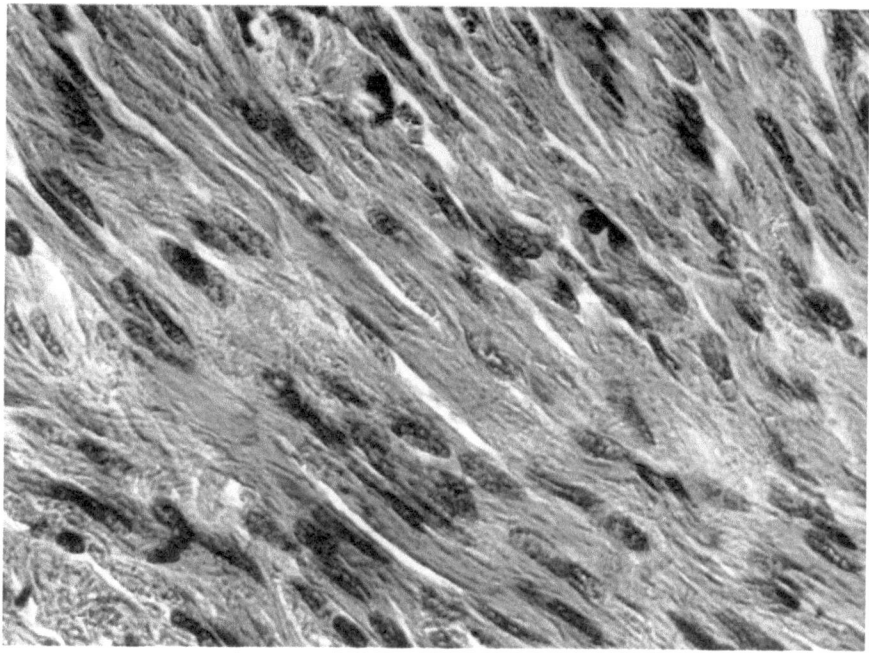

Fig. 253. × 650.   F 24 107—7

254   Papillary malignant
mesothelioma

     Papilläres bösartiges
Mesotheliom

Mésothéliome malin
papillaire

Mesotelioma maligno
papilífero

Папиллярная злокачест-
венная мезотелиома

Mesothelioma malignum
papilliferum

255   Tubular malignant
mesothelioma
Tubular malignant
endothelioma

     Tubuläres bösartiges
Mesotheliom
Tubuläres bösartiges
Endotheliom

Mésothéliome malin
tubuleux
Endothéliome malin
tubuleux

Mesotelioma maligno
tubular
Endotelioma maligno
tubular

Тубулярная злокачест-
венная мезотелиома
Тубулярная злокачест-
венная эндотелиома

Mesothelioma malignum
tubulare
Endothelioma malignum
tubulare

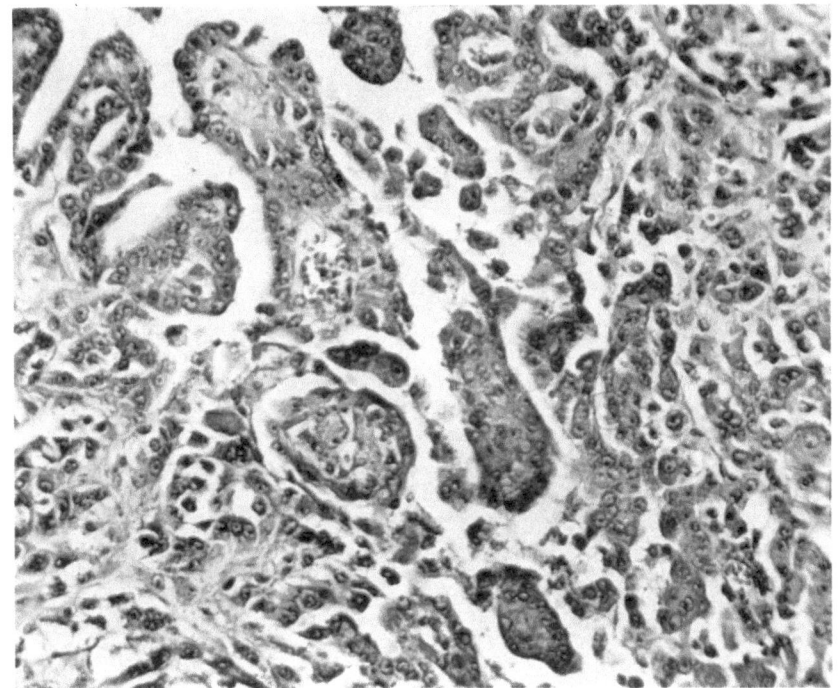

Fig. 254. × 360.   F 24 113—79

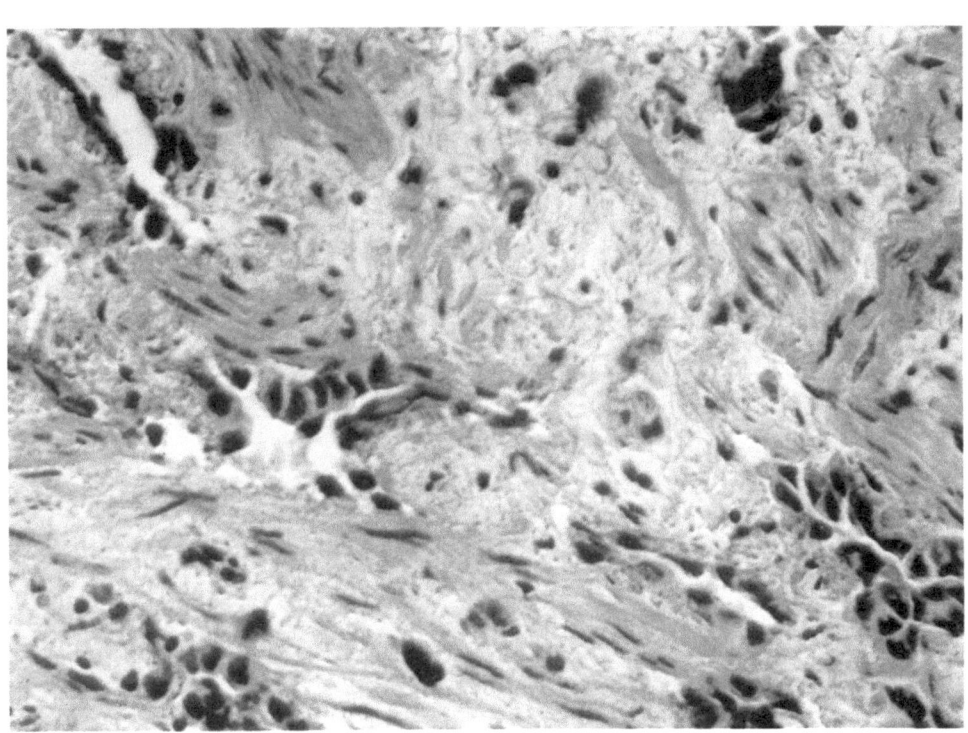

Fig. 255. × 410.   F 24 117—84

17   Nomenclature, 2. Edit.

VI.

Tumors of hematopoietic and lymphoid tissues and leucoses

Tumeurs des tissus hémopoïétiques, lymphoïdes et leucoses

Опухоли кровеобразующей ткани, лимфатической ткани и лейкозы

Tumoren des blutbildenden Gewebes, des Lymphgewebes
 und Leukosen

Tumores de tejidos hematopoyéticos y linfoides y leucosis

Tumores systematis haematopoietici et lymphatici et leukaemiae

1. **Myeloid tissue**   Tissu myéloïde   **Миэлоидная система**

     Myeloisches System   Tejido mieloide   Systema myeloides   (205)

256   Myelocytic Leukemia *   Leucémie myéloïde *   Миелоцитарная лейкемия *
     Granulocytic Leukemia   Leucémie granulocytaire   Гранулоцитарная лейкемия

     Myelozytäre Leukämie *   Leucemia mieloide *   Leucemia myeloides
     Granulozytäre Leukämie   Leucemia granulocitica   Leucemia granulocytica

---

* This pattern is indistinguishable from "chloroma".
* Cet aspect n'est pas à distinguer de celui du « chlorome ».
* По строению не отличается от ,,хлоромы".
* Dieses Gewebsbild ist nicht unterscheidbar von dem des ,,Chloroms".
* Por su aspecto no se puede distinguir del "cloroma".

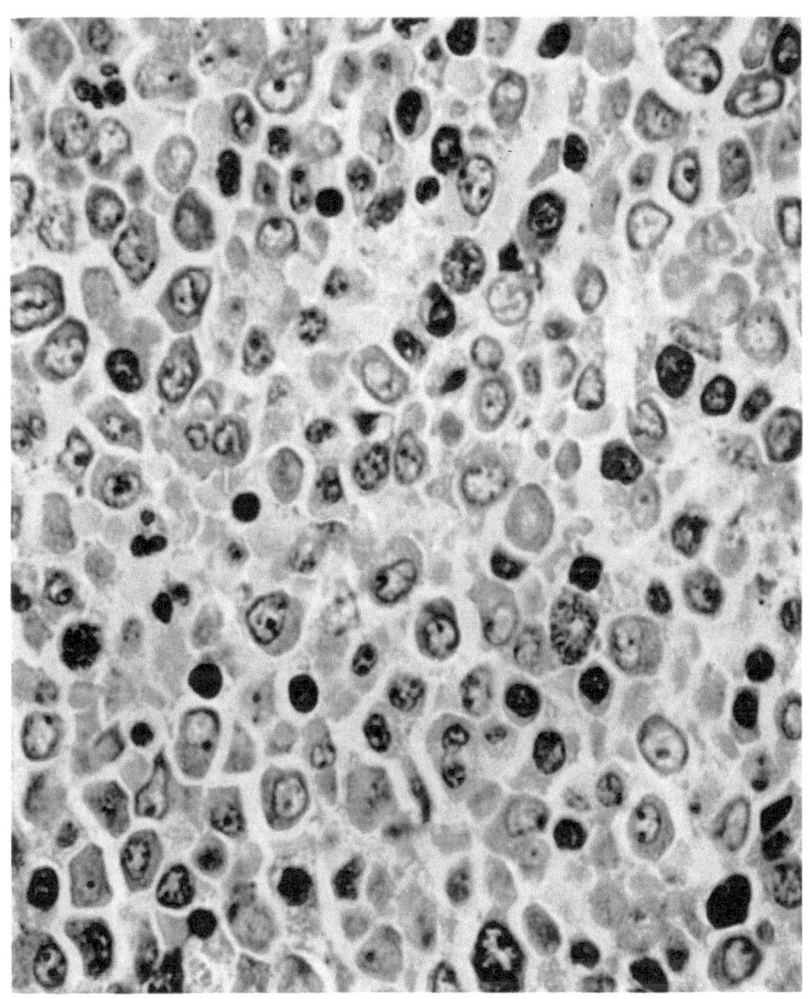

Fig. 256. × 1000.

2. **Lymphoid tissue**   Tissu lymphoïde   Лимфатическая система

   Lymphatisches System   Tejido linfoide   Systema lymphoides   (200, 202)

257   Giant follicular Lymphoma   Lymphome gigantofollicu-   Гигантофоликулярная
                                         laire   лнмфома

   Nodular Lymphoma   Lymphome nodulaire   Нодулярная лимфома
      (lymphocitic type)   (type lymphocytique)   (лимфоцитарный тип)
      well differentiated *   bien differencié *   высокодифференцирован-
                                                                           ная*

   (Brill-Symmers disease)   (Maladie de Brill-Symmers)   (Болезнь Брмлль-
                                                                          Симмерса)

   Großfollikuläres Lymphom   Linfoma giganto-folicular   Lymphoma giganto-
                                                                         folliculare

   Noduläre Lymphom   Linfoma nodular   Lymphoma nodulare
      (lymphozytärer Typ)   (de tipo linfocitico)   lymphocyticum
      ausdifferenziert *   bien deferenciado *   differentiatum
   (Brill-Symmerssche   (enfermedad de Brill-   (Morbus Brill-Symmers)
      Krankheit)   Symmers)

---

* This nodular pattern may also be found in lymphomas of poorly differentiated and reticulum type.
* Cet aspect nodulaire peut être rencontré dans les lymphomes peu differenciés et ceux à cellules réticulaires.
* Подобные нодулярные структуры также могут обнаруживаться в лимфомах низкодифференцированного и ретикулярноклеточного типа.
* Dieses noduläre Gewebsbild kann auch in wenig differenzierten Lymphomen und solchen des Reticulumzell-Typs gefunden werden.
* Este caracter nodular puede encontrarse tambien en linfomas poco diferenciados y en linfomas de celulas reticulares.

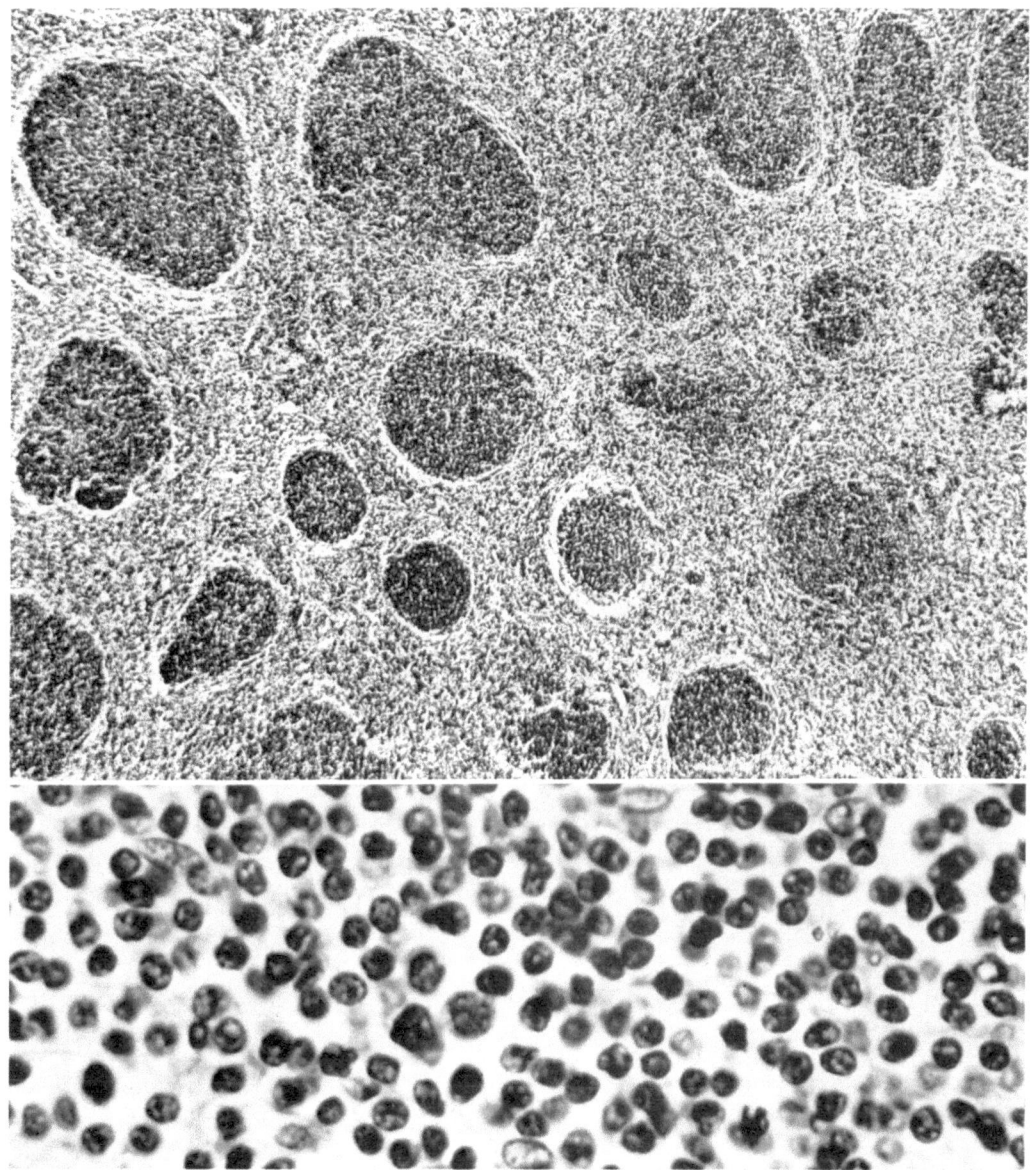

Fig. 257. × 42. × 1000.

F 8 153—157, 159

264

258 Lymphosarcoma *
Malignant Lymphoma
(lymphocytic type)
poorly differentiated

Lymphosarcome *
Lymphome malin
(lymphocytique)
peu differencié

Лимфосаркома*
Злокачественная лимфома
(лимфоцитарный тип)
низкодиффернцированная

Lymphosarkom *
Malignes Lymphom
(lymphozytärer Typ)
undifferenziert

Linfosarcoma *
Linfoma maligno
(de tipo linfocitico)
poco diferendiado

Lymphosarcoma
lymphocyticum
anaplasticum

---

* This pattern is indistinguishable from the pattern found in chronic lymphocytic leukemia.
* Cet aspect n'est pas à distinguer de celui qu'on trouve dans la leucémie lymphoide chronique.
* По характеру строения не отличается от хронической лимфоцитарной лейкемии.
* Dieses Gewebsbild ist nicht unterscheidbar von demjenigen der chronischen lymphozytären Leukämie.
* Por su aspecto no se puede distinguir de una leucemia linfoide cronica.

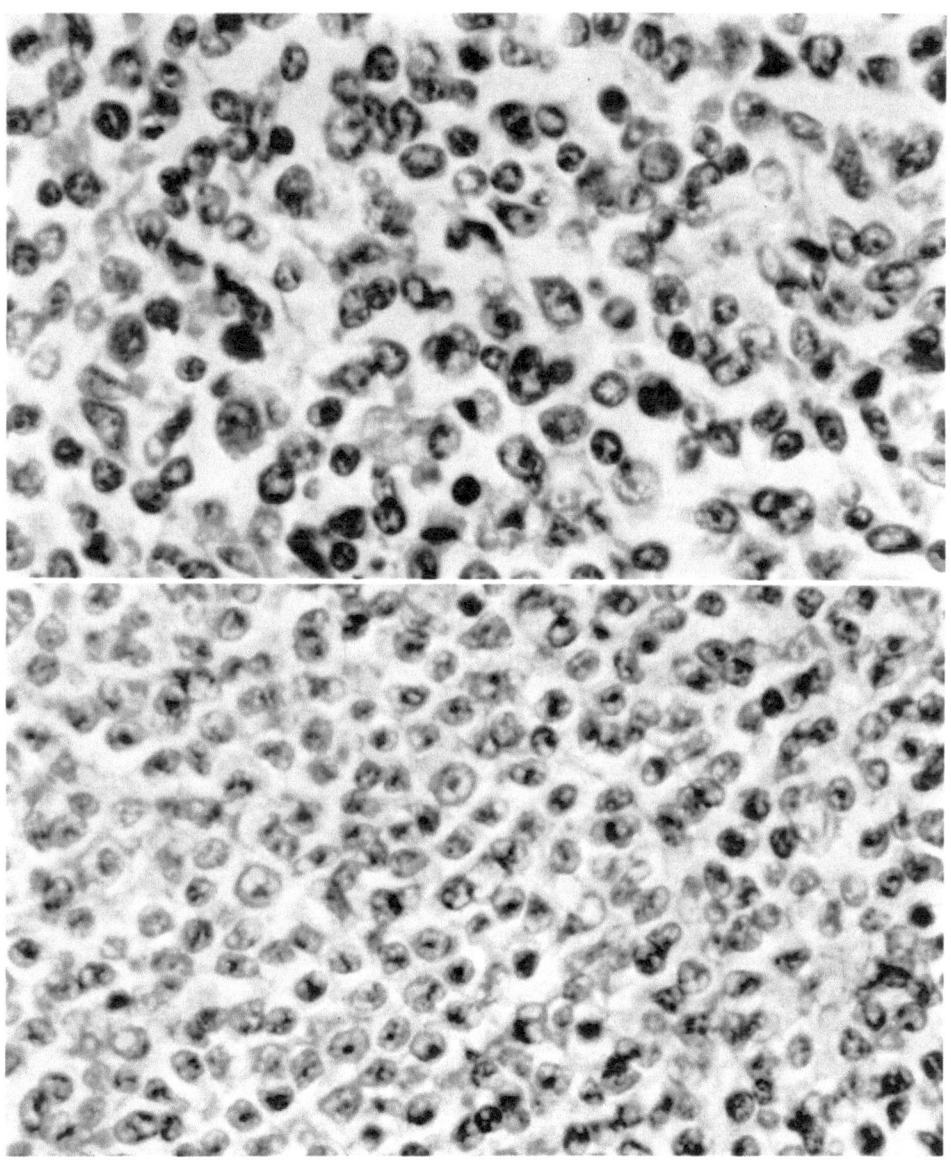

Fig. 258. × 1000.   F 8 143—143; 133—127

259 Malignant Lymphoma
mixed cell type

Lymphome malin
à cellules mixtes

Злокачественная лимфома
смешанного типа

Malignes Lymphom
vom gemischtzelligen Typ

Linfoma maligno
de tipo mixto

Lymphoma malignum
mixtum

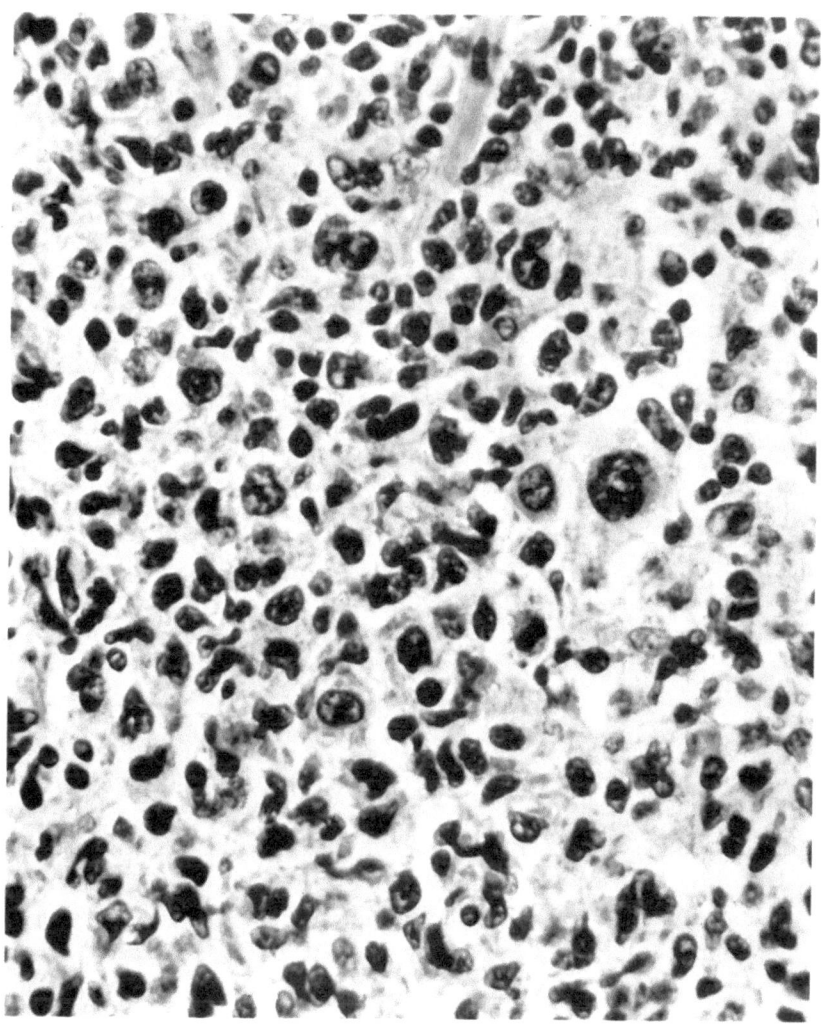

Fig. 259. × 1000.   F 8 125—116

3.	Reticular tissue and plasma cells	Tissu réticulaire et plasmocytes	**Ретикулярная ткань и плазматические клетки**
	Reticuläres Gewebe und Plasmazellen	Tejido reticular y células plasmáticas	Thela reticularis et plasmacytis (200, 201)

260   Extraosseous plasmocytoma (benign or malignant)

Plasmocytome extra-osseux (bénin ou malin)

Экстраоссальная плазмоцитома (доброкачественная или злокачественная)

Extraossales Plasmocytom (gutartiges oder bösartiges)

Plasmocitoma extraóseo (benigno o maligno)

Plasmocytoma extra-ossium (benignum s. malignum)

261   Malignant osseous plasmocytoma
Plasma cell myeloma
Multiple myeloma

Plasmocytome osseux malin
Myélome plasmocytaire
Myélome multiple

Злокачественная костная плазмоцитома
Миэлома из плазматических клеток
Множественная миэлома

Bösartiges ossäres Plasmocytom
Plasmazellmyelom
Multiples Myelom

Plasmocitoma óseo maligno
Mieloma de células plasmáticas
Mieloma múltiple

Plasmocytoma ossium malignum
Myeloma plasmocyticum
Myeloma multiplex

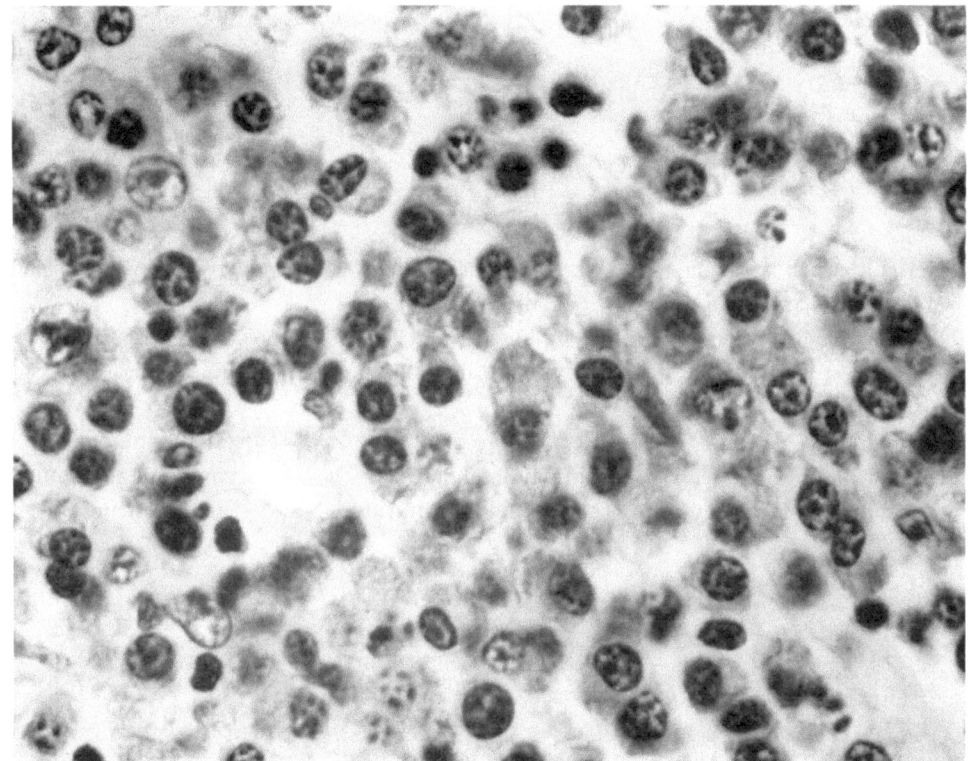

Fig. 260. × 1130.   F 5 109—68

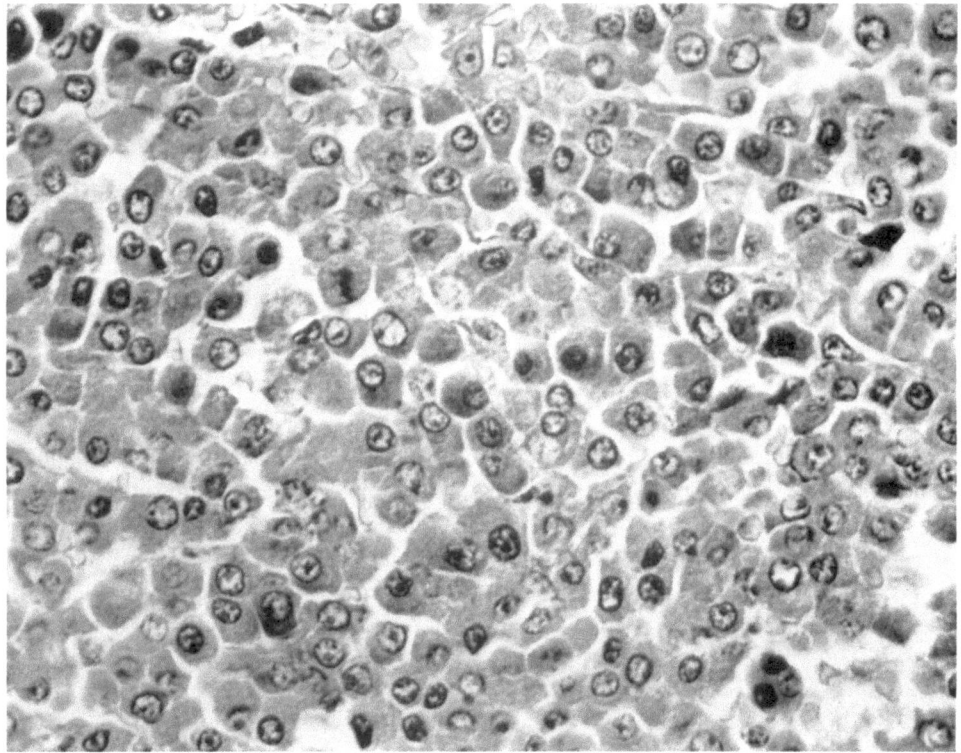

Fig. 261. × 660.   F 4 173—170

262   Reticulum Cell Sarcoma   Sarcome à cellules réti-   Ретикулярноклеточная
        Malignant Lymphoma   culaires   саркома
        of Histiocytic Type   Lymphome malin   Злокачественная лимфома
           type histiocytaire   гистиоцитарного типа

Reticulumzell Sarkom   Reticulosarcoma   Reticulosarcoma
Malignes Lymphom   Linfoma maligno   Lymphoma malignum
    von histiozytärem Typ   de tipo histiocitario   histiocyticum

263   Hodgkins Granuloma   Granuloma Hodgkinien   Гранулома Ходжкина
        a) with lymphocytic   a) à prédominance   a) с лимфоцитарным (или
           (and focal histiocytic)   lymphocytique (et   очаговым гистиоцитар-
           predominance in-   histiocytose focale) y   ным) преобладанием,
           cluding paragranuloma   compris le para-   включая
                                            granulome   парагранулёму

Hodgkins Granulom   Granuloma de Hodgkin   Granuloma Hodgkin
   a) mit Überwiegen der   a) de predominio linfo-   a) imprimis lymphocyti-
       Lymphozyten (und   citico (y en focos   cum (et histio-
       herdweise der Histio-   histiocitario), in-   cyticum) inclusive
       zyten), einschließlich   cluyendo el para-   paragranuloma
       Paragranulom   granuloma

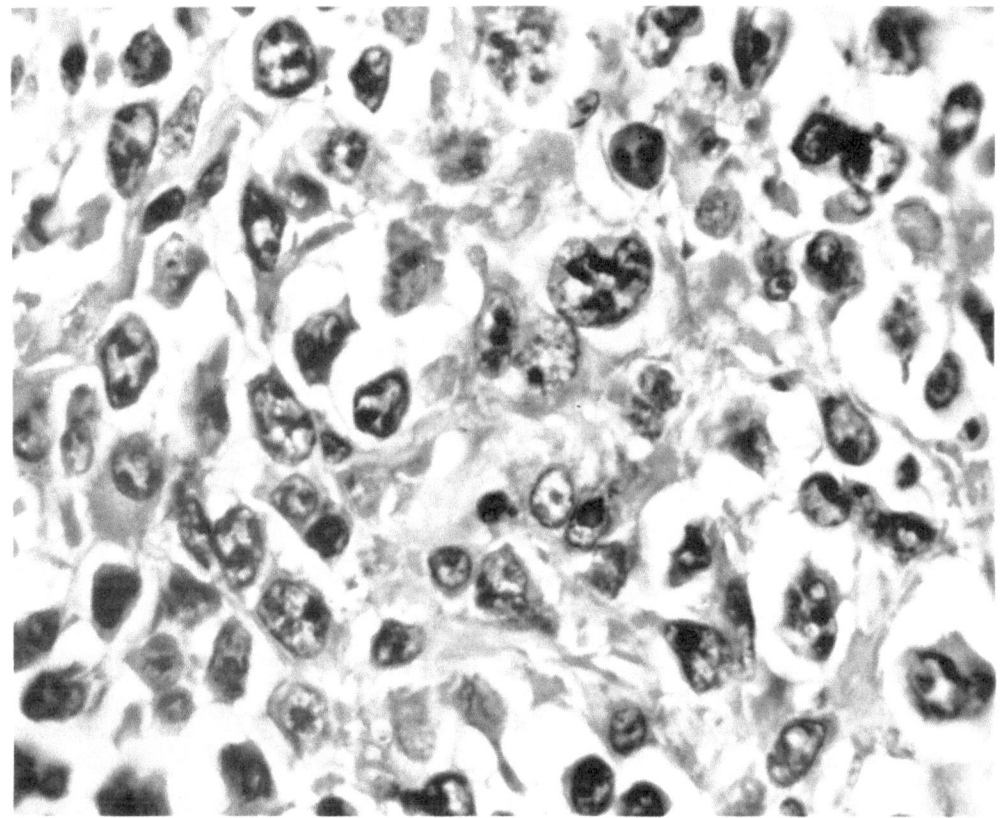

Fig. 262. × 1000.   F 8 115—100

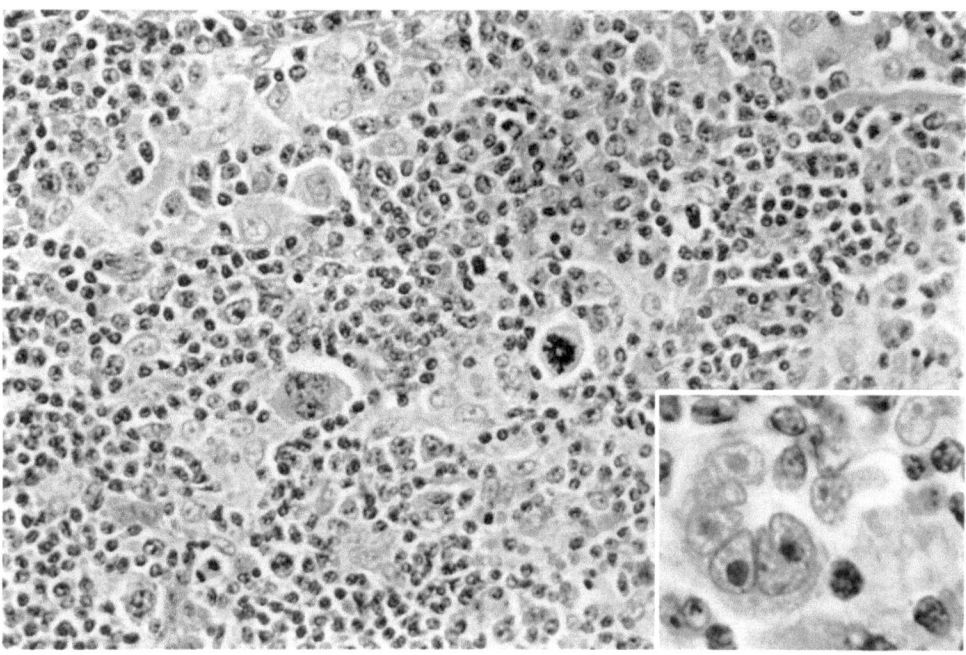

Fig. 263a. × 1000.   F 8 185—188

263 Hodgkins Granuloma

    b) with mixed cellularity

    c) with nodular sclerosis

Hodgkins Granulom

    b) mit gemischten Zell-
       formen

    c) mit nodulärer Sklerose

Granuloma de Hodgkinien

    b) à population
       cellulaire mixte

    c) à sclérose nodulaire

Granuloma de Hodgkin

    b) de celularidad mixta

    c) con esclerosis nodular

Грапулома Ходжкина

    б) со смешанным
       клеточным составом

    в) с нодулярным склёрозом

Granuloma Hodgkin

    b) mixtum

    c) cum sclerosi nodulare

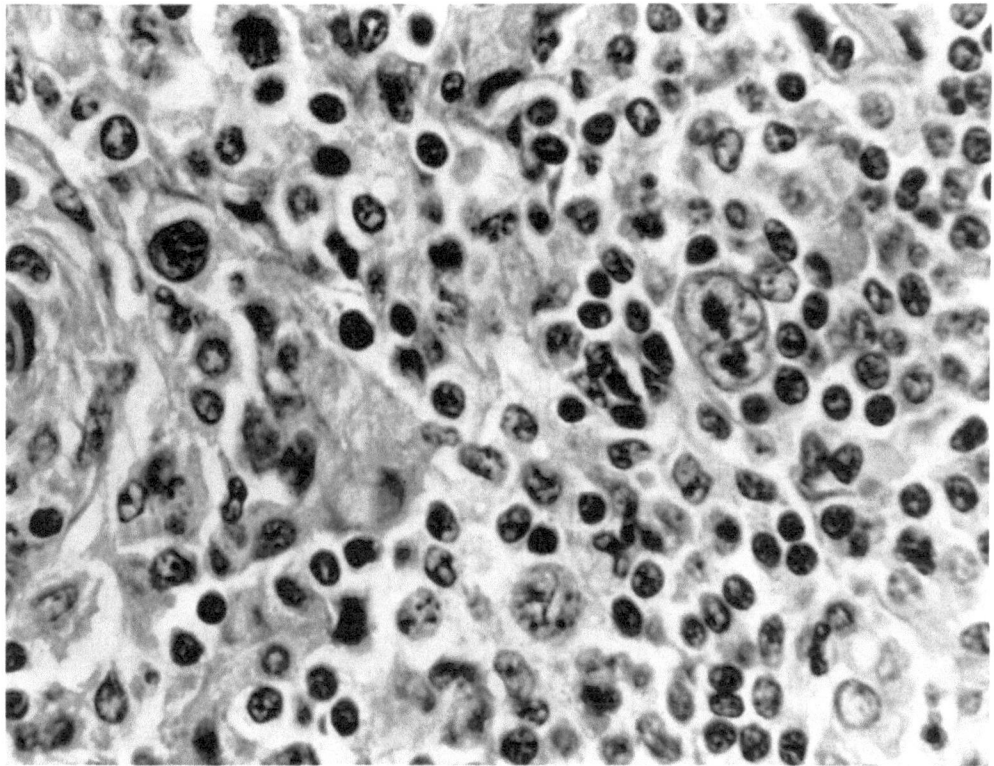

Fig. 263b. × 1000.   F 8 181—182

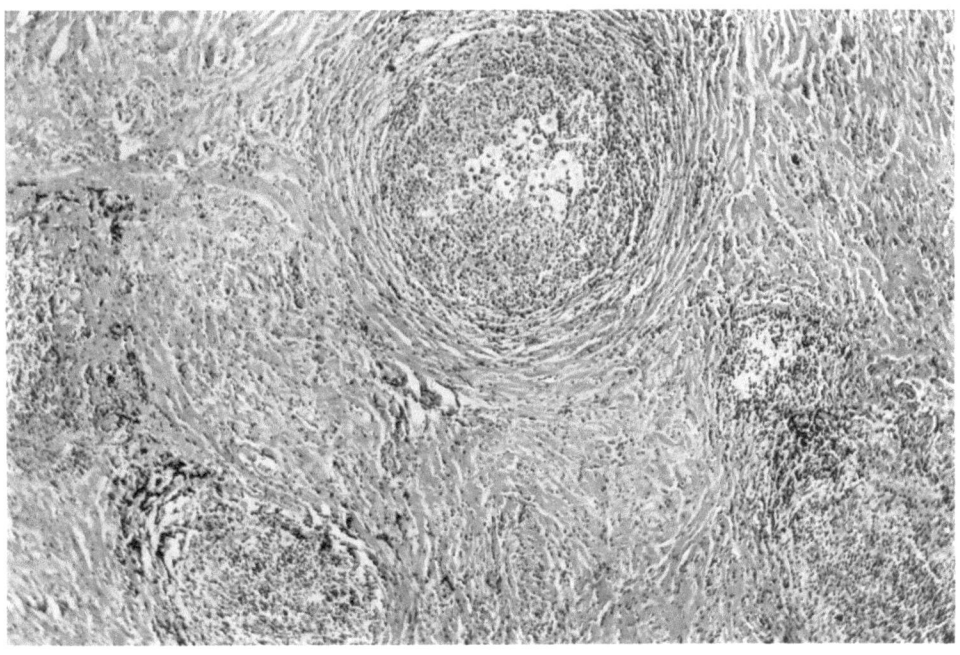

Fig. 263c. × 75.   F 8 183—184

18a Nomenclature, 2. Edit.

263 Hodgkins Granuloma
    d) with lymphocytic
       depletion

Granuloma Hodgkinien
   d) avec rarefaction
     lymphocytique

Гранулома Ходжкина
   г) с лимфоцитарным
     истощением

Hodgkins Granulom
   d) lymphozytenarm

Granuloma de Hodgkin
   d) con deplecion linfo-
     citica

Granuloma Hodgkin
   d) lymphocyticum

264 Monocytic leukemia
    Malignant reticulosis

Leucémie monocytaire
Réticulose maligne

Моноцитарная лейкемия
Злокачественный ретикулоз

Monocytenleukämie
Bösartige Retikulose

Leucemia monocítica
Reticulosis maligna

Leukaemia monocytica
Reticulosis maligna

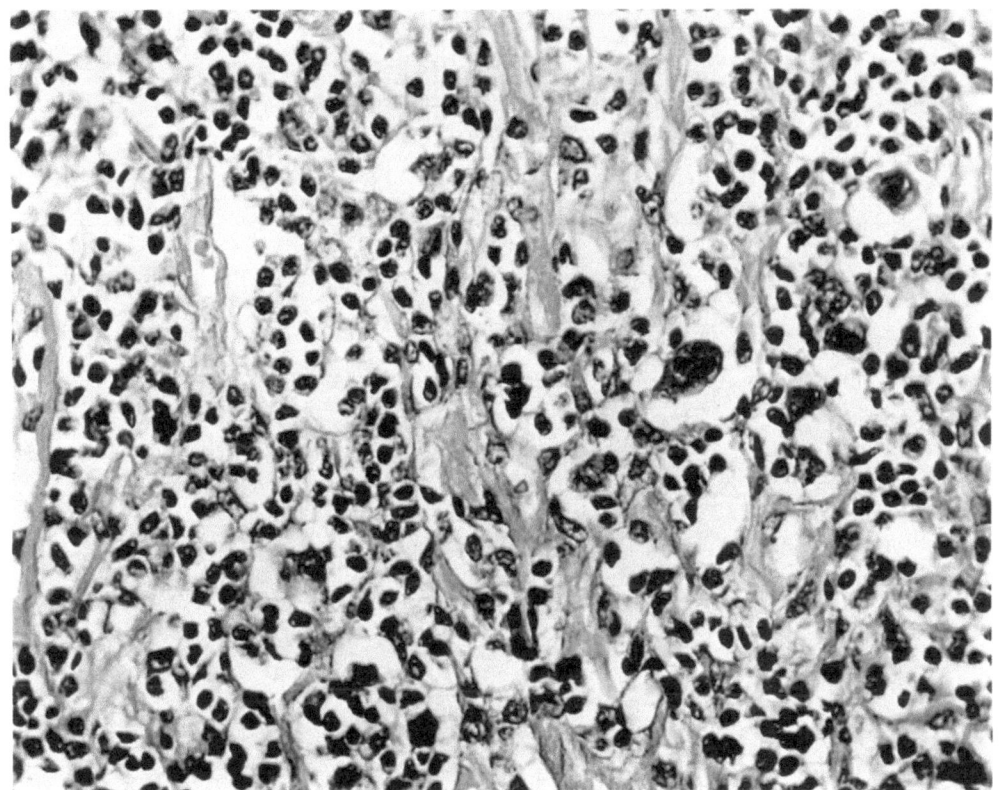

Fig. 263d. × 500.   F 8 173—171

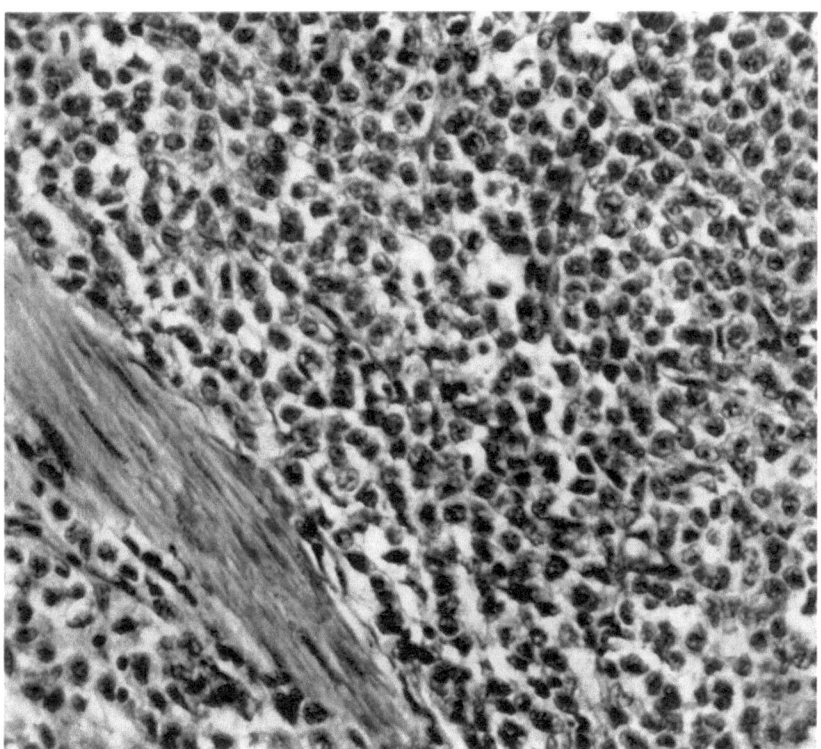

Fig. 264. × 355.   F 2 327—263

4. Thymus   Thymus   **Загрудинный узел (Тимус)**

     Thymus   Timo   Thymus   (194.2)

265   Lymphoepithelial thymoma

     Lymphoepitheliales Thymom

     Thymome lympho-épithélial

     Timoma linfoepitelial

     Лимфоэпителиальная Тимома

     Thymoma lymphoepitheliale

266   Epithelial thymoma

     Epitheliales Thymom

     Thymome épithélial

     Timoma epitelial

     Эпителиальная Тимома

     Thymoma epitheliale

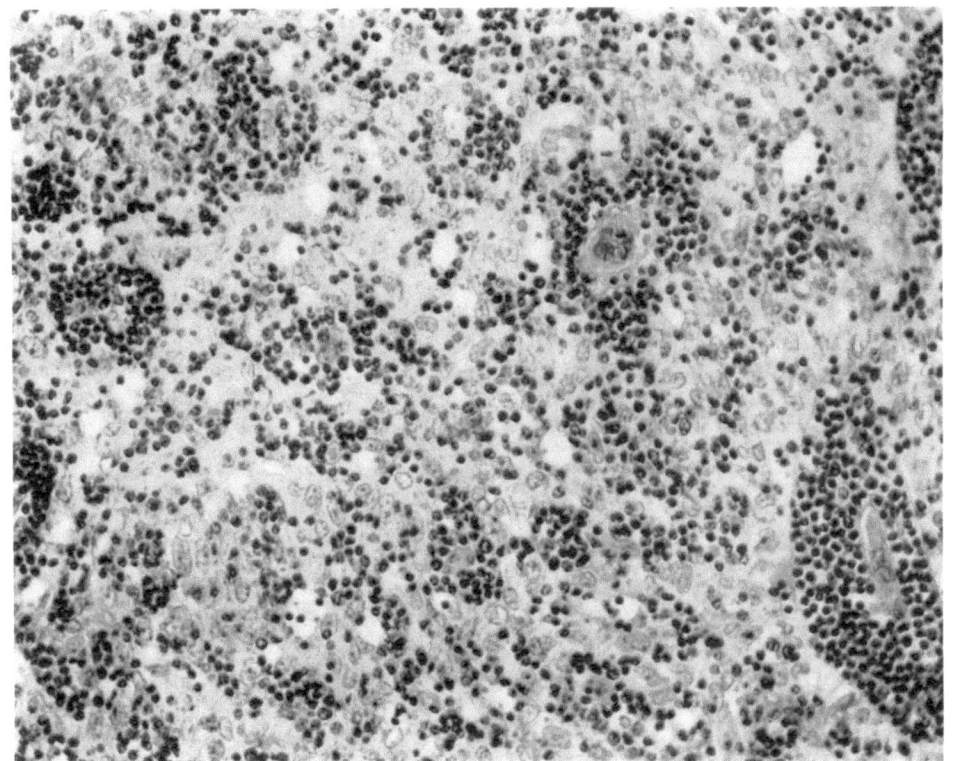

Fig. 265. × 300. F 19 39—32

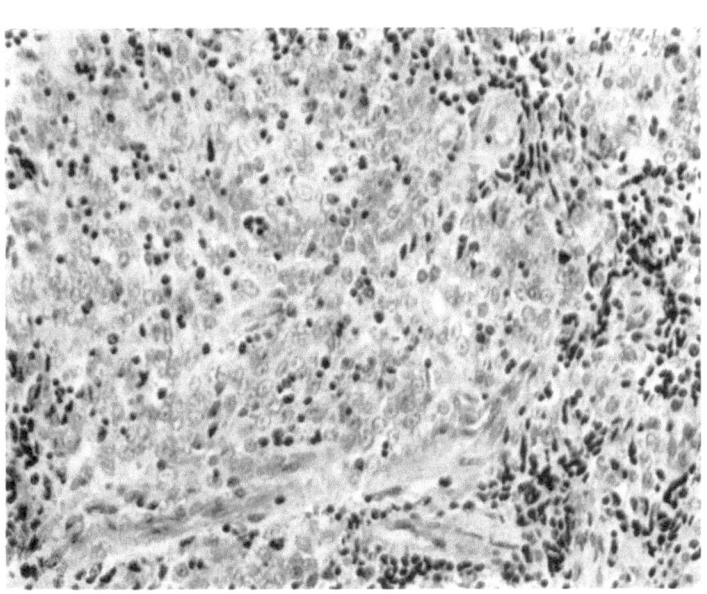

Fig. 266. × 200. F 19 35—28

267   Spindle cell thymoma   Thymome à cellules   Веретеноклегочная   Тимома
                                           fusiformes

      Spindelzelliges Thymom   Timoma fusocelular   Thymoma fusicellulare

268   Carcinoma   Epithélioma   Рак

      Carcinom   Carcinoma   Carcinoma

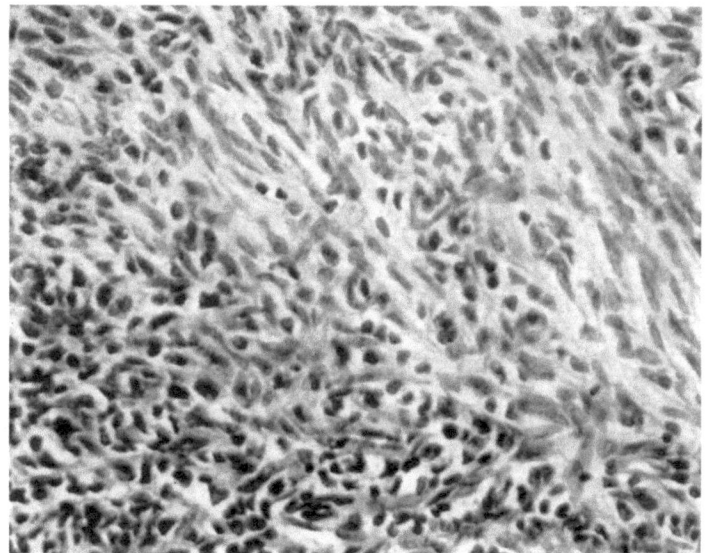

Fig. 267.   F 19 47—45

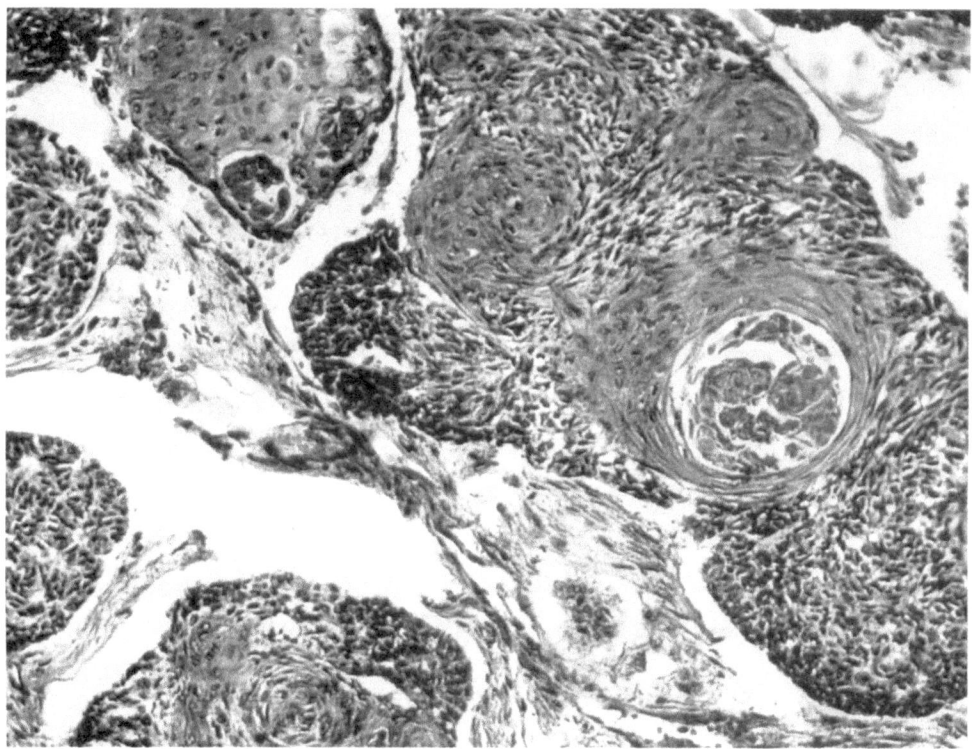

Fig. 268.   × 185.   F 19 51—50

VII.

Teratomas

Tératomes

Тератомы

Teratome

Teratomas

Teratomata

269　Differentiated teratoma　　Tératome différencié　　Зрелая тератома

Reifes Teratom　　Teratoma diferenciado　　Teratoma differentiatum

270　Malignant teratoma　　Tératome malin　　Злокачественная тератома

Bösartiges Teratom　　Teratoma maligno　　Teratoma malignum

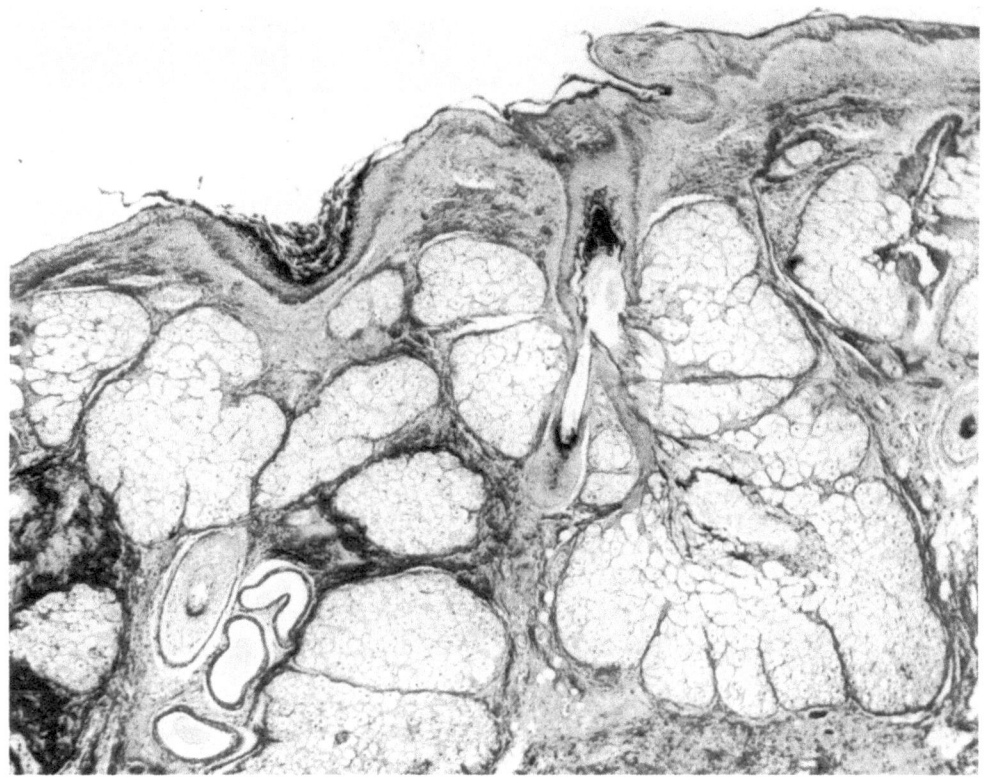

Fig. 269. × 55.   F 18 59—42

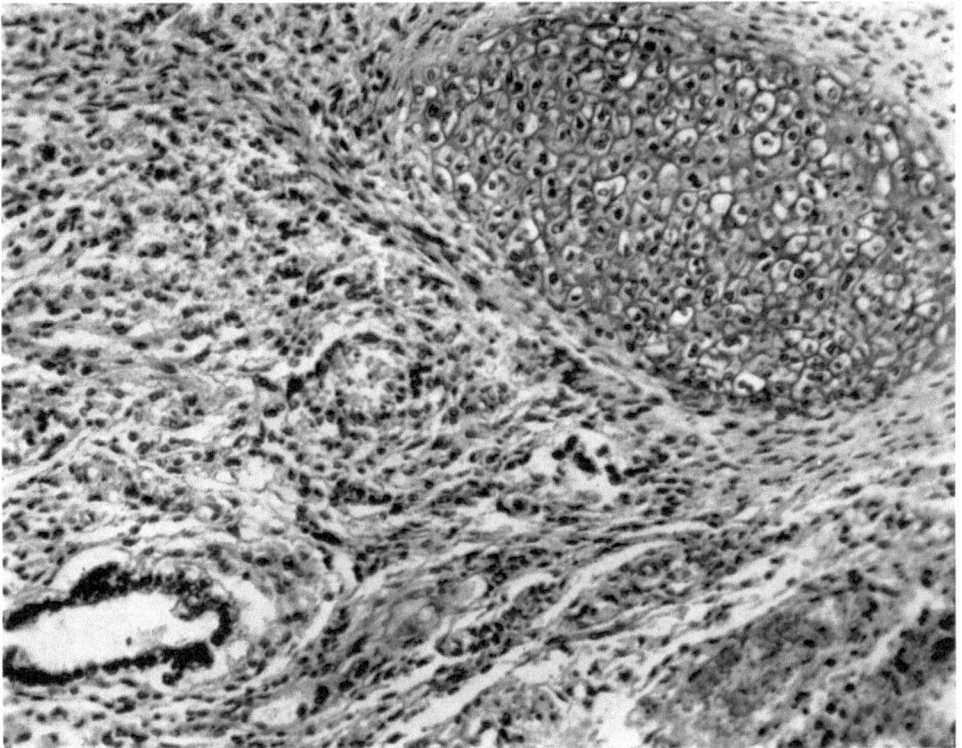

Fig. 270. × 145.   F 18 71—57